SINCE 1820

Founded in 1820, the **U.S.P. Convention** is responsible for establishing legally recognized drug quality standards in the United States—and for disseminating authoritative information for the use of medicines and related articles by health care professionals, patients and consumers. Over 1000 experts serve on USP Subcommittees and Advisory Panels and as *ad hoc* reviewers to ensure the accuracy and current relevance of USP standards and information.

THE

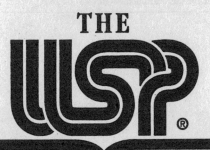

GUIDE TO
HEART
MEDICINES

FIRST EDITION

By authority of U. S. PHARMACOPEIA

AVON BOOKS ◆ NEW YORK

The information on page v constitutes an extension of this copyright page.

AVON BOOKS
A division of
The Hearst Corporation
1350 Avenue of the Americas
New York, New York 10019

Copyright © 1996 by The United States Pharmacopeial Convention, Inc.
Published by arrangement with The United States Pharmacopeial Convention, Inc.
Library of Congress Catalog Card Number: 95-94927
ISBN: 0-380-78094-1

First Avon Books Printing: March 1996

AVON TRADEMARK REG. U.S. PAT. OFF. AND IN OTHER COUNTRIES, MARCA REGISTRADA, HECHO EN U.S.A.

Printed in the U.S.A.

RA   10 9 8 7 6 5 4 3 2 1

Acknowledgments

The information in this book has been created primarily through the work of the USP Expert Advisory Panel on Cardiovascular and Renal Drugs, chaired by Burton E. Sobel, M.D. Doris Lee, DID Drug Information Specialist, served as staff liaison to the Panel and has been responsible for the development of the information. Ellen Loeb (Editorial Associate) also has contributed to the development of the information in this book.

For a complete listing of Panel and staff members, see Contributors section, pages 565–607.

CONTENTS

Contents

INTRODUCTION

Organization of This Book

The purpose of this book is to provide information about medicines used in the treatment of certain heart conditions. Individual discussions (monographs) of these medicines are arranged in alphabetical order by generic name only. By looking in the index, however, you can find either the brand name or the generic name of your medicine and the page listing for the monograph.

Preceding the drug monographs, there are general discussions of different heart conditions and their treatments and general information about use of medicines.

TO THE READER

When purchasing a medicine, whether over-the-counter (non-prescription) or with a doctor's prescription, you may have questions about its usefulness to you, the best way to take it, possible side effects, and precautions to take to avoid complications. For instance, some medicines should be taken with meals, others between meals. Some may make you drowsy while others may tend to keep you awake. Alcoholic or other beverages, other medicines, certain foods, or smoking may affect the way your medicine works. As for side effects, some are merely bothersome and may go away while others may require medical attention.

The USP Guide to Heart Medicines contains information which may provide general answers to some of your questions as well as suggestions for the correct use of your medicine. *It is important to remember, however, that the human body is very complex and medicines may act differently on different people—and even in the same person at different times. If you want additional information about your medicine or its possible side effects, ask your doctor, nurse, or pharmacist. They are there to help you.*

How to Use This Book

The USP Guide to Heart Medicines contains a section of general information about the correct use of any medicine, as well as individual discussions of a wide variety of commonly and not so commonly used medicines. *You should read both the general information and the information specific to the medicine you are taking.*

Each medicine has a generic name that all manufacturers who make that medicine must use. Some manufacturers also create a brand name to put on the label and to use in advertising. *Look in the index* for the generic name or the brand name of the medicine about which you have questions. We have put the generic names and common brand names in the same index, so you do not have to know whether the name you have is a generic name or a brand name. However, it is a good idea for you to learn both the generic and the brand names of the medicines you are using and to write them down and keep them for future use.

Although the informational entries generally appear in alphabetical order by generic name, there are numerous occasions when closely related medicines are grouped under a family name. Therefore, the surest way to quickly find the page number of the information about each medicine is to *look in the index first.*

The information for each medicine is presented according to the area of the body which is affected. As a general rule, information for one type of use will not be the same as for other types of use. For example, if you take tetracycline capsules by mouth for their systemic effect in treating an infection, the information will not be the same as for tetracycline ointment, which is applied directly to the skin for its topical effects. And both of these will be different from the information for tetracyclines used in the eye. Some common divisions are:

- *BUCCAL*—For general effects throughout the body when a medicine is placed in the cheek pocket and slowly absorbed.
- *DENTAL*—For local effects when applied to the teeth or gums.
- *INHALATION*—For local, and in some cases systemic, effects when inhaled into the lungs.
- *INTRA-AMNIOTIC*—For local effects when a medicine is injected into the sac that contains the fetus and amniotic fluid.
- *INTRACAVERNOSAL*—For local effects in the penis when a medicine is given by injection.
- *LINGUAL*—For general effects throughout the body when a medicine is absorbed through the lining of the mouth.
- *MUCOSAL*—For local effects when applied directly to mucous membranes (for example, the inside of the mouth).
- *NASAL*—For local effects when used in the nose.
- *OPHTHALMIC*—For local effects when applied directly to the eyes.
- *ORAL-LOCAL*—For local effects in the gastrointestinal

tract when taken by mouth (i.e., not absorbed into the body).

- *OTIC*—For local effects when used in the ear.
- *PARENTERAL-LOCAL*—For local effects in a specific area of the body when given by injection.
- *RECTAL*—For local, and in some cases systemic, effects when used in the rectum.
- *SUBLINGUAL*—For general effects throughout the body when a medicine is placed under the tongue and slowly absorbed.
- *SYSTEMIC*—For general effects throughout the body; applies to most medicines when taken by mouth or given by injection.
- *TOPICAL*—For local effects when applied directly to the skin.
- *VAGINAL*—For local, and in some cases systemic, effects when used in the vagina.

About USP

The information in this volume is prepared by the United States Pharmacopeia (USP), the organization that sets the official standards of strength, quality, purity, packaging, and labeling for medical products used in the United States.

The United States Pharmacopeia is an independent, not-for-profit corporation composed of delegates from the accredited colleges of medicine and pharmacy in the U.S.; state medical and pharmaceutical associations; many national associations concerned with medicines, such as the American Medical Association, the American Nurses Association, the American Dental Association, the National Association of Retail Druggists, and the American Pharmaceutical Association; and various departments of the federal government, including the Food and Drug Administration. In addition, four members have been appointed by the Board of Trustees specifically to represent the public. USP was established 175 years ago, and is the only national body that represents the professions of both pharmacy and medicine.

The first convention came into being on January 1, 1820, and within the year published the first national drug formulary of the United States. The *U.S. Pharmacopeia* of 1820

Notice:

The information about the drugs contained herein is general in nature and is intended to be used in consultation with your health care providers. It is not intended to replace specific instructions or directions or warnings given to you by your physician or other prescriber or accompanying a particular product. The information is selective and it is not claimed that it includes all known precautions, contraindications, effects, or interactions possibly related to the use of a drug. The information may differ from that contained in the product labeling which is required by law. The information is not sufficient to make an evaluation as to the risks and benefits of taking a particular drug in a particular case and is not medical advice for individual problems and should not alone be relied upon for these purposes. Since the inclusion or exclusion of particular information about a drug is judgmental in nature and since opinion as to drug usage may differ, you may wish to consult additional sources. Should you desire additional information or if you have any questions as to how this information may relate to you in particular, ask your doctor, nurse, pharmacist, or other health care provider.

Since new drugs are constantly being marketed and since previously unreported side effects, newly recognized precautions, or other new information for any given drug may come to light at any time, continuously updated drug information sources should be consulted as necessary.

There are many brands of drugs on the market. The listing of selected brand names is intended only for ease of reference. The inclusion of a brand name does not mean the USP has any particular knowledge that the brand listed has properties different from other brands of the same drug, nor should it be interpreted as an endorsement by the USP. Similarly, the fact that a brand name has not been included does not indicate that that particular brand has been judged to be unsatisfactory or unacceptable.

If any of the information in this book causes you special concern, do not decide against taking any medicine prescribed for you without first checking with your doctor.

contained 217 drug names, divided into two groups according to the level of general acceptance and usage.

When Congress passed the first major drug safety law in 1906, the standards recognized by that statute were those set forth in the *United States Pharmacopeia* and in the *National Formulary*. Today, the *USP* and *NF* continue to be the official U.S. compendia for standards for drugs and for the inactive ingredients in drug dosage forms. The *United States Pharmacopeia* is the world's oldest regularly revised national pharmacopeia and is generally accepted as being the most influential.

The work of the USP is carried out by the Committee of Revision. This committee of experts is elected by the members and currently consists of 114 outstanding physicians, pharmacists, dentists, nurses, chemists, microbiologists, and other individuals particularly qualified to judge the merits of drugs and the standards and information that should apply to them. Committee members serve without pay and are assisted by numerous advisory panels, other outside reviewers, and USP staff.

About *USP DI*

The USP Guide to Heart Medicines contains information extracted from *Advice for the Patient* (Volume II of *USP DI*). Volume I contains drug use information in technical language for the physician, dentist, pharmacist, nurse, or other health care provider, and Volume II is its lay language counterpart for use by consumers. Volume III provides information on approved drug products and legal requirements. The monthly *USP DI Update* keeps all volumes up-to-date with selected new drug entries and related information. Together, the volumes form the foundation of a coordinated approach to drug-use education. Many health care providers, institutions, and associations in the United States and Canada provide individual drug leaflets based on *Advice for the Patient*. Spanish translations for many medicines are also available.

USP DI was first published in 1980. It is continuously reviewed and revised and is intended for use by prescribers, dispensers, and consumers of medications. The information is developed by the consensus of the USP Committee of Revision and its Advisory Panels and anyone, including users of medicines, may contribute through review and comment on drafts of the monographs when they are published for comment in *USP DI Review*, a part of the monthly *USP DI Update*.

For further information about *USP DI* or to comment on how the information published in this volume might better meet your information needs, please contact:

USP Division of Information Development
12601 Twinbrook Parkway
Rockville, Maryland 20852
(301) 816-8351

GENERAL INFORMATION ABOUT USE OF MEDICINES

Information about the proper use of medicines is of two types. One type is drug specific and applies to a certain medicine or group of medicines only. The other type is general in nature and applies to the use of any medicine.

The information that follows is general in nature. For your own safety, health, and well-being, however, it is important that you learn about the proper use of your specific medicines as well. You can get this information from your health care professional, or find it in the individual listings of this book.

Before Using Your Medicine

Before you use any medicine, your health care professional should be told:

—if you have ever had an allergic or unusual reaction to any medicine, food, or other substance, such as yellow dye or sulfites.

—if you are on a low-salt, low-sugar, or any other special diet. Most medicines contain more than their active ingredient, and many liquid medicines contain alcohol.

—*if you are pregnant or if you plan to become pregnant.* Certain medicines may cause birth defects or other problems in the unborn child. For other medicines, safe use during pregnancy has not been established. *The use of any medicine during pregnancy must be carefully considered* and should be discussed with a health care professional.

—*if you are breast-feeding.* Some medicines may pass into the breast milk and cause unwanted effects in the baby.

—if you are now taking or have taken any medicines or dietary supplements in the recent past. Do not forget over-the-counter (nonprescription) medicines such as pain relievers, laxatives, and antacids or dietary supplements.

—if you have any medical problems other than the one(s) for which your medicine was prescribed.

—if you have difficulty remembering things or reading labels.

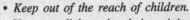

Storage of Your Medicine

It is important to store your medicines properly. Guidelines for proper storage include:

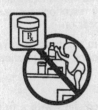

- *Keep out of the reach of children.*
- Keep medicines in their original containers.
- Store away from heat and direct light.
- Do not store capsules or tablets in the bathroom, near the kitchen sink, or in other damp places. Heat or moisture may cause the medicine to break down. Also, do not leave the cotton plug in a medicine container that has been opened, since it may draw moisture into the container.
- Keep liquid medicines from freezing.
- Do not store medicines in the refrigerator unless directed to do so.
- Do not leave your medicines in an automobile for long periods of time.
- Do not keep outdated medicine or medicine that is no longer needed. Be sure that any discarded medicine is out of the reach of children.

Proper Use of Your Medicine

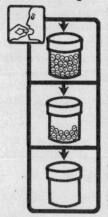

Take medicine only as directed, at the right time, and for the full length of your prescribed treatment. If you are using an over-the-counter (nonprescription) medicine, follow the directions on the label unless otherwise directed by your health care professional. If you feel that your medicine is not working for you, check with your health care professional.

Unless your pharmacist has packaged different medicines together in a "bubble-pack," different medicines should never be mixed in one container. It is best to keep your medicines tightly capped in their original containers when not in use. Do not remove the label since directions for use and other important information may appear on it.

To avoid mistakes, do not take medicine in the dark. Always read the label before taking, especially noting the expiration date and any directions for use.

For oral (by mouth) medicines:

- In general, it is best to take oral medicines with a full glass of water. However, follow your health care professional's directions. Some medicines should be taken with food, while others should be taken on an empty stomach.

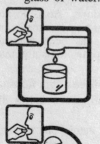

- When taking most long-acting forms of a medicine, each dose should be swallowed whole. Do not break, crush, or chew before swallowing unless you have been specifically told that it is all right to do so.

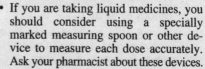

- If you are taking liquid medicines, you should consider using a specially marked measuring spoon or other device to measure each dose accurately. Ask your pharmacist about these devices.

The average household teaspoon may not hold the right amount of liquid.

• Oral medicine may come in a number of different dosage forms, such as tablets, capsules, and liquids. If you have trouble swallowing the dosage form prescribed for you, check with your health care professional. Another dosage form that you can swallow more easily may be available.

• Child-resistant caps on medicine containers have decreased greatly the number of accidental poisonings that occur each year. Use of these caps is required by law. However, if you find it hard to open such caps, you may ask your pharmacist for a regular, easier-to-open cap. He or she can provide you with a regular cap if you request it. However, you must make this request each time you get a prescription filled.

For skin patches:
• Apply the patch to a clean, dry skin area with little or no hair and free of scars, cuts, or irritation. Remove the previous patch before applying a new one.

• Apply a new patch if the first one becomes loose or falls off.

• Apply each patch to a different area of skin to prevent skin irritation or other problems.

• Do not try to trim or cut the adhesive patch to adjust the dosage. Check with your health care professional if you think the medicine is not working as it should.

For inhalers:
• Medicines that come in inhalers usually come with patient directions. *Read the directions carefully before using the medicine.* If you do not understand the directions, or if you are not sure how to use the inhaler, check with your health care professional.

• Since different types of inhalers may be used in different ways, it is very important to follow carefully the directions given to you.

For ophthalmic (eye) drops:
• To prevent contamination, do not let the tip of the eye drop applicator touch any surface (including the eye) and keep the container tightly closed.

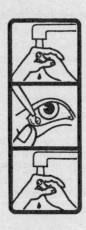

- The bottle may not be full; this is to provide proper drop control.
- How to apply: First, wash your hands. Tilt your head back and, with the index finger, pull the lower eyelid away from the eye to form a pouch. Drop the medicine into the pouch and gently close your eyes. Do not blink. Keep your eyes closed for 1 to 2 minutes.
- If your medicine is for glaucoma or inflammation of the eye: Follow the directions for application that are listed above. However, immediately after placing the drops in your eye, apply pressure to the inside corner of the eye with your middle finger. Continue to apply pressure for 1 to 2 minutes after the medicine has been placed in the eye. This will help prevent the medicine from being absorbed into the body and causing side effects.
- After applying the eye drops, wash your hands to remove any medicine.

For ophthalmic (eye) ointments:

- To prevent contamination of the eye ointment, do not let the tip of the applicator touch any surface (including the eye). After using, wipe the tip of the ointment tube with a clean tissue and keep the tube tightly closed.
- How to apply: First, wash your hands. Pull the lower eyelid away from the eye to form a pouch. Squeeze a thin strip of ointment into the pouch. A 1-cm (approximately ⅓-inch) strip of ointment is usually enough unless otherwise directed. Gently close your eyes and keep them closed for 1 to 2 minutes.
- After applying the eye ointment, wash your hands to remove any medicine.

For nasal (nose) drops:

- How to use: Blow your nose gently, without squeezing. Tilt your head back while standing or sitting up, or lie down on your back on a bed and hang your head over the side. Place the drops into each nostril and keep

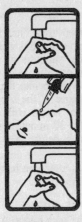

your head tilted back for a few minutes to allow the medicine to spread throughout the nose.

• Rinse the dropper with hot water and dry with a clean tissue. Replace the cap right after use. To avoid the spread of infection, do not use the container for more than one person.

For nasal (nose) spray:

• How to use: Blow your nose gently, without squeezing. With your head upright, spray the medicine into each nostril. Sniff briskly while squeezing the bottle quickly and firmly.

• Rinse the tip of the spray bottle with hot water, taking care not to suck water into the bottle, and dry with a clean tissue. Replace the cap right after cleaning. To avoid the spread of infection, do not use the container for more than one person.

For otic (ear) drops:

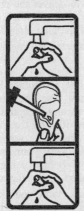

• To prevent contamination of the ear drops, do not touch the applicator tip to any surface (including the ear).

• The bottle may not be full; this is to provide proper drop control.

• How to apply: Lie down or tilt the head so that the ear that needs treatment faces up. For adults, gently pull the earlobe up and back to straighten the ear canal. (For children, gently pull the earlobe down and back.) Drop the medicine into the ear canal. Keep the ear facing up for about 5 minutes to allow the medicine to run to the bottom of the ear canal. (For young children and other patients who cannot stay still for 5 minutes, try to keep the ear facing up for at least 1 or 2 minutes.)

• Do not rinse the dropper after use. Wipe the tip of the dropper with a clean tissue and keep the container tightly closed.

For rectal suppositories:

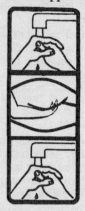

- How to insert suppository: First, wash your hands. Remove the foil wrapper and moisten the suppository with water. Lie down on your side. Push the suppository well up into the rectum with your finger. If the suppository is too soft to insert, chill it in the refrigerator for 30 minutes or run cold water over it before removing the foil wrapper.
- Wash your hands after you have inserted the suppository.

For rectal cream or ointment:

- Bathe and dry the rectal area. Apply a small amount of cream or ointment and rub it in gently.
- If your health care professional wants you to insert the medicine into the rectum: First, attach the plastic applicator tip onto the opened tube. Insert the applicator tip into the rectum and gently squeeze the tube to deliver the cream. Remove the applicator tip from the tube and wash with hot, soapy water. Replace the cap of the tube after use.
- Wash your hands after you have inserted the medicine.

For vaginal medicines:

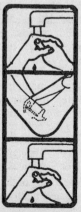

- How to insert the medicine: First, wash your hands. Use the special applicator. Follow any special directions that are provided by the manufacturer. However, if you are pregnant, check with your health care professional before using the applicator to insert the medicine.
- Lie on your back, with your knees drawn up. Using the applicator, insert the medicine into the vagina as far as you can without using force or causing discomfort. Release the medicine by pushing on the plunger. Wait several minutes before getting up.

• Wash the applicator and your hands with soap and warm water.

Precautions While Using Your Medicine

Never give your medicine to anyone else. It has been prescribed for your personal medical problem and may not be the correct treatment for or may even be harmful to another person.

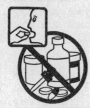

Many medicines should not be taken with other medicines or with alcoholic beverages. Follow your health care professional's directions to help avoid problems.

Before having any kind of surgery (including dental surgery) or emergency treatment, tell the physician or dentist about any medicine you are taking.

If you think you have taken an overdose of any medicine or if a child has taken a medicine by accident: Call your poison control center or your health care professional at once. Keep those telephone numbers handy. Also, keep a bottle of Ipecac Syrup safely stored in your home in case you are told to cause vomiting. Read the directions on the label of Ipecac Syrup before using.

Side Effects of Your Medicine

Along with its intended effects, a medicine may cause some unwanted effects. Some of these side effects may need medical attention, while others may not. It is important for you to know what side effects may occur and what you should do if you notice signs of them. Check with your health care professional about the possible side effects of the medicines you are taking, or if you notice any unusual reactions or side effects.

Additional Information

 It is a good idea for you to learn both the generic and brand names of your medicine and even to write them down and keep them for future use.

Many prescriptions may not be refilled until your pharmacist checks with your health care professional. *To save time, do not wait until you have run out of medicine before requesting a refill.* This is especially important if you must take your medicine every day.

When traveling:

- Carry your medicine with you rather than putting it in your checked luggage. Checked luggage may get lost or misplaced or may be stored in very cold or very hot areas.

- Make sure a source of medicine is available where you are traveling, or take a large enough supply to last during your visit. It is also a good idea to take a copy of your written prescription with you.

If you want more information about your medicines, ask your health care professional. *Do not be embarrassed to ask questions* about any medicine you are taking. To help you remember, it may be helpful to write down any questions and bring them with you on your next visit to your health care professional.

AVOIDING MEDICINE MISHAPS

Tips Against Tampering

Over-the-counter (OTC) or nonprescription medicines are now packaged so that it will be easier to notice signs of tampering. A tamper-evident package is required either to be unique so that it cannot be copied easily, or to have a barrier or indicator (that has an identifying characteristic, such as a pattern, picture, or logo) that will be easily noticed if it is broken. For two-piece, unsealed, hard gelatin capsules, two tamper-evident features are required. Improved packaging also includes the use of special wrappers, seals, or caps on the outer and/or inner containers, or sealing each dose in its own pouch.

Even with such packaging, however, no system is completely safe. It is important that you do your part by checking for signs of tampering whenever you buy or use a medicine.

The following information may help you detect possible signs of tampering.

Protecting yourself

General common sense suggestions include the following:

• When buying a drug product, *consider* the dosage form (for example, capsules, tablets, syrup), the type of packaging, and the tamper-evident features. Ask yourself: Would it be easy for someone to tamper with this product? Will I be able to determine whether or not this product has been tampered with?

• *Look very carefully* at the outer packaging of the drug product before you buy it. After you buy it, also check the inner packaging as soon as possible.

• If the medicine has a protective packaging feature, it should be described in the labeling. This description is required to be placed so that it will not be affected if the feature is broken or missing. If the feature is broken or missing, *do not buy or use* the product. If you have already purchased the product, return it to the store. Always be sure to tell someone in charge about any problems.

• *Do not take* medicines that show even the slightest signs of tampering or don't seem quite right.

• Never take medicines in the dark or in poor lighting. *Read* the label and check each dose of medicine before you take it.

What to look for

Packaging

• Are there breaks, cracks, or holes in the outer or inner wrapping or protective cover or seal?

• Does the outer or inner covering appear to have been disturbed, unwrapped, or replaced?

• Does a plastic or other shrink band (tight-fitting wrap) around the top of the bottle appear distorted or stretched, as though it had been rolled down and then put back into place? Is the band missing? Has the band been slit and retaped?

• Is the bottom of the container intact?

• Does the container appear to be too full or not full enough?

• Is the cap on tight?

• Are there bits of paper or glue stuck on the rim of the container that make it seem the container once had a bottle seal?

• Is the cotton plug or filler in the bottle torn, sticky, or stained, or does it appear to have been taken out and put back?

• Do eye drops have a protective seal? All eye drops must be sealed when they are made, in order to keep them germ-free. Do not use if there is any sign of a broken or removed seal.

• Check the bottom as well as the top of a tube. Is the tube properly sealed? Metal tubes crimped up from the bottom like a tube of toothpaste should be firmly sealed.

• Are the expiration date, lot number, and other information the same on both the container and its outer wrapping or box?

Liquids

• Is the medicine the usual color? Thickness?

• Is a normally clear liquid cloudy or colored?

• Are there particles (small pieces) in the bottom of the bottle or floating in the solution? For some liquids, called suspensions, floating particles are normal.

• Does the medicine have a strange or different taste or odor (for example, bleach, acid, gasoline-like, or other pungent or sharp odor)? Do not taste the medicine if it has a strange odor.

Tablets

• Do the tablets look different than they usually do? Do they have unusual spots or markings? If they normally are shiny and smooth, are some dull or rough? Is there anything unusual about the color?

• Are the tablets all the same size and thickness?

• If there is printing on the tablets, do they all have the same imprint? Is the imprint missing from any?

• Do the tablets have a strange or different odor or taste?

• Are any of the tablets broken?

Capsules

• Do the capsules look different than they usually do? Are any cracked or dented? Are they all the same size and color?

• Do they have their normal shiny appearance or are some dull or have fingerprints on them as though they have been handled?

• Are the capsules all the same length?

• If there is printing on the capsules, do they all have the same imprint? Is the imprint missing from any? Do the imprints all line up the same way?

• Do the capsules have an unexpected or unusual odor or taste?

Tubes and jars (ointments, creams, pastes, etc.)

• Does the product or container look different than usual?

• Are ointments and creams smooth and non-gritty? Have they separated?

Be a wise consumer. Look for signs of tampering before you buy a medicine and again each time you take a dose. Also, pay attention to the daily news in order to learn about any reported tampering.

It is important to understand that a change in the appearance or condition of a product may not mean that the package has been tampered with. The manufacturer may have changed the color of a medicine or its packaging. Also, the product may be breaking down with age or it may have had rough or unusual handling in shipping. In addition, some minor product variations may be normal.

Whenever you suspect that something is unusual about a medicine or its packaging, take it to your pharmacist. He or she is familiar with most products and their packaging. If there are serious concerns or problems, your pharmacist should report it to the USP Practitioners' Reporting Network^sm (USP PRN) at 1-800-487-7776, or other appropriate authorities.

Unintentional Poisoning

According to information provided by the American Association of Poison Control Centers, nearly one million children 6 years of age and under were unintentionally poisoned in 1993; 27 children 6 years of age and younger died as a result of poisoning.

Adults also may be unintentionally poisoned. This happens most often through carelessness or lack of information. For example, the sleepy adult who takes a medicine in the dark and winds up getting the wrong one, or the adult who decides to take the medicine prescribed for a friend to treat "the same symptoms."

Drug poisoning from an unintentional overdose is one type of accidental poisoning that contributes to these figures. Other causes include household chemical poisoning from unintentional ingestion or contact, and inhaled poisoning—for example, carbon monoxide, usually from a car.

Children are ready victims

The natural curiosity of children makes them ready victims of poisoning. Children explore everywhere and investigate their environment. What they find frequently goes into their mouths. They do not understand danger and possibly cannot read warning labels.

Accidental poisoning from medicine is especially dangerous in small children because the strength of most medicines that may be ingested is often based on their use in adults. Even a small quantity of an adult dose can sometimes poison a child.

Preventing poisoning from medicines

• Store medicines out of the sight and reach of children, preferably in a locked cabinet—not in the bathroom medicine cabinet or in a food cabinet.

• If you have children living with you or only as occasional guests, you should have child-resistant caps on your medicine containers. These will help to ensure that an accidental poisoning does not occur in your home. Always store your medicines in a secure place.

• Adults who have difficulty opening child-resistant closures may request traditional, easy-to-open packaging for their medicines.

• Always replace lids and return medicines to their storage place after use, even if you will be using them again soon.

• If you are called to the telephone or to answer the door while you are taking medicine, take the container with you or put the medicine out of the reach of small children. Children act quickly—usually when no one is watching.

• Date medicines when purchased and clean out your medicines periodically. Discard prescription medicines that are past their expiration or ''beyond use'' date. As medicines grow old, the chemicals in them may change. In general, medicines that do not have an expiration date should not be kept for more than 1 year. Carefully discard any medicines so that children cannot get them. Rinse containers well before discarding in the trash.

• Take only those medicines prescribed for you and give medicines only to those for whom prescribed. A medicine that worked well for one person may harm another.

• It is best to keep all medicines in their original containers with their labels intact. The label contains valuable information for taking the medicine properly. Also, in case of accidental poisoning, it is important to know the ingredients in a drug product and any emergency instructions from the manufacturer. While prescription medicines usually do not list ingredients, information on the label makes it possible for your pharmacist to identify the contents.

• Ask your pharmacist to include on the label the number of tablets or capsules that he or she put in the container. In case of poisoning, it may be important to know roughly how many tablets or capsules were taken.

• Do not trust your memory—read the label before using the medicine, and take it as directed.

• If a medicine container has no label or the label has been defaced so that you are not absolutely sure what it says, do not use it.

• Turn on a light when taking or giving medicines at night or in a dark room.

• Label medicine containers with poison symbols, especially if you have children, individuals with poor vision, or other persons in your home who cannot read well.

• Teach children that medicine is not candy by calling each medicine by its proper name.

• Do not take medicines in front of children. They may wish to imitate you.

• Communicate these safety rules to any babysitters you have and remember them if you babysit or are visiting a house with children. Children are naturally curious and can get into a pocketbook, briefcase, or overnight bag that contains medicines.

What to do if a poisoning happens

Remember:

• There may be no immediate, significant symptoms or warning signs, particularly in a child.

• Nothing you can give will work equally well in all cases of poisoning. In fact, one "antidote" may counteract the effects of another.

• Many poisons act quickly, leaving little time for treatment.

Therefore:

• If you think someone has swallowed medicine or a household product, and the person is unconscious, having seizures (convulsions), or is not breathing, immediately call for an ambulance. Otherwise, do not wait to see what effect the poison will have or if symptoms of overdose develop. Immediately call a Poison Control Center (listed in the white pages of your telephone book under "Poison Control" or inside the front cover with other emergency numbers). These numbers should be posted beside every telephone in the house, as should those of your pharmacist, the police, the fire department, and ambulance services. (Some poison control centers have TTY capability for the deaf. Check with your local center if you or someone in your family requires this service.)

• Have the container with you when you call so you can read the label on the product for ingredients.

• Describe what, when, and how much was taken and the age and condition of the person poisoned—for example, if the person is vomiting, choking, drowsy, shows a change in color or temperature of skin, is conscious or unconscious, or is convulsing.

• *Do not induce vomiting* unless instructed by medical personnel. *Do not induce vomiting or force liquids* into a person who is convulsing, unconscious, or very drowsy.

• Stay calm and in control of the situation.

Keep a bottle of Ipecac Syrup stored in a secure place in your home for emergency use. It is available at pharmacies in 1 ounce bottles without prescription. Ipecac Syrup is often recommended to induce vomiting in cases of poisoning.

Activated Charcoal also is sometimes recommended in certain types of poisoning and you may wish to add a supply to your emergency medicines. It is available without a prescription. Before using this medicine for poisoning, however, call a poison control center for advice.

GETTING THE MOST OUT OF YOUR MEDICINES

To get the most out of your medicines, there are certain things that you must do. Although your health care professionals will be working with you, you also have a responsibility for your own health.

Communicating with Your Health Care Provider

Communication between you and your health care professional is central to good medical care. Your health care professional needs to know about you, your medical history, and your current problems. In turn, you need to understand the recommendations he or she is making and what you will need to do to follow the treatment. You will have to ask questions—and answer some too. Communication is a two-way street.

Giving information

To provide effective care, your health care professional needs to know some details about your past and present medical history. In discussing these details, you should always be completely open and honest. Your health professional's diagnosis and treatment will be based in part on the information that you provide. A complete list of the details that should be included in a full medical history is provided below.

"Medical history" checklist

A "medical history" checklist covers the following information:

• All the serious illnesses you have ever had and the approximate dates.

• Your current symptoms, if any.

• All the medicines and dietary supplements you are taking or have taken in the recent past. This includes prescription and nonprescription medicines (such as pain relievers, antacids, laxatives, and cold medicines, etc.) and home remedies. This is especially important if you are seeing more than one health care professional; if you are having surgery, including dental or emergency treatment; or if you get your medicines from more than one source.

• Any allergies or sensitivities to medicines, foods, or other substances.

• Your smoking, drinking, and exercise habits.

• Any recent changes in your life-style or personal habits. New job? Retired? Change of residence? Death in family? Married? Divorced? Other?

• Any special diet you are on—low-sugar, low-sodium, low-fat, or a diet to lose or gain weight.

• If you are pregnant, plan to become pregnant, or if you are breast-feeding.

• All the vaccinations and vaccination boosters you have had, with dates if possible.

• Any operations you have had, including dental and those performed on an outpatient basis, and any accidents that have required hospitalization.

• Illnesses or conditions that run in your family.

• Cause of death of closest relatives.

Remember, be sure to tell your health care professional at each visit if there have been any changes since your last visit.

Many health care professionals have a standard "medical history" form they will ask you to fill out when they see you for the first time. Some may ask the questions and write down the answers for you. If you will be visiting a health care professional for the first time, prepare yourself before you go by thinking about the questions that might be asked and jotting down the answers—including dates—so that you will not forget an important detail. Once your "medical history" is in the files, subsequent visits will take less time.

You will have to supply each health care professional you see—every time you see one—with complete information about what happened since your last visit. It is important that your records are updated so he or she can make sound recommendations for your continued treatment, or treatment of any new problems.

It will simplify things if you develop a "medical history" file at home for yourself and each family member for whom you are responsible. Setting up the file will take time. However, once it is established, you need only to keep it up-to-date and remember to take it with you when you see a health care professional. This will be easier than having to repeat the information each time and running the risk of confusing or forgetting details.

It is also a good idea to carry in your wallet a card that summarizes your chronic medical conditions, the medicines you are taking, and your allergies and drug sensitivities. You should keep this card as up-to-date as possible. Many pharmacists provide these cards as a service.

Getting information

For your health care professional to be able to serve you well, you must communicate all that you know about your present health condition at every visit. In order to benefit from the advice for which you have paid, your health care professional must communicate full instructions for your care. More importantly, you must understand completely everything that he or she tells you. Do not be embarrassed to ask questions, or to ask him or her to explain again any instruction or detail that you do not understand. Then it is up to you to carry out those instructions precisely. If there is a failure in any part of this system, you will pay an even higher price—physically and financially—for your health care.

Your health care professional may provide instructions to you in written form. If he or she does not, you may want to write them down or ask the health care professional to write them down for you. If you do not have time to jot down everything while you are still with your health care professional, sit down in the waiting room before you leave and write down the information while it is still fresh in your mind and you can still ask questions. If you have been given a prescription, ask for written information about the drug and how to take it. Your pharmacist can also answer questions when you have your prescription filled.

Before starting treatment for your heart condition, there are several important things that you should remember—

You must decide whether you are willing to commit yourself to getting your condition under control. Whether it is controlled or not depends on you. Your doctor can prescribe medicine and suggest treatment. Only you can decide to follow through.

Treating your condition may necessitate some changes in your life-style which will probably last the rest of your life. You may have to make some changes in your diet and daily routine. By learning about your condition and becoming a partner with your doctor in your treatment, *you can be the decision-maker in your own care.*

Never change the dose of your medicine or stop taking it or change your nondrug treatment without discussing it with your doctor. You must decide together on the best thing to do.

Your chances of living an active, healthy life are good if you treat your condition wisely.

What you need to know about your medicines

There are a number of things that you should know about each medicine you are taking. These include:

• The medicine's generic and brand name. Can this prescription be written as a generic name instead of a brand name to save money?

• How the medicine will help you and the expected results. How it makes you feel. How long it takes to begin working.

• How much to take at one time.

• How often to take the medicine.

• How long it will be necessary to take the medicine.

• When to take it. Before, during, after meals? At bedtime? At any other special times?

• How to take it. With water? With fruit juice?

• What to do if you forget to take it (miss a dose).

• Foods, drinks, or other medicines that you should not take while taking the medicine.

• Can this medicine be taken during pregnancy or if you are breast-feeding?

• Restrictions on activities while taking the medicine. May I drive a car or operate other motor vehicles?

• Possible side effects. What to do if they appear. How to minimize the side effects. How soon they will go away.

• When to seek help if there are problems.

• How long to wait before reporting no change in symptoms.

• How to store the medicine.

• The expiration date.

• The cost of the medicine.

• How to have your prescription refilled, if necessary.

Other information

Following are some other issues and information that you may want to consider:

• Ask your health care professional about the ingredients in the medicines (both prescription and over-the-counter [OTC]) you are taking and whether there may be a conflict with other medicines. Your health care professional can help you avoid dangerous combinations or drug products that contain ingredients to which you are allergic or sensitive.

• Ask your health care professional for help in developing a system for taking your medicines properly, particularly if you are taking a number of them on a daily basis. (When you are a patient in a hospital, ask for instructions before you are discharged.) Do not hesitate or be embarrassed to ask questions or ask for help.

• If you are over 60 years of age, ask your health care professional if the dose of the medicine prescribed is right for you. Some medicines should be given in lower doses to certain older individuals.

• If you are taking several different medicines, ask your health care professional if all of them are necessary for you. You should take only those medicines that you need.

• Medicines should be kept in the container they came in. If this is not possible when you are at work or away from home, ask your pharmacist to provide or recommend a container to transport your medicines safely. The use of "pill boxes" can also cause some problems, such as broken or chipped tablets, mistaking one medicine for another, and even interactions between the medicine and the metal of these boxes.

• Some people have trouble taking tablets or capsules. Your health care professional will know if another dosage form is available, and if tablets or capsule contents can be taken in a liquid. If this is an ongoing problem, ask your prescriber to write the prescription for the dosage form you can take most comfortably.

• Child-resistant caps are required by law on most prescription medicines for oral use to protect children from accidental poisoning. These containers are designed so that children will have difficulty opening them. Since many adults also find these containers hard to open, the law allows consumers to request traditional, easy-to-open packaging for their drugs. If you do not use child-resistant packaging, make sure that your medicines are stored where small children cannot see or reach them. If you use child-resistant containers, ask your pharmacist to show you how to open them.

Consumer education is one of the most important responsibilities of your health care professional. To supplement what you learn during your visit, ask if there is any written information about your medicines that you can take home with you. Your health care professional may also have available various reference books or computerized drug information that you can consult for details about precautions, side effects, and proper use of your medicines.

Your Health Care Team

Your health care team will be made up of several different health care professionals. Each of these individuals will play an important part in the overall provision of your health care. It is important that you understand the roles of each of these providers and what you should be able to expect from each of them.

Your dentist

In addition to providing care and maintenance of your mouth, teeth, and gums, your dentist is also an essential member of your overall health care team since your oral health and general health often affect one another.

In providing dental treatment, your dentist should base his or her decisions upon an extensive knowledge of your current condition and past medical and dental history. Because the dentist is a prescriber of medications, it is very important that he or she is aware of your full medical and dental history. A complete medical and dental history should include the information that is listed in the "Medical history checklist" section above. Even if you do not consider this information important, you should inform your dentist as fully as possible.

In the treatment of any dental/oral problem your dentist should make every effort to inform you as fully as possible about the nature of the problem. He or she should explain why this problem has occurred, the advantages and disadvantages of available treatments (including no treatment), and what types of preventive measures can be employed to avoid future problems. These measures may include periodic visits to the dentist, and a general awareness of the manner in which dental and overall health may affect one another. In any type of treatment, your dentist should always allow you to ask questions, and should be willing to answer them to your satisfaction.

In selecting a dentist, it is important to keep in mind the role of the dentist as a member of the health care team, and the extent of the information that he or she should be asking for and providing. There are also several practical issues that you should consider, such as:

- Is the dentist a specialist or general practitioner?
- What are the office hours?
- Is the dentist or his/her associates available after office hours by phone? In emergencies, will you be able to contact a dentist?
- What is the office policy on cancellations?
- What types of payment are accepted at the office?

- What is the office policy on x-ray procedures?
- Is the dentist willing to work with other medical and/or dental specialists that you may be seeing?

Your dentist should be an integral part of your health care team. In treating problems and providing general maintenance of your oral health, your dentist should base decisions upon a full dental and medical history. He or she should also be willing to answer any questions that you have regarding your oral health, any medications prescribed, and preventive measures to avoid future problems.

Your nurse

Depending upon the setting, type of therapy being administered, and state regulations, the role of the nurse in your health care team may vary. Registered nurses practice in diverse health care settings, such as hospitals, out-patient clinics or physicians' offices, schools, workplaces, homes, and long-term care facilities like nursing homes and retirement centers. Some nurses, including certified nurse practitioners and midwives, hold a master's degree in nursing and may assume the role of primary health care professional, either in practice by themselves or in joint practices with physicians. In most states, nurse practitioners may prescribe selected medications. Clinical nurse specialists also have a master's degree in nursing and specialize in a particular area of health care. In some hospitals, long-term care facilities, and out-patient care settings, licensed practical nurses (LPNs) have certain responsibilities in administering medication to patients. LPNs usually work under the supervision of an RN or physician. Nursing aides assist RNs and LPNs with different kinds of patient care activities. In most places where people receive health care, RNs may be the primary source of information for drug therapies and other medical treatments. It is important that you be aware of the roles and responsibilities of the nurses participating in your health care.

Professional nurses participate with other health professionals, such as physicians and pharmacists, to ensure that your medication therapy is safe and effective and to monitor any effects (both desired and negative) from the medication. You may be admitted to the hospital so that nurses can administer medications and monitor your response to therapy. In hospitals or long-term care facilities, nurses are responsible for administering your medications in their proper dosage form and dose, and at correct time intervals, as well as monitoring your response to these medications. At home or in outpatient settings, nurses should ensure that you have the proper information and support of others, if needed, to get the medication and take it as prescribed. When nurses administer medication, they should explain why you are receiving this medication, how it works, any possible side effects, special precautions or actions that you must take while using the medication, and any potential interactions with other medications.

If you experience any side effects or symptoms from a medication, you should always tell your health care provider. It is important that these reactions be detected before they become serious or permanent. You can seek advice about possible ways to minimize these side effects from your nurse. Your health care professional should also be made aware of any additional medical problems or conditions (such as pregnancy) that you may have, since these can also affect the safety and effectiveness of a medication.

The professional nurse is someone who can help to clarify drug information. In most health care settings, nurses are accessible and can answer your questions or direct you to others who can assist you. Professional nurses are skilled in the process of patient teaching. To make sure that patients learn important information about their health problem and its treatment, RNs often use a combination of teaching methods, such as verbal instruction, written materials, demonstration, and audio-visual instructions. Above all, professional nurses should teach at a pace and level that are appropriate for you. RNs can also help you design a medication schedule that fits your life-style and may be less likely to cause unwanted side effects.

Your pharmacist

Your pharmacist is an important member of your health care team. In addition to performing traditional services, such as dispensing medications, your pharmacist can help you understand your medications and how to take them safely and effectively. By keeping accurate and up-to-date records and monitoring your use of medications, your pharmacist can help to protect you from improper medication therapy, unwanted side effects, and dangerous drug interactions. Because your pharmacist can play a vital role in protecting and improving your health, you should seek a pharmacist who will provide these services.

To provide you with the best possible care, your pharmacist should be informed about your current condition and medication history. Your personal medication history should include the information that is listed in the "Medical history checklist" section above. Your pharmacist should also be aware of any special packaging needs that you may have (such as child-resistant or easy-to-open containers). Your pharmacist should keep accurate and up-to-date records that contain this information. If you visit a new pharmacy that does not have access to your medication records, it is important that you inform that pharmacist as fully as possible about your medical history or provide him or her with a copy of your medication records from your previous pharmacy. In general, in order to get the most out of your pharmacy services, it is best to get all of your medications (including OTCs) from the same pharmacy.

Your pharmacist should be a knowledgeable and approachable source of information about your medications. Some of the information that your pharmacist should explain to you about your medications is listed in the "What you need to know about your medicines" section above. Ideally, this information should also be provided in written form, so that you may refer to it later if you have any questions or problems. The pharmacist should always be willing to answer any questions that you have regarding your medications, and should also be willing to contact your physician or other health care professionals (dentist, nurses, etc.) on your behalf if necessary.

Your pharmacist can also help you with information on the costs of your medicines. Many medicines are available from more than one company. They may have equal effects, but may have different costs. Your insurance company, HMO, or other third-party payment group may reimburse you for only some of these medications or only for part of their costs. Your pharmacist will be able to tell you which of these medications are covered by your payment plan or which cost less.

In selecting a pharmacist, it is important that you understand the role of the pharmacist as a member of your health care team and the extent of information that he or she should be asking for and providing. Because pharmacies can offer different types of services and have different policies regarding patient information, some of the issues that you should consider in selecting a pharmacist also relate to the pharmacy where that person practices. There are several issues regarding the pharmacist and pharmacy that you should consider, such as:

• Does the pharmacy offer written information that you can take home? Home delivery?

• Are you able to talk to your pharmacist without other people hearing you?

• Can the pharmacist be reached easily by phone? In an emergency, is a pharmacist available twenty-four hours a day (including weekends and holidays) by phone?

• What types of payment are accepted in the pharmacy?

• Does the pharmacy accept your HMO or third-party payment plan?

• Does the pharmacy offer any specialized services, such as diabetes education?

You should select your pharmacist and pharmacy as carefully as you select your physician, and stay with the same pharmacy so that all of your medication records are in the same place. This will help to ensure that your records are accurate and up-to-date and will allow you to develop a beneficial relationship with your pharmacist.

Your physician

One of the most important health care decisions that you will make is your choice of a personal physician. The physician is central to your health care team, and is responsible for helping you maintain your overall health. In addition to detecting and treating ailments or adverse conditions, your physician and his or her coworkers should also serve as primary sources of health care information. Because the physician plays such an important role in your overall health care, it is important that you understand the full range of the physician's role as health care and information provider.

In providing any type of treatment or counseling, your physician should base his or her decisions upon an extensive knowledge of your current condition and past medical history. A complete medical history should include the information that is listed in the ''Medical history checklist'' section above. Your physician should keep accurate and comprehensive medical records containing this information. Because your treatment (and your health) is dependent upon a full disclosure of your medical history, as well as any factors that may currently be affecting your health (i.e., stress, smoking, drug use, etc.), it is important that you inform your physician as fully as possible, even if you might not consider this information important.

It is important that you inform your personal physician of any other physicians (such as specialists or subspecialists), dentists, or other health care professionals that you are seeing. You should also inform your physician of the pharmacy that you use or intend to use, so that he or she can contact the pharmacist if necessary.

In treating any health problem, your physician should make every effort to help you understand completely the nature of the problem and its treatment. He or she should take the time to explain the problem, why it may have occurred, and what preventive measures (if any) can be taken to avoid it in the future. Your physician should explain fully the reasons for any prescribed treatment. He or she should also be willing to discuss alternative therapies, especially if you are uncomfortable with the one that has been prescribed. Your physician should always be willing to answer all of your questions to your satisfaction.

In selecting a physician, you should look for one who will provide a full range of services. Asking for a full medical history and providing complete information about your treatment and medications are some of these services. There are several other issues that you may want to consider. Does your physician:

- Consult peers with specialty training for difficult problems?
- Inquire about your general health as well as specific problems?
- Have a good working relationship with your pharmacist? With the nurses and staff at his/her office?
- Periodically have you bring in bottles or labels from all of the medications (prescription and nonprescription) that you are taking or have at home?
- Periodically check the status of your vaccinations?

You may also want to consider your physician's medical credentials. Your local medical society should be able to provide specific facts about your physician's training, experience, and membership in professional societies.

One of the most important issues in contemporary health care is that of cost and payment. Your physician should be sensitive to the costs of your treatment and the manner in which you intend to pay for this and related medications. If you belong to an HMO or third-party payment plan, be sure that your physician is aware of your involvement in the plan. You should also be aware of the different types of payment that are accepted at the physician's office.

In prescribing medications, your physician should take into account the manner in which you intend to pay for your drugs, and should be aware of any specific concerns regarding the costs of your treatment and medication. He or she should also explain why brand or generic medication may be preferable in certain situations.

In selecting a physician, there are also several practical issues and matters of convenience that you should consider, such as:

- Is the office convenient to your home or work?
- What are the office hours?
- Is your physician or his/her associates or partners available (twenty-four hours a day) by phone? In emergencies, will you be able to contact a physician?

- Are you able to arrange appointments to fit your schedule? What is the office policy on cancellations?
- Is the physician well regarded in the community? Does he or she have a reputation for listening to patients and answering questions?
- Does the physician have admitting privileges at a hospital of your preference?
- Does he/she participate in your health plan?

In addition to the considerations already mentioned, your physician should be sensitive to the special concerns of treating the elderly. Older patients can present disease processes differently from younger adults, can react differently to certain drugs and dosages, and may have preexisting conditions that require special treatments to be prescribed.

There are also several special issues to consider in your selection of a pediatrician or family physician. If your child is not old enough to understand all instructions and information, it is important that your child's physician explain to you any information pertaining to the nature of a problem and all instructions for medications. When your child is of school age, the physician should speak directly to the child as well, asking and answering questions, and providing information about cause and prevention of medical problems and the use of medications. He or she should choose a dosage form and dose that is appropriate for your child's age and explain what to do if your child has certain symptoms, such as fever, vomiting, etc. (including the amount and type of medicine to give, if any, and when to call him or her for advice).

Your physician should be a primary source of information about your health and any medications that you are taking. In providing treatment for medical problems or conditions, the physician should base decisions upon a full medical history and be willing to answer any questions that you have regarding your health, treatment, and medications.

Managing Your Medicines

To get the full benefit and reduce risks in taking your prescribed medicines, it is important to take the right medicine and dose at correct time intervals for the length of time prescribed. Bad effects can result from taking too much or too little of a medicine, or taking it too often or not often enough.

Each patient is different and medicine may not act the same for everyone. If one medicine does not work well enough, your doctor may try another. Just because you start taking one medicine does not mean you will always take that same medicine.

Many patients, depending on the condition, need to take only one medicine. However, others may require two or more to bring their condition under control. Your doctor may have to try different medicines at different dosages until the combination that works best for you and causes you the fewest side effects is found. It may take months to find the right medicine or combination of medicines to control your condition.

In addition to their helpful effects, most medicines may have some side effects; some of these are serious while others are only bothersome. If you experience side effects, you and your doctor can decide together whether to change the dose of the medicine or to switch to another medicine. However, there may be some side effects that cannot be avoided.

Establishing a system

Whether you are taking one or several medicines, you should develop a system for taking them. It can be just as difficult to remember whether you took your once-a-day medicine as it can be to keep track of a number of medicines that need to be taken several times a day. Many medicines also have special instructions that can further complicate proper use.

Establish a way of knowing whether you took your medicines properly, then make that a part of your daily routine. If you take 1 or 2 medicines a day, you may only need to take them at the same time that you perform some other regular task, such as brushing your teeth or getting dressed.

By associating the time you take your medicine with other things you do, you may find it easier to remember to take it. Plan a routine that works for *you*. Your health care professional may be able to help you plan a convenient medication schedule. Some medicines have effects that may be particularly inconvenient at certain times of the day, such as drowsiness or frequent urination. Also, some medicines should be taken on an empty stomach. You and your doctor and pharmacist can work out the best time of day for you to take your medicine so that these effects will interfere with your life as little as possible.

For most people, a check-off record can also be a handy way of managing multiple medicines. Keep your medicine record in a handy, visible place next to where you take your medicines. Check off each dose as you take it. If you miss a dose, make a note about what happened and what you did on the back of the record or the bottom of the sheet.

Be sure to note any unwanted effects or anything unusual that you think may be connected with your medicines. Also note if a medicine does not do what you expect. Remember that some medicines take a while before they start having a noticeable effect.

If you keep a check-off record faithfully, you will know for sure whether or not you took your medicine. You will also have a complete record for your health care professionals to review when you visit them again. This information can help them determine if the medicine is working properly or causing unwanted side effects, or whether adjustments should be made in your medicines and/or doses.

If your medicines or the instructions for taking them are changed, correct your record or make a new one. Keep the old record until you are sure you or your health care professionals no longer need that information.

You might want to color code your medicine containers to help tell them apart. If you are having trouble reading labels or if you are color-blind, codes that can be recognized by touch (rubber bands, a cotton ball, or a piece of emery board, for instance) can be attached to the container. If you code your medicines, be sure these identifications are included on any medicine record you use. If necessary, ask your pharmacist to type medicine labels in large letters for easier reading.

A check-off list is not the only method to record medicine use. If this system does not work for you, ask your health care professional to help you develop an alternative. Be sure he or she knows all the medicines prescribed for you and any nonprescription medicines you take regularly, the hours you usually eat your meals, and any special diet you are following.

Informed management

Your medicines have been prescribed for you and your condition. Ask your health care professional what benefits to expect, what side effects may occur, and when to report any side effects. If your symptoms go away, do not decide you are well and stop taking your medicine. If you stop too soon, the symptoms may come back. Finish all of the medicine if you have been told to do so. However, if you develop diarrhea or other unpleasant side effects, do not continue with the medicine just because you were told to finish it. Call your health care professional and report these effects. A change in dose or in the kind of medicine you are taking may be necessary.

When you are given a prescription for a medicine, ask the person who wrote it to explain it to you. For example, does "four times a day" mean one in the morning, one at noon, one in the evening, and one at bedtime; or does it mean every six hours around the clock? When a prescription says "take as needed," ask how close together the doses can be taken and what the maximum number of doses you can take in one day should be. Does "take with liquids" mean with water, milk, or something else? Are there some liquids that should avoided? What does "take with food" mean? At every meal time (some people must eat six meals a day), or with a snack? Do not trust your memory—have the instructions written down. To follow the instructions for taking your medicines, you must understand exactly what the prescriber wants you to do in order to "take as directed."

When the pharmacist dispenses your medicine, you have another opportunity to clarify information or to ask other questions. Before you leave, check the label on your medicine to be sure it matches the prescription and your understanding of what you are to do. If it does not, ask more questions.

The key to getting the most from your prescribed treatments is following instructions accurately and intelligently. If you have questions or doubts about the prescribed treatment, do not decide not to take the medicine or fail to follow the prescribed regimen. Discuss your questions and doubts with your health care professional.

The time and effort put into setting up a system to manage your medicines and establish a routine for taking them will pay off by relieving anxiety and helping you get the most from your prescribed treatment.

Keep all of your medical appointments. Even if you feel well, it is important that your doctor check your progress at periodic intervals. This also gives you a chance to ask any questions you may have. If you can't make it to your appointment, let your doctor know and make a new appointment for the earliest time that is convenient for you. Once your condition is under control, visits to the doctor will become less frequent.

Ask questions. Knowing as much as possible about your condition and its treatment will help you in bringing it under control. Write down questions when you think of them so that you will remember to ask your doctor at your next visit. Don't be afraid to ask questions. If something is of special concern to you, call your health care professional. Health care professionals are interested in your care and want to know your feelings, concerns, fears, and questions. The best way to help is to be informed about your condition.

Make a medication calendar. This will help you to keep track of your own treatment and to remember to take your medicine.

Be a partner with your doctor, nurse, dietitian, and pharmacist. Getting your condition under control requires close teamwork, and you are a key member of the team. Make the decision to follow your treatment and work with your doctor, nurse, dietitian, and pharmacist to make it as successful as possible.

Enlist your family's or friends' help. Remember, they need you and want you to have the longest, healthiest life possible.

They can help you remember to take your medicine and follow your diet. Have them read this book so they can understand your condition. Put *them* on your team, too.

Taking Your Medicine

To take medicines safely and get the greatest benefit from them, it is important to establish regular habits so that you are less likely to make mistakes.

Before taking any medicine, read the label and any accompanying information. You can also consult books to learn more about the medicine. If you have unanswered questions, check with your health care professional.

The label on the container of a prescription medicine should bear your first and last name; the name of the prescriber; the pharmacy address and telephone number; the prescription number; the date of dispensing; and directions for use. Some states or provinces may have additional requirements. If the name of the drug product is not on the label, ask the pharmacist to include the brand (if any) and generic names. An expiration date may also appear. All of this information is important in identifying your medicines and using them properly. The labels on containers should never be removed and all medicines should be kept in their original containers.

Some tips for taking medicines safely and accurately include the following:

- Read the label of each medicine container three times:
  —before you remove it from its storage place,
  —before you take the lid off the container to remove the dose, and
  —before you replace the container in its storage place.
- Never take medicines in the dark, even if you think you know exactly where to find them.
- Use standard measuring devices to take your medicines (the household teaspoon, cup, or glass vary widely in the amount they hold). Ask your pharmacist for help with measuring.

• Set bottles and boxes of medicines on a clear area, well back from the edge of the surface to prevent containers and/or caps from being knocked to the floor.

• When pouring liquid medicines, pick up the container with the label against the palm of your hand to protect it from being stained by dripping medicine.

• Wipe off the top and neck of bottles of liquid medicines to keep labels from being obscured, and to make it less likely that the lid will stick.

• Shake all liquid suspensions of drug products before pouring so that ingredients are mixed thoroughly.

• If you are to take medicine with water, take a full, 8 ounce glassful, not just enough to get it down. Too little liquid with some medicines can prevent the medicine from working properly, and can cause throat irritation if the medicine does not get completely to the stomach.

• To avoid accidental confusion of lids, labels, and medicines, replace the lid on one container before opening another.

• When you are interrupted while taking your medicine, take the container with you or put the medicine up out of the reach of small children. It only takes a second for them to take an overdose. When you return, check the label of the medicine to be sure you have the right one before taking it.

• Only crush tablets or open capsules to take with food or beverages if your health care professional has told you that this will not affect the way the medicine works. If you have difficulty swallowing a tablet or capsule, check with your health care professional about the availability of a different dosage form.

• Follow any diet instructions or other treatment measures prescribed by your health care professional.

• If at any point you realize you have taken the wrong medicine or the wrong amount, call your health care professional immediately. In an emergency, call your local emergency number.

When you have finished taking your medicines, mark it down immediately on your medication calendar to avoid "double dosing." Also, make notes of any unusual changes in your body: change in weight, color or amount of urine, perspiration, or sputum; your pulse, temperature, or any other items you may have been instructed to observe for your condition or your medicine.

Try to take your medicines on time, but a half hour early or late will usually not upset your schedule. If you are more than several hours late and are getting close to your next scheduled dose, check any instructions that were given to you by your health care professional. If you did not receive instructions for what to do about a missed dose, check with your health care professional. You may also find missed dose information in the entries included in this book.

When your medicines are being managed by someone else (for example, when you are a patient in a hospital or nursing home), question what is happening to you and communicate what you know about your previous drug therapy or any other treatments. If you know you always take 1, not 2, of a certain tablet, say so and ask that your record be checked before you take the medicine. If you think you are receiving the wrong treatment or medication, do not hesitate to say so. You should always remain involved in your own therapy.

Many hospitals and nursing homes now offer counseling in medicine management as part of their discharge planning for patients. If you or a family member is getting ready to come home, ask your health care professional if you can be part of such instruction.

The "Expiration Date" on Medicine Labels

To assure that a drug product meets applicable standards of identity, strength, quality, and purity at the time of use, an "expiration date" is added by the manufacturer to the label of most prescription and nonprescription drug products.

The expiration date on a drug product is valid only as long as the product is stored in the original, unopened container under the storage conditions specified by the manufacturer.

Among other things, drugs can be affected by humidity, temperature, light, and even air. A medicine taken after the expiration date may have changed in potency or may have formed harmful material as it deteriorates. In other instances, contamination with germs may have occurred. The safest rule is not to use any medicine beyond the expiration date.

Preventing deterioration

A drug begins to deteriorate the minute it is made. This rate of deterioration is factored in by the manufacturer in calculating the expiration date. Keeping the drug product in the container supplied by the pharmacist helps slow down deterioration. Storing the drug in the prescribed manner—for example, in a light-resistant container or in a cool, dry place (not the bathroom medicine cabinet)—also helps. The need for medicines to be kept in their containers and stored properly cannot be overstressed.

Patients sometimes ask their health care professionals to prescribe a large quantity of a particular medicine in order to "economize." Although this may be all right in some cases, this practice may backfire. If you have a large supply of your medicine and it deteriorates before you can use it all, or if your doctor changes your medicine, you may lose out.

Sometimes deterioration can be recognized by physical changes in the drug, such as a change in odor or appearance. For example, aspirin tablets develop a vinegar odor when they break down. These changes are not true of all drugs, however, and the absence of physical changes should not be assumed to mean that no deterioration has occurred.

Some liquid medicines mixed at the pharmacy will have a "beyond use" date on the label. This is an expiration date that is calculated from the date of preparation in the pharmacy. This is a definite date, after which you should discard any of the medicine that remains.

If your prescription medicines do not bear an "expiration" or "beyond use" date, your dispensing pharmacist is the best person to advise you about how long they can be safely utilized.

ABOUT THE MEDICINES
YOU ARE TAKING

New Drugs—From Idea to Marketplace

To be sold legitimately in the United States, new drugs must pass through a rigorous system of approval specified in the Food, Drug, and Cosmetic Act and supervised by the Food and Drug Administration (FDA). Except for certain drugs subject to other regulatory provisions, no new drug for human use may be marketed in this country unless FDA has approved a "New Drug Application" (NDA) for it.

The idea

The creation of a new drug usually starts with an idea. Most likely that idea results from the study of a disease or group of symptoms. Ideas can also come from observations of clinical research. This may involve many years of study, or the idea may occur from an accidental discovery in a research laboratory. Some may be coincidental discoveries, as in the case of penicillin.

Idea development takes place most often in the laboratory of a pharmaceutical company, but may also happen in laboratories at research institutions like the National Institutes of Health, at medical centers and universities, or in the laboratory of a chemical company.

Animal testing

The idea for a new drug is first tested on animals to help determine how toxic the substance may be. Most drugs interfere in some way with normal body functions. These animal studies are designed to discover the degree of that interference and the extent of the toxic effects.

After successful animal testing, perhaps over several years, the sponsors of the new drug apply to the FDA for an Investigational New Drug (IND) application. This status allows the drug to be tested in humans. As part of their request, the sponsoring manufacturer must submit the results of the animal studies, plus a detailed outline of the proposed human testing and information about the researchers that will be involved.

Human testing

Drug testing in humans usually consists of three consecutive phases. "Informed consent" must be secured from all volunteers participating in this testing.

Phase I testing is most often done on young, healthy adults. This testing is done on a relatively small number of subjects, generally between 20 and 80. Its purpose is to learn more about the biochemistry of the drug: how it acts on the body, and how the body reacts to it. The procedure differs for some drugs, however. For example, Phase I testing of drugs used to treat cancer involves actual patients with the disease from the beginning of testing.

During Phase II, small controlled clinical studies are designed to test the effectiveness and relative safety of the drug. These are done on closely monitored patients who have the disease for which the drug is being tested. Their numbers seldom go beyond 100 to 200 patients. Some volunteers for Phase II testing who have severely complicating conditions may be excluded.

A "control" group of people of comparable physical and disease types is used to do double-blind, controlled experiments for most drugs. These are conducted by medical investigators thoroughly familiar with the disease and this type of research. In a double-blind experiment, the patient, the health care provider, and other personnel do not know whether the patient is receiving the drug being tested, another active drug, or no medicine at all (a placebo or "sugar pill"). This helps eliminate bias and assures the accuracy of results. The findings of these tests are statistically analyzed to determine whether they are "significant" or due to chance alone.

Phase III consists of larger studies. This testing is performed after effectiveness of the drug has been established and is intended to gather additional evidence of effectiveness for specific uses of the drug. These studies also help discover adverse drug reactions that may occur with the drug.

Phase III studies involve a few hundred to several thousand patients who have the disease the drug is intended to treat.

Patients with additional diseases or those receiving other therapy may be included in later Phase II and Phase III studies. They would be expected to be representative of certain segments of the population who would receive the drug following approval for marketing.

Final approval

When a sponsor believes the investigational studies on a drug have shown it to be safe and effective in treating specific conditions, a New Drug Application (NDA) is submitted to FDA. This application is accompanied by all the documentation from the company's research, including complete records of all the animal and human testing. This documentation can run to many thousands of pages.

The NDA application and its documentation must then be reviewed by FDA physicians, pharmacologists, chemists, statisticians, and other professionals experienced in evaluating new drugs. Proposed labeling information for the physician and pharmacist is also screened for accuracy, completeness, and conformity to FDA-approved wording.

Regulations call for the FDA to review an NDA within 180 days. This period may be extended and actually takes an average of 2 to 3 years. When all research phases are considered, the actual time it takes from idea to marketplace may be 8 to 10 years or even longer. However, for drugs representing major therapeutic advances, FDA may "fast-track" the approval process to try to get those drugs to patients who need them as soon as possible.

After approval

After a drug is marketed, the manufacturer must inform the FDA of any unexpected side effects or toxicity that comes to its attention. Consumers and health care professionals have an important role in helping to identify any previously unreported effects. If new evidence indicates that the drug may present an "imminent hazard," the FDA can withdraw approval for marketing or add new information to the drug's labeling at any time.

Generic drugs

After a new drug is approved for marketing, a patent will generally protect the financial interests of the drug's developer for a number of years. The traditional protection period is for 17 years. In reality, however, the period is much less due to the extended period of time needed to gain approval before marketing can begin. Recognizing that a considerable part of a drug's patent life may be tied up in the approval process, in 1984 Congress passed a law providing patent extension for drugs whose commercial sale may have been unduly delayed by the approval process.

Any manufacturer can apply for permission to produce and market a drug after the patent for the drug has expired. Following a procedure called an Abbreviated New Drug Application (ANDA), the applicant must show that its product is bioequivalent to the originator's product. Although the extensive clinical testing the originator had to complete during the drug's development does not have to be repeated, comparative testing between the products must be done to ensure that they will be therapeutically equivalent.

Drug Names

Every drug must have a nonproprietary name, a name that is available for each manufacturer to use. These names are commonly called generic names.

The FDA requires that the generic name of a drug product be placed on its labeling. However, manufacturers often coin brand (trade) names to use in promoting their products. In general, brand names are shorter, catchier, and easier to use than the corresponding generic name. The brand name manufacturer will then emphasize its brand name (which cannot be used by anyone else) in its advertising and other promotions. In many instances, the consumer may not recognize that a drug being sold under one particular brand name is indeed available under other brand names or by generic name. Ask your pharmacist if you have any questions about the names of your medicines.

Drug Quality

After an NDA or an ANDA has been approved for a product, the manufacturer must then meet all requirements relating to production. These include current Good Manufacturing Practice regulations of the Food and Drug Administration (FDA) and any applicable standards relating to strength, quality, purity, packaging, and labeling that are established by the *United States Pharmacopeia* (USP).

Simply placing a brand name on a label does not assure the quality of the product inside the container. Rather, the quality of a product depends on the manufacturer's ability to create a value product consistently from batch to batch.

Routine product testing by the manufacturer is required by the Good Manufacturing Practice regulations of the FDA (the FDA itself does not routinely test all products, except in cases where there is a suspicion that something might be wrong). In addition to governmental requirements, drug products must meet public standards of strength, quality, and purity that are published in the USP. In order to market their products, all manufacturers in the United States must meet USP-established standards unless they specifically choose not to meet the standards for a particular product. In this case, that product's label must state that it is "not USP" and how it differs from USP standards (this occurs very rarely).

Differences in Drug Products

Although standards to ensure strength, quality, purity, and bioequivalence exist for drug products, the standards allow for variations in certain factors that may produce other differences from product to product. These product variations may be important to some patients, since not all patients are "equivalent." For example, the size, shape, and coating may vary and, therefore, be harder or easier for some patients to swallow; an oral liquid will taste good to some patients and awful to others; one manufacturer may use lactose as an inactive ingredient in its product while a therapeutically equivalent product may use some other inactive ingredient; one product may contain sugar or alcohol while another product may not.

In deciding to use one therapeutically equivalent product over another, consumers should keep the following in mind:

- Consider convenience factors of drug products (for example, ease of taking a particular dosage form).
- Don't overlook the convenience of the package. The package must protect the drug in accordance with USP requirements, but packages can be quite different in their ease of carrying, storing, opening, and measuring.
- If you have a known allergy or any type of dietary restriction, you need to be aware of the pharmaceutic or "inactive" ingredients that may be present in medicines you have to take. These inactive ingredients may vary from product to product.
- Price is always a consideration. The price difference between products (e.g., different brands, or brands versus generics) may be a major factor in the overall price of a prescription. Talk to your pharmacist about price considerations. Some states require that the pharmacist dispense exactly what is prescribed. However, other states allow the pharmacist to dispense less expensive medicines when appropriate.

Aside from differences in the drug product, there are many other factors that may influence the effectiveness of a medicine. For example, your diet, body chemistry, medical conditions, or other drugs you are taking may affect how much of a dose of a particular medicine gets into the body.

For the majority of drugs, slight differences in the amount of drug made available to the body will not make any therapeutic difference. For other drugs, the precise amount that gets into the body is more critical. For example, some heart or epilepsy medicines may create problems for the patient if the dose delivered to the body varies for some reason.

For those drugs that fall in the critical category, it is a good idea to stay on the specific product you started on. Changes should only be made after consultation with the health care professional who prescribed the medicine for you. If you feel that a certain batch of your medicine is more potent or does not work as well as other batches, or if you have other questions, check with your health care professional.

CORONARY HEART DISEASE AND OTHER HEART PROBLEMS

Coronary heart disease or atherosclerosis of the coronary arteries is a hardening of the arteries that supply blood to the heart. Coronary heart disease is a continuing process and tends to get worse over a long period of time. This can lead to a variety of heart problems, including heart attacks, arrhythmias, and congestive heart failure.

The conditions covered by this book are: (1) angina (chest discomfort), which usually occurs as a result of coronary heart disease, but may have other causes; (2) risk factors for coronary heart disease (e.g., high blood cholesterol, high blood pressure); (3) other heart problems, which may occur as a result of coronary heart disease or may have other causes (e.g., congestive heart failure, arrhythmias).

The Heart

About your heart

Your heart is a muscle about the size of a large fist. It is located in the center of your chest behind the breastbone. The heart beats in order to pump blood and oxygen to all parts of your body. Blood circulates throughout your body by a system of *blood vessels*. *Arteries* deliver blood from the heart to other body organs. The blood is returned to the heart in *veins*.

When your heart muscle tightens up (contracts), blood is forced out of your heart and is sent through your arteries, circulating throughout your body. Your heart then relaxes and fills up with fresh blood, which then gets pumped out on the next beat. After your body has used up the oxygen from the blood, the "used" blood flows back to your heart in veins. From there, the "used" blood goes to the lungs where the blood is replenished with oxygen. This "fresh" blood is then forced back to your heart, which continues to pump fresh blood out into the arteries.

Your heart is like a complex machine. There are actually four chambers that work together to keep blood flowing throughout your body and into the lungs for replenishment. Your heart needs oxygen in order to do all of this work. As blood is being pumped out of the heart, some of it flows into the *coronary arteries*. The coronary arteries supply blood and oxygen to the heart muscle itself. These arteries are very important. They are the lifeline to your heart.

Angina

About angina

What is angina?

Angina is usually the first noticeable sign that coronary heart disease is present. Angina is a feeling of discomfort, pain, or pressure which usually occurs in the mid-chest. The feeling may also spread to the arms, neck, jaw, back, or abdominal area. This usually happens when the heart muscle is working harder than usual and therefore, temporarily, needs more blood and oxygen. Not everyone who has coronary heart disease has angina. Some people may not have any symptoms at all.

An episode of angina is not a heart attack. Angina is a temporary reduction in the oxygen supply, while a heart attack is a complete or partial cutoff of oxygen to a portion of the heart muscle. That part of the heart dies, resulting in permanent injury to the heart muscle. Angina, on the other hand, does not cause permanent injury to the heart muscle.

What causes angina?

The heart needs oxygen in order to pump blood efficiently. The oxygen is supplied to the heart by blood circulating through arteries located around the heart (coronary arteries). Angina occurs when the oxygen supply to the heart is not enough to meet the needs of the heart. During times of physical activity the heart needs more oxygen. Normally, the heart is able to provide the extra oxygen needed by pumping harder and faster. However, sometimes the heart may not be able to deliver enough oxygen to meet this increased need. There are different reasons why this may happen.

Angina is usually caused by cholesterol buildup (plaque) in the walls of the coronary arteries. Over time, this causes the coronary arteries to narrow and reduces the delivery of blood, and, thus, oxygen, to the heart.

Many patients have what is known as *chronic stable angina*. With this type of angina, the chest discomfort is often brought on by physical activity and only lasts for a short time, usually just a few minutes.

Angina also sometimes occurs in patients without coronary heart disease. It can be caused by spasm of the coronary arteries. The spasm causes the coronary arteries to narrow, which reduces the flow of blood and oxygen to the heart. This condition is known as *variant angina*. Sometimes, a mixture of chronic stable and variant angina can occur. This occurs when there is a spasm in an artery with an existing plaque.

Unstable angina is a condition in which the chest pain is more severe, occurs more frequently, or occurs for longer periods of time than in chronic stable angina. Chest pain may occur when an individual is at rest or with very little physical activity. Unstable angina usually occurs when chronic stable angina gets worse over time. The plaque buildup on the wall of the coronary artery may attract certain substances in the body responsible for clotting blood, such as platelets. When these substances attach to the plaque, a spasm of the artery may occur or a larger plaque may form. Sometimes a small blood clot that breaks loose from somewhere else in the body may get caught in the plaque. This further narrows an already narrowed artery. These events may reduce blood circulation through the coronary artery, causing severe chest pain. Sometimes, people without a previous history of coronary heart disease may experience unstable angina as a first sign that a problem exists.

Can angina be prevented?

Current evidence seems to show that the risk of chronic stable angina can be reduced, particularly in those people who are most likely to develop angina. This includes those individuals with a family history of heart disease, those who smoke, those who are over 60 years of age, and men. Increased risk is also associated with medical problems, such as diabetes, high blood cholesterol, or high blood pressure. Life-style changes may help lower the risk of angina. It is especially important to stop smoking since smoking adversely affects the heart and may also speed up the development of plaque in the arteries. Also, reducing dietary fat intake can help lower blood cholesterol, and controlling body weight and reducing sodium (salt) intake can help lower blood pressure.

The risk factors for variant angina are not as clear as those for chronic stable angina. However, patients with variant angina are often heavy smokers.

People who develop unstable angina often suffer from other forms of angina. If you already have angina, you may reduce your chance of getting unstable angina by following your doctor's instructions and taking your medicine as prescribed. Sometimes, however, unstable angina may occur despite your best efforts to prevent it.

Why does angina need to be treated?

There is no real cure for angina. However, angina needs to be treated in order to lower the number of angina episodes (attacks), to improve symptoms, and to prevent the development of more serious heart problems, such as a heart attack.

General approach to therapy

The general approach to therapy for angina is to prevent angina attacks and to control the symptoms. This is done through use of medicines as well as through modification of certain personal behaviors that may increase the severity of your coronary heart disease.

• **Diet**—It may be important for you to follow a low-fat diet, especially if you have high blood cholesterol. This may help prevent the plaques in your arteries from getting worse. It may even cause some of the plaques to become smaller, which may improve your condition. If you have high blood pressure, following a diet low in sodium (salt) may be important. Lowering sodium intake has been shown to lower blood pressure. This does not relate directly to angina, but lowering blood pressure may reduce your overall risk of serious complications due to coronary heart disease.

• **Smoking**—It is particularly important to stop smoking. Smoking may make your angina symptoms worse, increase plaque buildup, and increase the likelihood that you will have a heart attack or even die suddenly from a disturbance of your heart's rhythm. Therefore, it is extremely important to stop smoking right away.

• **Excess weight**—If you are very overweight, it is important for you to lose weight and keep the weight off. This may help improve symptoms of angina. A structured program for weight loss should be discussed with your doctor.

• **Avoiding potential causes of angina attacks**—It is important for you to recognize activities that lead to angina attacks. This may include eating large meals, drinking a large amount of alcohol, or performing unusually strenuous exercise. These activities should be avoided whenever possible. However, some patients can benefit from an individualized exercise program worked out with their doctor.

• **Treatment with medicines**—You will most likely have to take medicines to help control your symptoms. Most of the medicines used for angina will help prevent or decrease the number of angina attacks. They usually work by relaxing blood vessels and increasing the supply of blood and oxygen to your heart. You will probably also be given a medicine, nitroglycerin, that will relieve an angina attack once it has started. The major classes of medicines that may be used include nitrates (e.g., nitroglycerin, isosorbide), beta-blockers (e.g., atenolol, propranolol), and calcium channel blockers (e.g., diltiazem, nifedipine).

High Blood Cholesterol

About high blood cholesterol

What is cholesterol?

Cholesterol is a waxy substance that is produced naturally by the liver. Cholesterol is present in cell membranes and is needed by the body to make certain hormones and vitamin D. The body also uses cholesterol to make bile acids, which help digest the fat you eat. The amount of cholesterol in the bloodstream is determined partly by heredity and partly by other factors such as diet and physical activity.

Cholesterol travels in the blood attached to particles called lipoproteins. There are two kinds of lipoprotein complexes Low-density lipoproteins (LDL) carry most of the cholesterol in the blood. LDL-cholesterol is "bad" cholesterol. High-density lipoproteins (HDL) carry some of the cholesterol in the blood, but this cholesterol is taken back to the liver where it can be removed from the circulation. HDL-cholesterol is therefore known as "good" cholesterol.

From now on, when high blood cholesterol is mentioned, it will refer to the "bad" cholesterol (LDL).

Why is too much cholesterol bad?

When there is too much cholesterol in the blood, it begins to stick to the walls of the arteries, especially the coronary arteries that supply blood to the heart. As time goes by, the buildup of cholesterol (plaque) may cause atherosclerosis (hardening of the arteries). This causes narrowing of the arteries, which prevents the adequate delivery of blood and oxygen to the heart. After a while, the narrowing may become worse, leading to problems such as angina or even a heart attack.

What makes cholesterol high?

There are many factors that may determine whether your cholesterol level is high or low. These can include the family history, diet, weight, age, and gender. Heredity can determine the amount of cholesterol your body makes. Therefore, if you have a family history of high blood cholesterol, you may be more likely to have high blood cholesterol. A high dietary intake of fat and cholesterol can raise cholesterol levels. Excess body weight also tends to raise cholesterol levels.

Why does high blood cholesterol need to be treated?

Having high blood cholesterol increases your risk of getting coronary heart disease. Therefore, lowering your cholesterol levels, as well as controlling other risk factors for coronary heart disease, can lower your risk of getting coronary heart disease later in life. If you already have coronary heart disease, it is even more important for you to lower your cholesterol. A person with coronary heart disease has a much greater chance of having a heart attack than a person without coronary heart disease. In a person with coronary heart disease, lowering cholesterol levels can decrease the risk of a heart attack. However, high blood cholesterol levels in elderly individuals may not pose as great a risk as high cholesterol in younger individuals.

General approach to therapy

Lowering high blood cholesterol levels is not an end in itself. Rather, the aim of therapy is to prevent or at least delay the consequences of high blood cholesterol levels, namely, coronary heart disease. Therefore, along with lowering your blood cholesterol, it will be important for you to reduce other risk factors for coronary heart disease. Some risk factors, such as age, male gender, or family history, are uncontrollable. However, there are a number of risk factors that can be modified by changing your life-style. These include cigarette smoking, excess weight, physical inactivity, high blood pressure, and diabetes mellitus.

• **Smoking**—Cigarette smoking greatly increases the risk of coronary heart disease. Stopping smoking has been shown to reduce this risk. Even within the first year after a person stops smoking, the risk for coronary heart disease is significantly reduced. Changing to low-tar or low-nicotine cigarettes does not appear to help. Therefore, it is extremely important to stop smoking right away.

• **Excess weight**—Being overweight increases the risk of diabetes mellitus, high blood pressure, and high blood cholesterol, all of which increase the risk for coronary heart disease. Therefore, it is important for overweight people to lose weight under the supervision of a doctor and dietitian. This is especially important if you carry more weight in the abdominal region.

• **Physical inactivity**—Studies have shown that regular physical activity of moderate intensity can help reduce the risk of coronary heart disease. An example of moderate physical activity is walking briskly for 30 minutes three times a week. Increasing physical activity can help to increase the ''good'' cholesterol and also helps to control weight and improve blood pressure. In addition, physical activity may have a direct beneficial effect on the heart and arteries. Before increasing your amount of physical activity, you and your doctor should discuss a routine that is right for you.

• **High blood pressure**—Increased blood pressure that continues over a long period of time can increase the risk of coronary heart disease. Therefore, it is important that you follow carefully your doctor's instructions for control of your high blood pressure.

• **Diabetes mellitus**—Diabetes increases the risk for coronary heart disease. Diabetes can increase the risk of coronary heart disease in men by threefold, and in women the increased risk may be even greater. Therefore, if you have diabetes, it is important that you follow carefully your doctor's instructions for control of your diabetes.

• **Diet**—Diet modification is the cornerstone of cholesterol-lowering therapy. Your doctor will ask you to adhere to a strict diet designed specifically for you. Sometimes a dietitian may help you to select appropriate foods and help you tailor the diet to your needs. In general, you will be instructed to avoid foods high in saturated fat and cholesterol. An important goal is to lower your blood cholesterol levels without the need for medicine.

• **Treatment with medicines**—The decision to treat high cholesterol with medicines comes only after life-style changes and strict dietary measures have failed to lower blood cholesterol adequately. The decision to use medicine will also depend on how high your cholesterol level is and what other risk factors for heart disease you have. Sometimes individuals considered to be at very low risk for developing heart disease may be able to hold off taking medicines and continue on a strict diet. This is a decision you and your doctor will make. The major classes of medicines that may be used to treat high cholesterol include bile acid sequestrants (cholestyramine, colestipol), nicotinic acid (niacin), HMG-CoA reductase inhibitors (fluvastatin, lovastatin, pravastatin, simvastatin), fibric acids (gemfibrozil, clofibrate), and probucol.

The risk of heart disease is increased in women after menopause. This increase in risk may be related to reduced estrogen production after menopause. There is evidence that oral estrogen replacement may reduce this risk. Estrogens appear to lower cholesterol levels, and, in animals, estrogens appear to lower the amount of cholesterol that binds to the artery walls. The use of oral estrogen replacement therapy remains controversial, however, because estrogens may increase the risk of endometrial (lining of the uterus) or breast cancer. The risk of endometrial cancer may be reduced by taking a progestin with the estrogen. Postmenopausal women with high cholesterol levels should discuss this with their doctor.

High Blood Pressure

About high blood pressure

What is blood pressure?

When your heart beats, it pumps blood through your blood vessels. The force of the blood that is pumped out then pushes against the walls of these vessels and creates the force known as blood pressure. In fact, blood pressure is the force that keeps blood moving through the vessels.

Blood pressure is expressed as two values measured in terms of millimeters of mercury (mm Hg). For example, normal blood pressure for a young or middle-aged adult is usually around 120/80 mm Hg. The upper (first) value is called systolic blood pressure. It describes the force that occurs when the heart pumps, pushing blood out into the arteries. The lower (second) value is called diastolic blood pressure. It describes the pressure inside the blood vessels when the heart relaxes.

Blood pressure may vary even when it is normal. It is usually lowest when you are asleep, but it may increase if you are excited or nervous or when you are exercising. It may also be increased by a sudden injury or by smoking a cigarette or drinking coffee. However, these are only temporary increases and your blood pressure goes back down to its usual level after a short time.

What is high blood pressure?

High blood pressure is an abnormally elevated amount of pressure of the blood against the blood vessels. Blood pressure is elevated if your vessels narrow or tighten, making it harder for the blood to flow. This causes your blood pressure to rise in order to overcome the resistance.

Most doctors define high blood pressure as a systolic pressure of greater than 140 mm Hg and/or a diastolic pressure of greater than 90 mm Hg that occurs on more than two measurements in a row. High blood pressure is classified into four stages. All four stages of high blood pressure are associated with an increased risk of heart and kidney disease or stroke.

Hypertension is the medical term for high blood pressure. It does not refer to nervous tension. Primary or essential hypertension refers to the most common type of high blood pressure. The exact cause of this type of hypertension is unknown, although it tends to run in families. The term essential should not be understood to mean that the elevated pressure is necessary.

From now on, when the terms "high blood pressure" and "hypertension" are used in this book, they will refer to primary or essential hypertension.

What causes high blood pressure?

High blood pressure, contrary to popular belief, is not caused by tension or nervousness, although too much emotional upset may elevate blood pressure. Essential hypertension has no known cause and is the type that occurs in approximately 90 percent of patients having high blood pressure. For the remaining 10 percent, different causes may be responsible for the elevated blood pressure. For example, some cases may be the result of kidney disease or narrowing of one of the blood vessels to the kidney, disease of the adrenal gland, or other hormonal abnormalities.

Although the exact cause of essential hypertension is unknown, there are certain personal factors that may identify a person who is more likely to develop hypertension. In many people, a combination of these factors may be involved. For example, hypertension is generally more common in men, in blacks, in persons over 50 years of age, and in those who have a family history of hypertension. In addition, some people are overly sensitive to sodium (salt) and may be more likely to develop or aggravate hypertension.

Can high blood pressure be prevented?

Current evidence seems to show that high blood pressure can often be prevented, especially in those people who are most likely to develop high blood pressure. This includes individuals whose blood pressure is in the high-normal range, those with a family history of high blood pressure, members of some minority populations (such as blacks), and those who are overweight, eat too much sodium (salt), are physically inactive, or have a high alcohol intake. Therefore, primary prevention of high blood pressure is very important. The goal of primary prevention is to lower the blood pressure of the population as a whole and decrease the likelihood of getting high blood pressure. Life-style changes such as losing weight, reducing sodium (salt) intake, reducing alcohol intake, and exercising regularly can help reduce your risk of getting high blood pressure.

How is high blood pressure detected?

Hypertension usually does not produce any noticeable signs or symptoms until blood pressure is extremely high or has been present for a long time. Your doctor may discover that you have it by taking a routine blood pressure measurement before symptoms develop. However, one high measurement does not necessarily mean that you have high blood pressure. It could be due to emotional upset, anger, or recent exercise. Several measurements that are consistently high when you are lying down, sitting, and standing, however, may mean that you have hypertension.

Why does high blood pressure need to be treated?

Most doctors now recommend treatment of high blood pressure, even when it is not very much above normal. High blood pressure adds to the workload of the heart and arteries. If it continues for a long time, the heart and arteries may not function properly. Hypertension can damage the blood vessels of the brain, heart, and kidneys, and can cause a stroke, heart failure, or kidney failure. Hypertension is also a major risk factor underlying heart attacks. These problems may be less likely to occur if blood pressure is controlled.

The amount of damage that hypertension causes is related to how high the blood pressure is and how long it has been elevated. Therefore, it is best to treat hypertension early, before damage occurs or gets worse.

Myths about high blood pressure

Myth: If I feel well, then my blood pressure must be normal.

In most people, there are no symptoms of hypertension; it is detected through blood pressure measurements.

Myth: Only tense, anxious people get high blood pressure.

Anyone can have high blood pressure and the cause may not be known. There are approximately 58 million people in the United States who have high blood pressure. While emotional upset will raise your blood pressure temporarily, this does not cause the condition; even very calm, relaxed people can develop high blood pressure.

Myth: High blood pressure can be treated with tranquilizers.

Tranquilizers generally are not useful in treating hypertension since it is not caused by tension; tranquilizers do not lower blood pressure. What is useful is a program of proper diet, exercise, and medication that you and your doctor will work out together.

Myth: High blood pressure is a disease of old age.

People of all ages can develop high blood pressure, although people over 50 years of age are more likely to have it. Even children can have hypertension; however, the cause is often different in children than in adults.

Myth: Essential high blood pressure can be cured.

Essential hypertension is a condition that usually requires lifelong treatment; it can be controlled by proper life-style modification (weight reduction, increased physical activity, and limiting salt and alcohol intake) and medication, but it cannot be cured. If you stop your treatment when your blood pressure improves, it probably will go up again. However, some other types of hypertension can be cured.

Myth: High blood pressure significantly restricts my life.

This should not be true. With your participation in the planning and carrying out of your treatment, you can lead a normal life; however, early, proper, and continued treatment is necessary to prevent the damage that untreated high blood pressure can cause.

General approach to therapy

Treatment for high blood pressure requires that you make some changes in your life-style. You may have to make some changes in your diet and daily routine. Your doctor may suggest that you take your own blood pressure measurements. By measuring your own blood pressure, you can help manage your treatment program and watch your progress in bringing your high blood pressure under control. Your doctor or nurse can teach you the proper way and the best time to take a blood pressure measurement. Remember that your blood pressure may be slightly different at different times of day, or if you are sick or have a fever. Check with your doctor if you are concerned about a change in your blood pressure. Also, your blood pressure measurement equipment should be periodically checked to ensure that it is taking accurate measurements. Other life-style changes include:

• **Diet**—Your doctor may want you to follow a diet that is low in sodium (salt) and fats. Lowering sodium intake has been shown to help lower blood pressure, especially in patients who are salt-sensitive. Sodium (most commonly thought of as table salt or sodium chloride) is important in maintaining proper levels of fluid in your body. Other forms of sodium in our diet may be included in any number of salts (e.g., sodium ascorbate, sodium bicarbonate, sodium citrate, sodium glutamate) used to process and preserve canned, frozen, and processed foods. You need only about 200 mg of sodium a day, but many people take in much more than this. In general, highly processed foods contain large amounts of salt. Because salt is used in many ways in food processing, it often cannot be tasted and therefore may appear as "hidden" salt. If you are thinking about taking a salt substitute, check with your doctor first. Most salt substitutes contain potassium, which can cause problems when you are taking some high blood pressure medicines. Although dietary fat is not directly related to blood pressure, lowering fat intake may reduce the risk of heart disease and may also help you control your weight.

- **Alcohol**—Large amounts of alcohol can raise blood pressure. Therefore, you should limit the amount of alcohol you drink. In general, you should drink no more than 1 ounce of pure alcohol (8 ounces of wine, 24 ounces of beer, or 2 ounces of 100 proof whiskey) a day.

- **Physical activity**—Regular aerobic physical activity may help lower blood pressure and control weight. Physical activity does not have to be complicated or expensive. For most people, 30 to 45 minutes of brisk walking three to five times a week will be helpful. You should work closely with your doctor to safely increase your level of physical activity.

- **Smoking avoidance**—Smoking greatly increases the risks of heart and blood vessel disease associated with hypertension and should be avoided.

- **Stress reduction**—Stress reduction alone will probably not lower your blood pressure, but it may help the other methods of treatment to be more effective.

- **Weight reduction**—Being overweight is closely related to increased blood pressure. If you are overweight, a weight-loss diet prescribed by your doctor and dietitian may help bring your blood pressure under control. If you control your blood pressure by losing weight and making the other life-style changes mentioned above, you may not need to take medicines.

- **Treatment with medicines**—If treatment without medicine involving the above-mentioned changes in life-style is not sufficient, drug therapy may be added. Since there are many different kinds of high blood pressure medicine, your doctor will determine which is the best for your particular condition.

Congestive Heart Failure

About congestive heart failure

What is congestive heart failure?

Congestive heart failure is a condition or "syndrome" that results from a number of different diseases or problems. It occurs when the heart is unable to pump enough blood to body tissues and organs. When this happens over a long period of time, blood gets backed up in the heart and lungs, leading to fluid overload or congestion. Congestive heart failure can occur when the heart muscle is damaged or weakened or it can occur when the amount of fluid (blood) being pumped is increased. "Heart failure" does not mean that the heart has stopped functioning altogether.

The symptoms of congestive heart failure include shortness of breath, particularly with physical activity (even walking), inability to lie flat (having to sleep on 2 or more pillows) without getting short of breath, sudden shortness of breath in the middle of the night, fluid buildup (accumulation) or backup in the feet and legs, and frequent urination during the night.

Congestive heart failure may make you short of breath with physical activity. The severity of congestive heart failure will vary among different people. Some patients will get short of breath even while performing regular daily activities such as walking or light housework. Other patients may get short of breath only with heavier exertion or exercise.

Although shortness of breath and fluid buildup in the feet and legs are expected with this condition, you must be aware of your level of disability. You must notify your doctor if you feel your symptoms are getting worse; for example, if last week you were able to walk a mile without getting short of breath, but this week you can only walk half a mile before getting short of breath.

What causes congestive heart failure?

Congestive heart failure can be caused by a number of different diseases. Most commonly, it is caused by coronary heart disease with heart attack, high blood pressure, cardiomyopathy (disease of the heart muscle), or heart valve problems.

Can congestive heart failure be prevented?

Congestive heart failure can sometimes be prevented or the onset delayed by preventing or controlling the problems that cause heart disease (e.g., high blood cholesterol, high blood pressure).

General approach to therapy

Treatment of congestive heart failure is aimed at treating the underlying cause, relieving the symptoms of heart failure, and prolonging life. Successful management of congestive heart failure often requires life-style changes. You should understand that you will get short of breath with physical activity and you will feel tired. These symptoms are expected with congestive heart failure. However, it is important that you recognize when the symptoms are getting worse so that you can notify your doctor. Your doctor may ask you to weigh yourself each morning. This will keep track of any fluid accumulation. If you have gained more than 4 pounds since your last medical appointment, your doctor should be notified.

- **Diet**—You may be asked to limit your sodium (salt) intake. This usually means not adding salt to foods after cooking and avoiding salty foods. However, in some cases, patients may be asked to limit salt intake more severely. You should discuss your individual situation with your doctor.

- **Alcohol**—Alcohol use is not recommended. Alcohol may interfere with the pumping action of the heart in people with heart problems.

- **Physical exercise**—The idea of exercising in patients with congestive heart failure is somewhat controversial. Given the nature of the condition, strenuous exercise may make you feel worse. However, under the supervision of your doctor you may be able to take part in a mild exercise routine. Do not begin an exercise program without first discussing the risks and benefits with your doctor.

- **Treatment with medicines**—Treatment with medicines will help to relieve some of the symptoms of congestive heart failure, such as shortness of breath and swelling in the legs. Some medicines may also help slow down the worsening of heart failure and help you live longer. Several different classes of medicines may be used for heart failure.

You will probably be given an angiotensin-converting enzyme (ACE) inhibitor. These medicines have been shown to improve symptoms and may help you live longer. You should feel much better and be able to do more without getting short of breath (improved "functional capacity"). You may also be given a diuretic ("water pill"). This will help decrease the amount of fluid in your legs and will help your breathing. One of the oldest medicines used to treat congestive heart failure is digitalis. Digitalis medicines may help to improve your symptoms by increasing the force of pumping of the heart. Other medicines that may be used are vessel dilators (vasodilators), such as hydralazine and nitrates.

There are some medicines, used in the hospital setting, that increase the force of pumping of the heart. These medicines are primarily injected into a vein and may help improve symptoms. However, their long-term effect is not yet known.

Arrhythmias

About arrhythmias

What is a normal heartbeat?

The heart is made up of four chambers that normally work together to pump blood throughout the body. The pumping action of the heart depends on certain electrical impulses. A normal heart pumps blood at a regular rhythm and at a certain speed, usually between 60 and 100 beats per minute. A heartbeat that has a normal speed and normal rhythm is called "normal sinus rhythm."

What is an arrhythmia?

An arrhythmia is any change from the normal rhythm or rate of the heartbeat. There are many different kinds of arrhythmias. These can include a heart rate that is too slow or too fast, a rhythm that is irregular, or one with skipped beats. An arrhythmia can occur in any chamber of the heart. Some arrhythmias are more serious than others because they begin in a critical portion of the heart or because they allow the heart to beat very slowly, very quickly, or very erratically so that the heart is unable to pump blood effectively. Some arrhythmias may be less serious. Your doctor will evaluate the nature of your arrhythmia and suggest a course of treatment.

What causes arrhythmias?

Arrhythmias can have many different causes. They can occur after a heart attack. The damaged heart tissue after a heart attack makes it difficult for electrical impulses to get through. Arrhythmias can also be caused by imbalances of certain chemicals (ions) in the blood, such as potassium or magnesium. These chemicals are important for the electrical impulses. Sometimes arrhythmias can be caused by medications, and sometimes the cause may be unknown. Most adults over 50 years of age have occasional irregular beating of the heart. In most cases this is not serious.

General approach to therapy

Type of arrhythmia

The decision to treat an arrhythmia depends greatly on the type of arrhythmia. For instance, arrhythmias that are caused by an imbalance of potassium or magnesium in the blood can be treated simply by correcting that imbalance. These arrhythmias often do not need continuing treatment. However, some arrhythmias require treatment with antiarrhythmic medicines. In some cases arrhythmias can be very serious and even life-threatening.

Choice of antiarrhythmic treatment

If you have an arrhythmia that requires continuing medical treatment, your doctor may choose to treat the condition with medicines, with a device (e.g., implanted electrical device or pacemaker), or with a combination of the two. Your doctor may also change from one type of treatment to another if the initial treatment isn't working as well as it should.

Although antiarrhythmic medicines are often prescribed, they can have serious side effects in some patients. Most of the medicines used to treat arrhythmias can actually cause a new arrhythmia or make the existing arrhythmia worse. Arrhythmias caused by medicine are called "proarrhythmias." Although not common, proarrhythmias can happen in anyone taking an antiarrhythmic medicine. However, they may be more likely to occur in patients with more severe forms of arrhythmias or in patients who have other heart problems. The serious side effects associated with antiarrhythmic medicines, especially at higher doses, make the use of devices attractive. However, the devices are very expensive and may not be the best treatment for all patients.

Drug
Monographs

Entries appear alphabetically by generic or "family" names (groupings of closely related medicines). To find the location of brand name entries, refer to the index at the back of the book.

AMIODARONE Systemic

A commonly used brand name in the U.S. and Canada is Cordarone.

Description

Amiodarone (am-ee-OH-da-rone) belongs to the group of medicines known as antiarrhythmics. It is used to correct irregular heartbeats to a normal rhythm.

Amiodarone produces its helpful effects by slowing nerve impulses in the heart and acting directly on the heart tissues.

This medicine is available only with your doctor's prescription, in the following dosage form:

Oral

• Tablets (U.S. and Canada)

Before Using This Medicine

In deciding to use a medicine, the risks of taking the medicine must be weighed against the good it will do. This is a decision you and your doctor will make. For amiodarone, the following should be considered:

Allergies—Tell your doctor if you have ever had any unusual or allergic reaction to amiodarone. Also tell your health care professional if you are allergic to any other substances, such as foods, preservatives, or dyes.

Pregnancy—Amiodarone has been shown to cause thyroid problems in babies whose mothers took amiodarone when pregnant. In addition, there is concern that amiodarone could cause slow heartbeat in the newborn. However, this medicine may be needed in serious situations that threaten the mother's life. Be sure you have discussed this with your doctor before taking this medicine.

Breast-feeding—Although amiodarone passes into breast milk, it has not been shown to cause problems in nursing babies. However, amiodarone has been shown to cause growth problems in rats. It may be necessary for you to stop breast-feeding during treatment. Be sure you have discussed the risks and benefits of the medicine with your doctor.

Children—Amiodarone can cause serious side effects in any patient. Therefore, it is especially important that you discuss with the child's doctor the good that this medicine may do as well as the risks of using it.

Older adults—Elderly patients may be more likely to get thyroid problems with this medicine. Also, difficulty in walking and numbness, tingling, trembling, or weakness in hands or feet are more likely to occur in the elderly.

Other medicines—Although certain medicines should not be used together at all, in other cases two different medicines may be used together even if an interaction might occur. In these cases, your doctor may want to change the dose, or other precautions may be necessary. When you are taking amiodarone, it is especially important that your health care professional knows if you are taking any of the following:
- Anticoagulants (blood thinners) or
- Other heart medicine or
- Phenytoin (e.g., Dilantin)—Effects may be increased

Other medical problems—The presence of other medical problems may affect the use of amiodarone. Make sure you tell your doctor if you have any other medical problems, especially:
- Liver disease—Effects may be increased because of slower removal from the body
- Thyroid problems—Risk of overactive or underactive thyroid is increased

Proper Use of This Medicine

Take amiodarone exactly as directed by your doctor even though you may feel well. Do not take more medicine than ordered and do not miss any doses.

Dosing—The dose of amiodarone will be different for different patients. *Follow your doctor's orders or the directions on the label.* The following information includes only the average doses of amiodarone. *If your dose is different, do not change it* unless your doctor tells you to do so:

* For *oral* dosage form (tablets):

  —For treatment of *ventricular arrhythmias:*

    * Adults—At first, 800 to 1600 milligrams (mg) per day taken in divided doses. Then, 600 to 800 mg per day for one month. Then, 400 mg per day.
    * Children—Dose is based on body weight and must be determined by your doctor. The dose for the first ten days is usually 10 mg per kilogram (4.55 mg per pound) of body weight per day. Then, the dose is decreased to 5 mg per kilogram (2.27 mg per pound) of body weight per day. After several weeks, the dose is then decreased to 2.5 mg per kilogram (1.14 mg per pound) of body weight per day.

Missed dose—If you miss a dose of this medicine, do not take the missed dose at all and do not double the next one. Instead, go back to your regular dosing schedule. If you miss two or more doses in a row, check with your doctor.

Storage—To store this medicine:

* Keep out of the reach of children.
* Store away from heat and direct light.
* Do not store in the bathroom, near the kitchen sink, or in other damp places. Heat or moisture may cause the medicine to break down.

- Do not keep outdated medicine or medicine no longer needed. Be sure that any discarded medicine is out of the reach of children.

Precautions While Using This Medicine

It is important that your doctor check your progress at regular visits to make sure the medicine is working properly. This will allow for changes to be made in the amount of medicine you are taking, if necessary.

Your doctor may want you to carry a medical identification card or bracelet stating that you are taking this medicine.

Before having any kind of surgery (including dental surgery) or emergency treatment, tell the medical doctor or dentist in charge that you are taking this medicine.

Amiodarone increases the sensitivity of your skin to sunlight; too much exposure could cause a serious burn. Your skin may continue to be sensitive to sunlight for several months after treatment with this medicine is stopped. A burn can occur even through window glass or thin cotton clothing. If you must go out in the sunlight, *cover your skin and wear a wide-brimmed hat. A special sun-blocking cream should also be used;* it must contain zinc or titanium oxide because other sunscreens will not work. *In case of a severe burn, check with your doctor.*

After you have taken this medicine for a long time, it may cause a blue-gray color to appear on your skin, especially in areas exposed to the sun, such as your face, neck, and arms. This color will usually fade after treatment with amiodarone has ended, although it may take several months. However, check with your doctor if this effect occurs.

Side Effects of This Medicine

Along with its needed effects, a medicine may cause some
unwanted effects. Although not all of these side effects
may occur, if they do occur they may need medical attention. Also, some side effects may not appear until several
weeks or months, or even years, after you start taking
amiodarone.

Check with your doctor immediately if any of the following side effects occur:

   More common
      Cough; painful breathing; shortness of breath

Check with your doctor as soon as possible if any of the
following side effects occur:

   More common
      Fever (slight); numbness or tingling in fingers or toes;
         sensitivity of skin to sunlight; trembling or shaking of
         hands; trouble in walking; unusual and uncontrolled
         movements of the body; weakness of arms or legs

   Less common
      Blue-gray coloring of skin on face, neck, and arms; blurred
         vision or blue-green halos seen around objects; cold-
         ness; dry eyes; dry, puffy skin; fast or irregular heart-
         beat; nervousness; pain and swelling in scrotum;
         sensitivity of eyes to light; sensitivity to heat; slow
         heartbeat; sweating; swelling of feet or lower legs; trou-
         ble in sleeping; unusual tiredness; weight gain or loss

   Rare
      Skin rash; yellow eyes or skin

Other side effects may occur that usually do not need
medical attention. These side effects may go away during
treatment as your body adjusts to the medicine. However,
check with your doctor if any of the following side effects
continue or are bothersome:

   More common
      Constipation; headache; loss of appetite; nausea and
         vomiting

Less common

> Bitter or metallic taste; decreased sexual ability in males; decrease in sexual interest; dizziness; flushing of face

After you stop using this medicine, your body may need time to adjust. The length of time this takes depends on the amount of medicine you were using and how long you used it. During this period of time check with your doctor if you notice any of the following side effects:

> Cough; fever (slight); painful breathing; shortness of breath

Other side effects not listed above may also occur in some patients. If you notice any other effects, check with your doctor.

AMLODIPINE   Systemic†

A commonly used brand name in the U.S. is Norvasc.

†Not commercially available in Canada.

Description

Amlodipine (am-LOE-di-peen) is a calcium channel blocker used to treat angina (chest pain) and high blood pressure. Amlodipine affects the movement of calcium into the cells of the heart and blood vessels. As a result, amlodipine relaxes blood vessels and increases the supply of blood and oxygen to the heart while reducing its workload.

High blood pressure adds to the workload of the heart and arteries. If it continues for a long time, the heart and arteries may not function properly. This can damage the blood vessels of the brain, heart, and kidneys, resulting in a stroke, heart failure, or kidney failure. High blood pressure may also increase the risk of heart attacks. These problems may be less likely to occur if blood pressure is controlled.

This medicine is available only with your doctor's prescription, in the following dosage form:

Oral
• Tablets (U.S.)

Before Using This Medicine

In deciding to use a medicine, the risks of taking the medicine must be weighed against the good it will do. This is a decision you and your doctor will make. For amlodipine, the following should be considered:

Allergies—Tell your doctor if you have ever had any unusual or allergic reaction to amlodipine. Also tell your health care professional if you are allergic to any other substances, such as foods, preservatives, or dyes.

Pregnancy—Amlodipine has not been studied in pregnant women. However, studies in animals have shown that, at very high doses, amlodipine may cause fetal death. Before taking this medicine, make sure your doctor knows if you are pregnant or if you may become pregnant.

Breast-feeding—It is not known whether amlodipine passes into breast milk. Although most medicines pass into breast milk in small amounts, many of them may be used safely while breast-feeding. Mothers who are taking this medicine and who wish to breast-feed should discuss this with their doctor.

Children—Studies on this medicine have been done only in adult patients, and there is no specific information comparing use of amlodipine in children with use in other age groups.

Older adults—Elderly people may be especially sensitive to the effects of amlodipine. This may increase the chance of side effects during treatment.

Other medicines—Although certain medicines should not be used together at all, in other cases two different medicines may be used together even if an interaction might occur. In these cases, your doctor may want to change the dose, or other precautions may be necessary. Tell your health care professional if you are using any other prescription or nonprescription (over-the-counter [OTC]) medicine.

Other medical problems—The presence of other medical problems may affect the use of amlodipine. Make sure you tell your doctor if you have any other medical problems, especially:

- Congestive heart failure—There is a small chance that amlodipine may make this condition worse
- Liver disease—Higher blood levels of amlodipine may result and a smaller dose may be needed
- Very low blood pressure—Amlodipine may make this condition worse

---

Proper Use of This Medicine

Take this medicine exactly as directed even if you feel well and do not notice any chest pain. Do not take more of this medicine and do not take it more often than your doctor ordered. Do not miss any doses.

For patients taking this medicine *for high blood pressure:*

- In addition to the use of the medicine your doctor has prescribed, treatment for your high blood pressure may include weight control and care in the types of food you eat, especially foods high in sodium (salt). Your doctor will tell you which of these are most important for you. You should check with your doctor before changing your diet.
- Many patients who have high blood pressure will not notice any signs of the problem. In fact, many may feel normal. It is very important that you *take your medicine exactly as directed* and that you keep your appointments with your doctor even if you feel well.

- Remember that this medicine will not cure your high blood pressure but it does help control it. Therefore, you must continue to take it as directed if you expect to lower your blood pressure and keep it down. *You may have to take high blood pressure medicine for the rest of your life.* If high blood pressure is not treated, it can cause serious problems such as heart failure, blood vessel disease, stroke, or kidney disease.

Dosing—The dose of amlodipine will be different for different patients. *Follow your doctor's orders or the directions on the label.* The following information includes only the average doses of amlodipine. *If your dose is different, do not change it* unless your doctor tells you to do so.

The number of tablets that you take depends on the strength of the medicine.

- For *oral* dosage form (tablets):
  —For angina (chest pain):
    - Adults—5 to 10 milligrams (mg) once a day.
    - Children—Use must be determined by your doctor.
  —For high blood pressure:
    - Adults—2.5 to 10 mg once a day.
    - Children—Use must be determined by your doctor.

Missed dose—If you miss a dose of this medicine, take it as soon as possible. However, if it is almost time for your next dose, skip the missed dose and go back to your regular dosing schedule. Do not double doses.

Storage—To store this medicine:

- Keep out of the reach of children.
- Store away from heat and direct light.
- Do not store in the bathroom, near the kitchen sink, or in other damp places. Heat or moisture may cause the medicine to break down.

- Keep the medicine from freezing. Do not refrigerate.
- Do not keep outdated medicine or medicine no longer needed. Be sure that any discarded medicine is out of the reach of children.

Precautions While Using This Medicine

It is important that your doctor check your progress at regular visits. This will allow your doctor to make sure the medicine is working properly and to change the dosage if needed.

If you have been using this medicine regularly for several weeks, do not suddenly stop using it. Stopping suddenly may cause your chest pain or high blood pressure to come back or get worse. Check with your doctor for the best way to reduce gradually the amount you are taking before stopping completely.

Chest pain resulting from exercise or physical exertion usually is reduced or prevented by this medicine. This may tempt you to be too active. *Make sure you discuss with your doctor a safe amount of exercise for your medical problem.*

After taking a dose of this medicine you may get a headache that lasts for a short time. This should become less noticeable after you have taken this medicine for a while. If this effect continues, or if the headaches are severe, check with your doctor.

In some patients, tenderness, swelling, or bleeding of the gums may appear soon after treatment with this medicine is started. Brushing and flossing your teeth carefully and regularly and massaging your gums may help prevent this. *See your dentist regularly* to have your teeth cleaned. Check with your medical doctor or dentist if you have any questions about how to take care of your teeth and gums, or if you notice any tenderness, swelling, or bleeding of your gums.

For patients taking this medicine *for high blood pressure:*

- *Do not take other medicines unless they have been discussed with your doctor.* This especially includes over-the-counter (nonprescription) medicines for appetite control, asthma, colds, cough, hay fever, or sinus problems, since they may tend to increase your blood pressure.

Side Effects of This Medicine

Along with its needed effects, a medicine may cause some unwanted effects. Although not all of these side effects may occur, if they do occur they may need medical attention.

Check with your doctor as soon as possible if any of the following side effects occur:

More common
    Swelling of ankles or feet

Less common
    Dizziness; pounding heartbeat

Rare
    Chest pain; dizziness or lightheadedness when getting up from a lying or sitting position; slow heartbeat

Other side effects may occur that usually do not need medical attention. These side effects may go away during treatment as your body adjusts to the medicine. However, check with your doctor if any of the following side effects continue or are bothersome:

More common
    Flushing; headache

Less common
    Nausea; unusual tiredness or weakness

Other side effects not listed above may also occur in some patients. If you notice any other effects, check with your doctor.

AMYL NITRITE   Systemic

Generic name product available in the U.S. and Canada.

Description

Amyl nitrite (AM-il NYE-trite) is related to the nitrate medicines and is used by inhalation to relieve the pain of angina attacks. It works by relaxing blood vessels and increasing the supply of blood and oxygen to the heart while reducing its workload.

Amyl nitrite may also be used for other conditions as determined by your doctor.

This medicine comes in a glass capsule covered by a protective cloth. The cloth covering allows you to crush the glass capsule between your fingers without cutting yourself.

On the street, this medicine and others like it are sometimes called "poppers." They have been used by some people to cause a "high" or to improve sex. Use in this way is not recommended. Amyl nitrite can cause serious harmful effects if too much is inhaled.

Amyl nitrite is available only with your doctor's prescription, in the following dosage form:

Inhalation
- Glass capsules (U.S. and Canada)

Before Using This Medicine

In deciding to use a medicine, the risks of taking the medicine must be weighed against the good it will do.

This is a decision you and your doctor will make. For amyl nitrite, the following should be considered:

Allergies—Tell your doctor if you have ever had any unusual or allergic reaction to amyl nitrite or nitrates. Also tell your health care professional if you are allergic to any other substances, such as foods or dyes.

Pregnancy—Studies on effects in pregnancy have not been done in either humans or animals. However, use of amyl nitrite is not recommended during pregnancy because it could cause serious problems in the unborn baby.

Breast-feeding—It is not known whether amyl nitrite passes into breast milk. However, use of amyl nitrite is not recommended during breast-feeding, because it may cause unwanted effects in nursing babies.

Children—Studies on this medicine have been done only in adult patients and there is no specific information comparing use of amyl nitrite in children with use in other age groups.

Older adults—Dizziness or lightheadedness may be more likely to occur in the elderly, who are usually more sensitive to the effects of amyl nitrite.

Other medicines—Although certain medicines should not be used together at all, in other cases two different medicines may be used together even if an interaction might occur. In these cases, your doctor may want to change the dose, or other precautions may be necessary. When you are taking amyl nitrite, it is especially important that your health care professional knows if you are taking any of the following:

- Amantadine (e.g., Symmetrel) or
- Antidepressants (medicine for depression) or
- Antihypertensives (high blood pressure medicine) or
- Antipsychotics (medicine for mental illness) or
- Bromocriptine (e.g., Parlodel) or
- Diuretics (water pills) or
- Levodopa (e.g., Dopar) or

- Medicine for heart disease or
- Nabilone (e.g., Cesamet)—in high doses or
- Narcotic pain medicine or
- Nimodipine (e.g., Nimotop) or
- Pentamidine (e.g., Pentam) or
- Pimozide (e.g., Orap) or
- Promethazine (e.g., Phenergan) or
- Trimeprazine (e.g., Temaril)—May increase dizziness or lightheadedness when getting up from a lying or sitting position

It is also important that your health care professional knows if you are using any of the following medicines in the eye:

- Levobunolol (e.g., Betagan) or
- Metipranolol (e.g., Optipranolol) or
- Timolol (e.g., Timoptic)—May increase dizziness or lightheadedness when getting up from a lying or sitting position

Other medical problems—The presence of other medical problems may affect the use of amyl nitrite. Make sure you tell your doctor if you have any other medical problems, especially:

- Anemia (severe)
- Glaucoma—Amyl nitrite may make this condition worse
- Overactive thyroid
- Recent stroke, heart attack, or head injury

Proper Use of This Medicine

To use amyl nitrite:

- *When you begin to feel an attack of angina starting (chest pains or a tightness or squeezing in the chest), sit down. Then crush the cloth-covered glass capsule containing amyl nitrite between your finger and thumb. Pass it back and forth close to your nose and inhale the vapor several (1 to 6) times.* Since you may become dizzy, lightheaded, or faint soon after using amyl nitrite, it is best to sit or lie down rather than stand while the medicine is working. If you become dizzy or faint while sitting, take several deep breaths of air and either bend forward with your head between your knees or lie down with your feet elevated.

- Remain calm and you should feel better in a few minutes.

Use this medicine exactly as directed by your doctor, and do not use more than your doctor ordered. Using too much amyl nitrite may cause a dangerous overdose. If the medicine does not seem to be working as well after you have used it for a while, check with your doctor. *Do not increase the dose on your own.*

Dosing—*Follow your doctor's orders or the directions on the label.* The following information includes only the average doses of amyl nitrite:

- For *inhalation* dosage form:
  —Adults: 0.18 or 0.3 milliliter (1 ampul) taken by inhaling the vapor of amyl nitrite through the nose. Dose may be repeated within 1 to 5 minutes if pain is not relieved. *If you still have chest pain after a total of 2 doses in a 10-minute period, contact your doctor or have someone take you to a hospital emergency room without delay.*

Storage—To store this medicine:

- Keep out of the reach of children.
- Store away from heat and direct light.
- Do not store in the bathroom or in the kitchen. Heat may cause the medicine to break down.
- Do not keep outdated medicine or medicine no longer needed. Be sure that any discarded medicine is out of the reach of children.

Precautions While Using This Medicine

Amyl nitrite is extremely flammable. Keep it away from heat or any open flame, especially when crushing the capsule. Amyl nitrite can catch fire very easily and cause serious burns.

Dizziness or lightheadedness may occur, especially when you get up from a lying or sitting position. Getting up slowly may help, but if the problem continues or gets worse, check with your doctor.

Drinking alcohol while you are taking this medicine may make the dizziness or lightheadedness worse and may cause a serious drop in blood pressure. Check with your doctor before drinking alcoholic beverages.

After using a dose of amyl nitrite, you may get a mild headache that lasts for a short time. This is a common side effect and is no cause for alarm. However, if this effect continues, or if the headaches are severe, check with your doctor.

Side Effects of This Medicine

Along with its needed effects, a medicine may cause some unwanted effects. Although not all of these side effects may occur, if they do occur they may need medical attention.

Check with your doctor as soon as possible if any of the following side effects occur:

Rare

   Skin rash; unusual tiredness or weakness

Signs and symptoms of overdose

   Bluish-colored lips, fingernails, or palms of hands; dizziness (extreme) or fainting; feeling of extreme pressure in head; shortness of breath; unusual tiredness or weakness; weak and fast heartbeat

Other side effects may occur that usually do not need medical attention. These side effects may go away during treatment as your body adjusts to the medicine. However,

check with your doctor if any of the following side effects continue or are bothersome:

> *More common*
>> Dizziness or lightheadedness, especially when getting up from a lying or sitting position; fast pulse; flushing of face and neck; headache (mild); nausea or vomiting; restlessness

Other side effects not listed above may also occur in some patients. If you notice any other effects, check with your doctor.

ANGIOTENSIN-CONVERTING ENZYME (ACE) INHIBITORS
Systemic

Some commonly used brand names are:

In the U.S.—

Accupril[7]	Monopril[5]
Altace[8]	Prinivil[6]
Capoten[2]	Vasotec[3,4]
Lotensin[1]	Zestril[6]

In Canada—

Capoten[2]	Vasotec[3,4]
Prinivil[6]	Zestril[6]

Note: For quick reference, the following angiotensin-converting enzyme (ACE) inhibitors are numbered to match the corresponding brand names.

This information applies to the following medicines:

1. Benazepril (ben-AY-ze-pril)†
2. Captopril (KAP-toe-pril)
3. Enalapril (e-NAL-a-pril)
4. Enalaprilat (e-NAL-a-pril-at)
5. Fosinopril (foe-SIN-oh-pril)†
6. Lisinopril (lyse-IN-oh-pril)
7. Quinapril (KWIN-a-pril)†
8. Ramipril (ra-MI-pril)†

---

†Not commercially available in Canada.

Description

ACE inhibitors belong to the class of medicines called high blood pressure medicines (antihypertensives). They are used to treat high blood pressure (hypertension).

High blood pressure adds to the workload of the heart and arteries. If it continues for a long time, the heart and arteries may not function properly. This can damage the blood vessels of the brain, heart, and kidneys, resulting in a stroke, heart failure, or kidney failure. High blood pressure may also increase the risk of heart attacks. These problems may be less likely to occur if blood pressure is controlled.

Captopril is used in some patients after a heart attack. After a heart attack, some of the heart muscle is damaged and weakened. The heart muscle may continue to weaken as time goes by. This makes it more difficult for the heart to pump blood. Captopril helps slow down the further weakening of the heart.

Captopril is also used to treat kidney problems in some diabetic patients who use insulin to control their diabetes. Over time, these kidney problems may get worse. Captopril may help slow down the further worsening of kidney problems.

In addition, some ACE inhibitors are used to treat congestive heart failure, or may be used for other conditions as determined by your doctor.

The exact way that these medicines work is not known. They block an enzyme in the body that is necessary to produce a substance that causes blood vessels to tighten. As a result, they relax blood vessels. This lowers blood pressure and increases the supply of blood and oxygen to the heart.

These medicines are available only with your doctor's prescription, in the following dosage forms:

Oral

Benazepril
- Tablets (U.S.)

Captopril
- Tablets (U.S. and Canada)

Enalapril
- Tablets (U.S. and Canada)

Fosinopril
- Tablets (U.S.)

Lisinopril
- Tablets (U.S. and Canada)

Quinapril
- Tablets (U.S.)

Ramipril
- Capsules (U.S.)

Parenteral

Enalaprilat
- Injection (U.S. and Canada)

Before Using This Medicine

In deciding to use a medicine, the risks of taking the medicine must be weighed against the good it will do. This is a decision you and your doctor will make. For the angiotensin-converting enzyme (ACE) inhibitors, the following should be considered:

Allergies—Tell your doctor if you have ever had any unusual or allergic reaction to benazepril, captopril, enalapril, fosinopril, lisinopril, quinapril, or ramipril. Also tell your health care professional if you are allergic to any other substances, such as foods, preservatives, or dyes.

Pregnancy—Use of angiotensin-converting enzyme (ACE) inhibitors during pregnancy, especially in the second and third trimesters (after the first three months) can cause low blood pressure, severe kidney failure, too much potassium, or even death in the newborn. *Therefore, it is important that you check with your doctor immediately if you think* *that you may be pregnant.* Be sure that you have discussed this with your doctor before taking this medicine. In addition, if you are taking:

- *Benazepril*—Benazepril has not been shown to cause birth defects in animals when given in doses more than 3 times the highest recommended human dose.

- *Captopril*—Studies in rabbits and rats at doses up to 400 times the recommended human dose have shown that captopril causes an increase in deaths of the fetus and newborn. Also, captopril has caused deformed skulls in the offspring of rabbits given doses 2 to 70 times the recommended human dose.

- *Enalapril*—Studies in rats at doses many times the recommended human dose have shown that use of enalapril causes the fetus to be smaller than normal. Studies in rabbits have shown that enalapril causes an increase in fetal death. Enalapril has not been shown to cause birth defects in rats or rabbits.

- *Fosinopril*—Studies in rats have shown that fosinopril causes the fetus to be smaller than normal. Studies in rabbits have shown that fosinopril causes fetal death, probably due to extremely low blood pressure. In rats, birth defects such as skeletal and facial deformities were seen. However, it is not clear that the deformities were related to fosinopril. Birth defects were not seen in rabbits.

- *Lisinopril*—Studies in mice and rats at doses many times the recommended human dose have shown that use of lisinopril causes a decrease in successful pregnancies, a decrease in the weight of infants, and an increase in infant deaths. It has also caused a decrease in successful pregnancies and abnormal bone growth in rabbits. Lisinopril has not been shown to cause birth defects in mice, rats, or rabbits.

- *Quinapril*—Studies in rats have shown that quinapril causes lower birth weights and changes in kidney structure of the fetus. However, birth defects were not seen in rabbits given quinapril.

- *Ramipril*—Studies in animals have shown that ramipril causes lower birth weights.

Breast-feeding—

- *Benazepril, captopril, and fosinopril*—These medicines pass into breast milk.
- *Enalapril, lisinopril, quinapril, or ramipril*—It is not known whether these medicines pass into breast milk. However, these medicines have not been reported to cause problems in nursing babies.

Children—Children may be especially sensitive to the blood pressure–lowering effect of ACE inhibitors. This may increase the chance of side effects or other problems during treatment. Therefore, it is especially important that you discuss with the child's doctor the good that this medicine may do as well as the risks of using it.

Older adults—This medicine has been tested in a limited number of patients 65 years of age or older and has not been shown to cause different side effects or problems in older people than it does in younger adults.

Other medicines—Although certain medicines should not be used together at all, in other cases two different medicines may be used together even if an interaction might occur. In these cases, your doctor may want to change the dose, or other precautions may be necessary. When you are taking or receiving ACE inhibitors it is especially important that your health care professional know if you are taking any of the following:

- Diuretics (water pills)—Effects on blood pressure may be increased. In addition, some diuretics make the increase in potassium in the blood caused by ACE inhibitors even greater
- Potassium-containing medicines or supplements or
- Salt substitutes or
- Low-salt milk—Use of these substances with ACE inhibitors may result in an unusually high potassium level in the blood, which can lead to heart rhythm and other problems

Other medical problems—The presence of other medical problems may affect the use of the ACE inhibitors. Make sure you tell your doctor if you have any other medical problems, especially:

- Diabetes mellitus (sugar diabetes)—Increased risk of potassium levels in the body becoming too high
- Heart or blood vessel disease or
- Heart attack or stroke (recent)—Lowering blood pressure may make problems resulting from these conditions worse
- Kidney disease or
- Liver disease—Effects may be increased because of slower removal of medicine from the body
- Kidney transplant—Increased risk of kidney disease caused by ACE inhibitors
- Systemic lupus erythematosus (SLE)—Increased risk of blood problems caused by ACE inhibitors
- Previous reaction to any ACE inhibitor involving hoarseness; swelling of face, mouth, hands, or feet; or sudden trouble in breathing—Reaction is more likely to occur again

---

Proper Use of This Medicine

To help you remember to take your medicine, try to get into the habit of taking it at the same time each day.

For patients taking *captopril:*

- This medicine is best taken on an empty stomach 1 hour before meals, unless you are otherwise directed by your doctor.

For patients taking this medicine *for high blood pressure:*

- In addition to the use of the medicine your doctor has prescribed, treatment for your high blood pressure may include weight control and care in the types of foods you eat, especially foods high in sodium. Your doctor will tell you which of these are most important for you. You should check with your doctor before changing your diet.

- Many patients who have high blood pressure will not notice any signs of the problem. In fact, many may feel normal. It is very important that you *take your medicine exactly as directed* and that you keep your appointments with your doctor even if you feel well.

- Remember that this medicine will not cure your high blood pressure but it does help control it. Therefore, you must continue to take it as directed if you expect to lower your blood pressure and keep it down. *You may have to take high blood pressure medicine for the rest of your life.* If high blood pressure is not treated, it can cause serious problems such as heart failure, blood vessel disease, stroke, or kidney disease.

Dosing—The dose of the ACE inhibitor will be different for different patients. *Follow your doctor's orders or the directions on the label.* The following information includes only the average doses. *If your dose is different, do not change it* unless your doctor tells you to do so.

The number of capsules or tablets that you take depends on the strength of the medicine. Also, *the number of doses you take each day, the time allowed between doses, and the length of time you take the medicine depend on the medical problem for which you are taking the ACE inhibitor.*

For benazepril
- For *oral* dosage form (tablets):
    —For high blood pressure:
        - Adults—10 milligrams (mg) once a day at first. Then, your doctor may increase your dose to 20 to 40 mg a day taken as a single dose or divided into two doses.
        - Children—Use and dose must be determined by your doctor.

For captopril
- For *oral* dosage form (tablets):

—For congestive heart failure:

• Adults—12.5 to 100 mg two or three times a day.

• Children—Dose must be determined by your doctor.

—For high blood pressure:

• Adults—12.5 to 25 mg two or three times a day.

• Children—Dose must be determined by your doctor.

—For kidney problems related to diabetes:

• Adults—25 mg three times a day.

—For treatment after a heart attack:

• Adults—12.5 to 50 mg three times a day.

For enalapril

• For *oral* dosage form (tablets):

—For congestive heart failure:

• Adults—2.5 mg once a day or two times a day at first. Your doctor may increase your dose to 5 to 20 mg a day taken as a single dose or divided into two doses.

• Children—Use and dose must be determined by your doctor.

—For high blood pressure:

• Adults—5 mg once a day at first. Then, your doctor may increase your dose to 10 to 40 mg a day taken as a single dose or divided into two doses.

• Children—Use and dose must be determined by your doctor.

—For treating weakened heart muscle:

• Adults—2.5 mg two times a day at first. Then, your doctor may increase your dose up to 20 mg a day taken in divided doses.

- For *injection* dosage form:
  - —For high blood pressure:
    - Adults—1.25 mg every six hours injected into a vein.
    - Children—Use and dose must be determined by your doctor.

For fosinopril

- For *oral* dosage form (tablets):
  - —For high blood pressure:
    - Adults—10 to 40 mg once a day.
    - Children—Use and dose must be determined by your doctor.

For lisinopril

- For *oral* dosage form (tablets):
  - —For congestive heart failure:
    - Adults—2.5 to 20 mg once a day.
    - Children—Use and dose must be determined by your doctor.
  - —For high blood pressure:
    - Adults—10 to 40 mg once a day.
    - Children—Use and dose must be determined by your doctor.

For quinapril

- For *oral* dosage form (tablets):
  - —For high blood pressure:
    - Adults—10 mg once a day at first. Then, your doctor may increase your dose to 20 to 80 mg a day taken as a single dose or divided into two doses.
    - Children—Use and dose must be determined by your doctor.

For ramipril

- For *oral* dosage form (capsules):
  - —For high blood pressure:

- Adults—2.5 mg once a day at first. Then, your doctor may increase your dose up to 20 mg a day taken as a single dose or divided into two doses.
- Children—Use and dose must be determined by your doctor.

Missed dose—If you miss a dose of this medicine, take it as soon as possible. However, if it is almost time for your next dose, skip the missed dose and go back to your regular dosing schedule. Do not double doses.

Storage—To store this medicine:

- Keep out of the reach of children.
- Store away from heat and direct light.
- Do not store in the bathroom, near the kitchen sink, or in other damp places. Heat or moisture may cause the medicine to break down.
- Do not keep outdated medicine or medicine no longer needed. Be sure that any discarded medicine is out of the reach of children.

Precautions While Using This Medicine

It is important that your doctor check your progress at regular visits to make sure that this medicine is working properly and to check for unwanted effects.

For patients taking this medicine *for high blood pressure:*

- *Do not take other medicines unless they have been discussed with your doctor.* This especially includes over-the-counter (nonprescription) medicines for appetite control, asthma, colds, cough, hay fever, or sinus problems, since they may tend to increase your blood pressure.

Dizziness or lightheadedness may occur after the first dose of this medicine, especially if you have been taking a diuretic (water pill). Make sure you know how you react to this medicine before you drive, use machines, or do anything else that could be dangerous if you are dizzy.

Check with your doctor right away if you become sick while taking this medicine, especially with severe or continuing nausea and vomiting or diarrhea. These conditions may cause you to lose too much water and lead to low blood pressure.

Dizziness, lightheadedness, or fainting may also occur if you exercise or if the weather is hot. Heavy sweating can cause loss of too much water and low blood pressure. Use extra care during exercise or hot weather.

Avoid alcoholic beverages until you have discussed their use with your doctor. Alcohol may make the low blood pressure effect worse and/or increase the possibility of dizziness or fainting.

Before having any kind of surgery (including dental surgery) or emergency treatment, tell the medical doctor or dentist in charge that you are taking this medicine.

For patients taking *captopril or fosinopril:*
- Before you have any medical tests, tell the doctor in charge that you are taking this medicine. The results of some tests may be affected by this medicine.

Side Effects of This Medicine

Along with its needed effects, a medicine may cause some unwanted effects. Although not all of these side effects may occur, if they do occur they may need medical attention.

Check with your doctor immediately if any of the following side effects occur:

> *Rare*
>> Fever and chills; hoarseness; swelling of face, mouth, hands, or feet; trouble in swallowing or breathing (sud-

den); stomach pain, itching of skin, or yellow eyes or skin

Check with your doctor as soon as possible if any of the following side effects occur:

Less common

Dizziness, lightheadedness, or fainting; skin rash, with or without itching, fever, or joint pain

Rare

Abdominal pain, abdominal distention, fever, nausea, or vomiting; chest pain

Signs and symptoms of too much potassium in the body

Confusion; irregular heartbeat; nervousness; numbness or tingling in hands, feet, or lips; shortness of breath or difficulty breathing; weakness or heaviness of legs

Other side effects may occur that usually do not need medical attention. These side effects may go away during treatment as your body adjusts to the medicine. However, check with your doctor if any of the following side effects continue or are bothersome:

More common

Cough (dry, continuing)

Less common

Diarrhea; headache; loss of taste; nausea; unusual tiredness

Other side effects not listed above may also occur in some patients. If you notice any other effects, check with your doctor.

Additional Information

Once a medicine has been approved for marketing for a certain use, experience may show that it is also useful for other medical problems. Although these uses are not included in product labeling, ACE inhibitors are used in certain patients with the following medical conditions:

• Hypertension in scleroderma (high blood pressure in patients with hardening and thickening of the skin)

- Renal crisis in scleroderma (kidney problems in patients with hardening and thickening of the skin)

Other than the above information, there is no additional information relating to proper use, precautions, or side effects for these uses.

ANGIOTENSIN-CONVERTING ENZYME (ACE) INHIBITORS AND HYDROCHLOROTHIAZIDE
Systemic†

Some commonly used brand names are:

In the U.S.—

Capozide[1]	Vaseretic[2]
Prinzide[3]	Zestoretic[3]

Note: For quick reference, the following medicines are numbered to match the corresponding brand names.

This information applies to the following medicines:

1. Captopril (KAP-toe-pril) and Hydrochlorothiazide (hye-droe-klor-oh-THYE-a-zide)†
2. Enalapril (e-NAL-a-pril) and Hydrochlorothiazide†
3. Lisinopril (lyse-IN-oh-pril) and Hydrochlorothiazide†

†Not commercially available in Canada.

Description

This combination belongs to the class of medicines called high blood pressure medicines (antihypertensives). It is used to treat high blood pressure (hypertension).

High blood pressure adds to the workload of the heart and arteries. If it continues for a long time, the heart and arteries may not function properly. This can damage the blood vessels of the brain, heart, and kidneys, resulting in a stroke, heart failure, or kidney failure. High blood pressure may also increase the risk of heart attacks. These problems may be less likely to occur if blood pressure is controlled.

The exact way in which captopril, enalapril, and lisinopril work is not known. They block an enzyme in the body that is necessary to produce a substance that causes blood vessels to tighten. As a result, they relax blood vessels. This lowers blood pressure and increases the supply of blood and oxygen to the heart. Hydrochlorothiazide helps reduce the amount of salt and water in the body by acting on the kidneys to increase the flow of urine; this also helps to lower blood pressure.

This combination may also be used for other conditions as determined by your doctor.

This medicine is available only with doctor's prescription, in the following dosage forms:

Oral

Captopril and Hydrochlorothiazide
 • Tablets (U.S.)
Enalapril and Hydrochlorothiazide
 • Tablets (U.S.)
Lisinopril and Hydrochlorothiazide
 • Tablets (U.S.)

Before Using This Medicine

In deciding to use a medicine, the risks of taking the medicine must be weighed against the good it will do. This is a decision you and your doctor will make. For the angiotensin-converting enzyme (ACE) inhibitors and hydrochlorothiazide, the following should be considered:

Allergies—Tell your doctor if you have ever had any unusual or allergic reaction to enalapril, captopril, lisinopril, sulfonamides (sulfa drugs), bumetanide, furosemide, acetazolamide, dichlorphenamide, or methazolamide or to hydrochlorothiazide or any of the other thiazide diuretics (water pills). Also tell your health care professional if you are allergic to any other substances, such as foods, sulfites or other preservatives, or dyes.

Pregnancy—Studies with this combination medicine have not been done in pregnant women. However, use of any of the ACE inhibitors (captopril, enalapril, lisinopril) during pregnancy, especially in the second and third trimesters (after the first three months) can cause low blood pressure, kidney failure, too much potassium, or even death in newborns. *Therefore, it is important that you check with your doctor immediately if you think that you may be pregnant.* Be sure that you have discussed this with your doctor before taking this medicine. In addition, if your medicine contains:

- *Captopril*—Studies in rabbits and rats at doses up to 400 times the recommended human dose have shown that captopril causes an increase in death of the fetus and newborn. Also, captopril has caused deformed skulls in the offspring of rabbits given doses 2 to 70 times the recommended human dose.

- *Enalapril*—Studies in rats at doses many times the recommended human dose have shown that use of enalapril causes the fetus to be smaller than normal. Studies in rabbits have shown that enalapril causes an increase in fetal death. Enalapril has not been shown to cause birth defects in rats or rabbits.

- *Lisinopril*—Studies in mice and rats at doses many times the recommended human dose have shown that use of lisinopril causes a decrease in successful pregnancies, a decrease in the weight of infants, and an increase in infant deaths. It has also caused a decrease in successful pregnancies and abnormal bone growth in rabbits. Lisinopril has not been shown to cause birth defects in mice, rats, or rabbits.

- *Hydrochlorothiazide*—Hydrochlorothiazide has not been shown to cause birth defects or other problems in animal studies. However, when hydrochlorothiazide is used during pregnancy, it may cause side effects including jaundice, blood problems, and low potassium in the newborn baby.

Breast-feeding—

- *Captopril*—Passes into breast milk. However, this medicine has not been reported to cause problems in nursing babies.

- *Enalapril or lisinopril*—It is not known whether enalapril or lisinopril passes into breast milk. However, these medicines have not been reported to cause problems in nursing babies.

- *Hydrochlorothiazide*—Passes into breast milk. However, this medicine has not been reported to cause problems in nursing babies.

Children—Children may be especially sensitive to the blood pressure–lowering effect of ACE inhibitors. This may increase the chance of side effects or other problems during treatment. Extra caution may be necessary when using hydrochlorothiazide in infants with jaundice because it can make this condition worse. Therefore, it is especially important that you discuss with the child's doctor the good that this medicine may do as well as the risks of using it.

Older adults—Dizziness or lightheadedness and symptoms of too much potassium loss may be more likely to occur in the elderly, who may be more sensitive to the effects of this medicine.

Other medicines—Although certain medicines should not be used together at all, in other cases two different medicines may be used together even if an interaction might occur. In these cases, your doctor may want to change the dose, or other precautions may be necessary. When taking ACE inhibitors and hydrochlorothiazide it is especially important that your health care professional know if you are taking any of the following:

- Cholestyramine or
- Colestipol—Use with thiazide diuretics may prevent the diuretic from working properly; the diuretic should be taken at least 1 hour before or 4 hours after cholestyramine or colestipol
- Digitalis glycosides (heart medicine)—If potassium levels

in the body are decreased, symptoms of digitalis toxicity may occur

- Diuretics (water pills)—Effects on blood pressure may be increased
- Lithium (e.g., Lithane)—Risk of lithium overdose, even at low doses, may be increased
- Potassium-containing medicines or supplements or
- Salt substitutes or
- Low-salt milk—Use of these substances with ACE inhibitors may result in an unusually high potassium level in the blood, which can lead to heart rhythm and other problems

Other medical problems—The presence of other medical problems may affect the use of the ACE inhibitors. Make sure you tell your doctor if you have any other medical problems, especially:

- Diabetes mellitus (sugar diabetes)—Increased risk of potassium levels in the body becoming too high
- Gout (or history of)—Hydrochlorothiazide may increase the amount of uric acid in the body, which can lead to gout
- Heart or blood vessel disease or
- Heart attack or stroke (recent)—Lowering blood pressure may make problems resulting from these conditions worse
- Kidney disease or
- Liver disease—Effects may be increased because of slower removal from the body
- Kidney transplant—Increased risk of kidney disease caused by ACE inhibitors
- Pancreatitis (inflammation of the pancreas)—Hydrochlorothiazide can make this condition worse
- Systemic lupus erythematosus (SLE) (or history of)—Hydrochlorothiazide may worsen the condition, and there is an increased risk of blood problems caused by ACE inhibitors
- Previous reaction to captopril, enalapril, or lisinopril involving hoarseness; swelling of face, mouth, hands, or feet; or sudden trouble in breathing—Reaction is more likely to occur again

Proper Use of This Medicine

To help you remember to take your medicine, try to get into the habit of taking it at the same time each day.

For patients taking *captopril and hydrochlorothiazide:*

- This medicine is best taken on an empty stomach 1 hour before meals, unless you are otherwise directed by your doctor.

For patients taking this medicine *for high blood pressure:*

- In addition to the use of the medicine your doctor has prescribed, treatment for your high blood pressure may include weight control and care in the types of foods you eat, especially foods high in sodium. Your doctor will tell you which of these are most important for you. You should check with your doctor before changing your diet.

- Many patients who have high blood pressure will not notice any signs of the problem. In fact, many may feel normal. It is very important that you *take your medicine exactly as directed* and that you keep your appointments with your doctor even if you feel well.

- Remember that this medicine will not cure your high blood pressure, but it does help control it. Therefore, you must continue to take it as directed if you expect to lower your blood pressure and keep it down. *You may have to take high blood pressure medicine for the rest of your life.* If high blood pressure is not treated, it can cause serious problems such as heart failure, blood vessel disease, stroke, or kidney disease.

This medicine may cause you to have an unusual feeling of tiredness when you begin to take it. You may also notice an increase in the amount of urine or in your frequency of urination. After you have taken the medicine for a while, these effects should lessen. In general, to keep the increase in urine from affecting your sleep:

- If you are to take a single dose a day, take it in the morning after breakfast.
- If you are to take more than one dose a day, take the last dose no later than 6 p.m., unless otherwise directed by your doctor.

However, it is best to plan your dose or doses according to a schedule that will least affect your personal activities and sleep. Ask your health care professional to help you plan the best time to take this medicine.

Dosing—The dose of these medicines will be different for different patients. *Follow your doctor's orders or the directions on the label.* The following information includes only the average doses of these medicines. *If your dose is different, do not change it* unless your doctor tells you to do so.

The number of tablets that you take depends on the strength of the medicine.

For captopril and hydrochlorothiazide combination
- For *oral* dosage form (tablets):
  —For high blood pressure:
    - Adults—1 tablet two or three times a day.
    - Children—Dose is based on body weight and must be determined by your doctor.

For enalapril and hydrochlorothiazide combination
- For *oral* dosage form (tablets):
  —For high blood pressure:
    - Adults—1 tablet once a day.
    - Children—Dose is based on body weight and must be determined by your doctor.

For lisinopril and hydrochlorothiazide combination
- For *oral* dosage form (tablets):
  —For high blood pressure:
    - Adults—1 or 2 tablets once a day.
    - Children—Dose must be determined by your doctor.

Missed dose—If you miss a dose of this medicine, take it as soon as possible. However, if it is almost time for your next dose, skip the missed dose and go back to your regular dosing schedule. Do not double doses.

Storage—To store this medicine:

- Keep out of the reach of children.
- Store away from heat and direct light.
- Do not store in the bathroom, near the kitchen sink, or in other damp places. Heat or moisture may cause the medicine to break down.
- Do not keep outdated medicine or medicine no longer needed. Be sure that any discarded medicine is out of the reach of children.

Precautions While Using This Medicine

It is important that your doctor check your progress at regular visits to make sure that this medicine is working properly and to check for unwanted effects.

Dizziness or lightheadedness may occur, especially after the first dose of this medicine. Make sure you know how you react to the medicine before you drive, use machines, or do anything else that could be dangerous if you are dizzy.

Check with your doctor right away if you become sick while taking this medicine, especially with severe or continuing nausea and vomiting or diarrhea. These conditions may cause you to lose too much water and lead to low blood pressure.

Dizziness, lightheadedness, or fainting may also occur if you exercise or if the weather is hot. Heavy sweating can cause loss of too much water and low blood pressure. Use extra care during exercise or hot weather.

Avoid alcoholic beverages until you have discussed their use with your doctor. Alcohol may make the low blood pressure effect worse and/or increase the possibility of dizziness or fainting.

Before having any kind of surgery (including dental surgery) or emergency treatment, tell the medical doctor or dentist in charge that you are taking this medicine.

For patients taking *captopril and hydrochlorothiazide:*

- Before you have any medical tests, tell the doctor in charge that you are taking this medicine. The results of some tests may be affected by this medicine.

For patients taking this medicine *for high blood pressure:*

- *Do not take other medicines unless they have been discussed with your doctor.* This especially includes over-the-counter (nonprescription) medicines for appetite control, asthma, colds, cough, hay fever, or sinus problems, since they may tend to increase your blood pressure.

For *diabetic patients:*

- Hydrochlorothiazide (contained in this combination medicine) may raise blood sugar levels. While you are taking this medicine, be especially careful in testing for sugar in your urine.

Hydrochlorothiazide (contained in this combination medicine) may cause your skin to be more sensitive to sunlight than it is normally. Exposure to sunlight, even for brief periods of time, may cause a skin rash, itching, redness or other discoloration of the skin, or a severe sunburn. When you first begin taking this medicine:

- Stay out of direct sunlight, especially between the hours of 10:00 a.m. and 3:00 p.m., if possible.
- Wear protective clothing, including a hat. Also, wear sunglasses.
- Apply a sun block product that has a skin protection factor (SPF) of at least 15. Some patients may require

a product with a higher SPF number, especially if they have a fair complexion. If you have any questions about this, check with your health care professional.

- Apply a sun block lipstick that has an SPF of at least 15 to protect your lips.
- Do not use a sunlamp or tanning bed or booth.

If you have a severe reaction from the sun, check with your doctor.

Before you have any medical tests, tell the doctor in charge that you are taking this medicine. The results of some tests may be affected by this medicine.

Side Effects of This Medicine

Along with its needed effects, a medicine may cause some unwanted effects. Although not all of these side effects may occur, if they do occur they may need medical attention.

Check with your doctor immediately if any of the following side effects occur:

Rare

Fever and chills; hoarseness; swelling of face, mouth, hands, or feet; trouble in swallowing or breathing (sudden)

Check with your doctor as soon as possible if any of the following side effects occur:

Less common

Dizziness, lightheadedness, or fainting; skin rash, with or without itching, fever, or joint pain

Rare

Chest pain; joint pain; lower back or side pain; stomach pain (severe) with nausea and vomiting; unusual bleeding or bruising; yellow eyes or skin

Signs and symptoms of too much or too little potassium in the body

Dryness of mouth; increased thirst; irregular heartbeats; mood or mental changes; muscle cramps or pain; numbness or tingling in hands, feet, or lips; weakness or heaviness of legs; weak pulse

Other side effects may occur that usually do not need medical attention. These side effects may go away during treatment as your body adjusts to the medicine. However, check with your doctor if any of the following side effects continue or are bothersome:

More common

Cough (dry, continuing)

Less common

Diarrhea; headache; increased sensitivity of skin to sunlight (skin rash, itching, redness or other discoloration of skin or severe sunburn after exposure to sunlight); loss of appetite; loss of taste; stomach upset; unusual tiredness

Other side effects not listed above may also occur in some patients. If you notice any other effects, check with your doctor.

Additional Information

Once a medicine has been approved for marketing for a certain use, experience may show that it is also useful for other medical problems. Although this use is not included in product labeling, ACE inhibitors and hydrochlorothiazide are used in certain patients with the following medical condition:

• Congestive heart failure

Other than the above information, there is no additional information relating to proper use, precautions, or side effects for this use.

ANTICOAGULANTS   Systemic

Some commonly used brand names are:

In the U.S.—
    Coumadin[3]   Panwarfin[3]
    Miradon[1]   Sofarin[3]

In Canada—
    Coumadin[3]   Warfilone[3]

Note: For quick reference, the following anticoagulants are numbered to match the corresponding brand names.

This information applies to the following medicines:

1. Anisindione (an-iss-in-DYE-one)[†]
2. Dicumarol (dye-KOO-ma-role)[†][‡]
3. Warfarin (WAR-far-in)[‡]

This information does *not* apply to heparin.

[†]Not commercially available in Canada.
[‡]Generic name product may also be available in the U.S.

Description

Anticoagulants decrease the clotting ability of the blood and therefore help to prevent harmful clots from forming in the blood vessels. These medicines are sometimes called blood thinners, although they do not actually thin the blood. They also will not dissolve clots that have already formed, but they may prevent the clots from becoming larger and causing more serious problems. They are often used as treatment for certain blood vessel, heart, and lung conditions.

In order for an anticoagulant to help you without causing serious bleeding, it must be used properly and all of the precautions concerning its use must be followed exactly. Be sure that you have discussed the use of this medicine with your doctor. It is very important that you understand all of your doctor's orders and that you are willing and able to follow them exactly.

Anticoagulants are available only with your doctor's prescription, in the following dosage forms:

Oral

   Anisindione
      • Tablets (U.S.)
   Dicumarol
      • Tablets (U.S.)
   Warfarin
      • Tablets (U.S. and Canada)

Parenteral

   Warfarin
      • Injection (U.S.)

Before Using This Medicine

In deciding to use a medicine, the risks of taking the medicine must be weighed against the good it will do. This is a decision you and your doctor will make. For anticoagulants, the following should be considered:

Allergies—Tell your doctor if you have ever had any unusual or allergic reaction to an anticoagulant. Also tell your health care professional if you are allergic to any other substances, such as foods, preservatives, or dyes.

Pregnancy—Anticoagulants may cause birth defects. They may also cause other problems affecting the physical or mental growth of the fetus or newborn baby. In addition, use of this medicine during the last 6 months of pregnancy may increase the chance of severe, possibly fatal, bleeding in the fetus. If taken during the last few weeks of pregnancy, anticoagulants may cause severe bleeding in both the fetus and the mother before or during delivery and in the newborn infant.

Do not begin taking this medicine during pregnancy, and do not become pregnant while taking it, unless you have first discussed the possible effects of this medicine with your doctor. Also, if you suspect that you may be pregnant and you are already taking an anticoagulant, check with your doctor at once. Your doctor may suggest that you take a different anticoagulant that is less likely to harm the fetus or the newborn infant during all or part of your pregnancy. Anticoagulants may also cause severe bleeding in the mother if taken soon after the baby is born.

Breast-feeding—Warfarin is not likely to cause problems in nursing babies. Other anticoagulants may pass into the breast milk. A blood test can be done to see if unwanted effects are occurring in the nursing baby. If necessary, another medicine that will overcome any unwanted effects of the anticoagulant can be given to the baby.

Children—Very young babies may be especially sensitive to the effects of anticoagulants. This may increase the chance of bleeding during treatment.

Older adults—Elderly people are especially sensitive to the effects of anticoagulants. This may increase the chance of bleeding during treatment.

Other medicines—Although certain medicines should not be used together at all, in other cases two different medicines may be used together even if an interaction might occur. In these cases, your doctor may want to change the dose, or other precautions may be necessary. *Many different medicines can affect the way anticoagulants work in your body.* Therefore, it is very important that your health care professional knows if you are taking *any* other prescription or nonprescription (over-the-counter [OTC]) medicine, even aspirin, laxatives, vitamins, or antacids.

Other medical problems—The presence of other medical problems may affect the use of anticoagulants. Make sure you tell your doctor if you have *any* other medical problems, or if you are now being treated by any other medical doctor or dentist. Many medical problems and treatments will affect the way your body responds to this medicine.

Also, it is important that you tell your doctor if you have recently had any of the following conditions or medical procedures:

- Childbirth or
- Falls or blows to the body or head or
- Fever lasting more than a couple of days or
- Heavy or unusual menstrual bleeding or
- Insertion of intrauterine device (IUD) or
- Medical or dental surgery or
- Severe or continuing diarrhea or
- Spinal anesthesia or
- X-ray (radiation) treatment—The risk of serious bleeding may be increased

---

Proper Use of This Medicine

Take this medicine only as directed by your doctor. Do not take more or less of it, do not take it more often, and do not take it for a longer time than your doctor ordered. This is especially important for elderly patients, who are especially sensitive to the effects of anticoagulants.

Your doctor should check your progress at regular visits. A blood test must be taken regularly to see how fast your blood is clotting. This will help your doctor decide on the proper amount of anticoagulant you should be taking each day.

Dosing—The dose of these medicines will be different for different patients. *Follow your doctor's orders or the directions on the label.* The following information includes only the average doses of these medicines. *If your dose is different, do not change it* unless your doctor tells you to do so.

For anisindione

- For *oral* dosage form (tablets):

  —For preventing harmful blood clots:

  - Adults and teenagers—The usual dose is 25 to 250 milligrams (mg) per day.
  - Children—Dose must be determined by your doctor.

For dicumarol
- For *oral* dosage form (tablets):
  —For preventing harmful blood clots:
    - Adults and teenagers—The usual dose is 25 to 200 milligrams (mg) per day.
    - Children—Dose must be determined by your doctor.

For warfarin
- For *oral* dosage form (tablets):
  —For preventing harmful blood clots:
    - Adults and teenagers—The starting dose is usually 10 to 15 milligrams (mg) per day for two to four days. Then, your doctor may decrease the dose to 2 to 10 mg per day, depending on your condition.
    - Children—Dose must be determined by your doctor.
- For *injection* dosage form:
  —For preventing harmful blood clots:
    - Adults and teenagers—The starting dose is usually 10 to 15 mg, injected into a muscle or a vein, once a day for two to four days. Then, your doctor may decrease the dose to 2 to 10 mg per day, depending on your condition.
    - Children—Dose must be determined by your doctor.

Missed dose—If you miss a dose of this medicine, take it as soon as possible. Then go back to your regular dosing schedule. If you do not remember until the next day, do not take the missed dose at all and do not double the next one. *Doubling the dose may cause bleeding.* Instead, go back to your regular dosing schedule. It is recommended that you keep a record of each dose as you take it to avoid mistakes. Also, be sure to give your doctor a record of any doses you miss. If you have any questions about this, check with your doctor.

Storage—To store this medicine:

- Keep out of the reach of children.
- Store away from heat and direct light.
- Do not store this medicine in the bathroom, near the kitchen sink, or in other damp places. Heat or moisture may cause the medicine to break down.
- Do not keep outdated medicine or medicine no longer needed. Be sure that any discarded medicine is out of the reach of children.

Precautions While Using This Medicine

Tell all medical doctors, dentists, and pharmacists you go to that you are taking this medicine.

Check with your health care professional before you start or stop taking any other medicine. This includes any nonprescription (over-the-counter [OTC]) medicine, even aspirin or acetaminophen. Many medicines change the way this medicine affects your body. You may not be able to take the other medicine, or the dose of your anticoagulant may need to be changed.

It is important that you carry identification stating that you are using this medicine. If you have any questions about what kind of identification to carry, check with your health care professional.

While you are taking this medicine, it is very important that you avoid sports and activities that may cause you to be injured. Report to your doctor any falls, blows to the body or head, or other injuries, since serious internal bleeding may occur without your knowing about it.

Be careful to avoid cutting yourself. This includes taking special care in brushing your teeth and in shaving. Use a soft toothbrush and floss gently. Also, it is best to use an electric shaver rather than a blade.

Drinking too much alcohol may change the way this anti-coagulant affects your body. You should not drink regularly on a daily basis or take more than 1 or 2 drinks at any time. If you have any questions about this, check with your doctor.

The foods that you eat may also affect the way this medicine affects your body. Eat a normal, balanced diet while you are taking this medicine. Do not go on a reducing diet, make other changes in your eating habits, start taking vitamins, or begin using other nutrition supplements unless you have first checked with your health care professional. Also, check with your doctor if you are unable to eat for several days or if you have continuing stomach upset, diarrhea, or fever. These precautions are important because the effects of the anticoagulant depend on the amount of vitamin K in your body. Therefore, it is best to have the same amount of vitamin K in your body every day. Some multiple vitamins and some nutrition supplements contain vitamin K. Vitamin K is also present in meats, dairy products (such as milk, cheese, and yogurt), and green, leafy vegetables (such as broccoli, cabbage, collard greens, kale, lettuce, and spinach). It is especially important that you do not make large changes in the amounts of these foods that you eat every day while you are taking an anticoagulant.

After you stop taking this medicine, your body will need time to recover before your blood clotting ability returns to normal. Your health care professional can tell you how long this will take depending on which anticoagulant you were taking. Use the same caution during this period of time as you did while you were taking the anticoagulant.

Side Effects of This Medicine

Along with its needed effects, a medicine may cause some unwanted effects. Although not all of these side effects

may occur, if they do occur they may need medical attention.

Check with your doctor immediately if any of the following side effects occur:

Less common or rare

Blue or purple color of toes and pain in toes; cloudy or dark urine; difficult or painful urination; sores, ulcers, or white spots in mouth or throat; sore throat and fever or chills; sudden decrease in amount of urine; swelling of face, feet, or lower legs; unusual tiredness or weakness; unusual weight gain; yellow eyes or skin

Since many things can affect the way your body reacts to this medicine, you should always watch for signs of unusual bleeding. Unusual bleeding may mean that your body is getting more medicine than it needs. *Check with your doctor immediately if any of the following signs of overdose occur:*

Bleeding from gums when brushing teeth; unexplained bruising or purplish areas on skin; unexplained nosebleeds; unusually heavy bleeding or oozing from cuts or wounds; unusually heavy or unexpected menstrual bleeding

Signs and symptoms of bleeding inside the body

Abdominal or stomach pain or swelling; back pain or backaches; blood in urine; bloody or black tarry stools; constipation; coughing up blood; dizziness; headache (severe or continuing); joint pain, stiffness, or swelling; vomiting blood or material that looks like coffee grounds

Also, check with your doctor as soon as possible if any of the following side effects occur:

Less common or rare

Diarrhea (more common with dicumarol); nausea or vomiting; skin rash, hives, or itching; stomach cramps or pain

For patients taking *anisindione* (e.g., Miradon):

• Depending on your diet, this medicine may cause your urine to turn orange. Since it may be hard to tell the difference between blood in the urine and this normal color change, check with your doctor if you notice any color change in your urine.

Other side effects may occur that usually do not need medical attention. These side effects may go away during treatment as your body adjusts to the medicine. However, check with your doctor if any of the following side effects continue or are bothersome:

More common
> Bloated feeling or gas (with dicumarol)

Less common
> Blurred vision or other vision problems (with anisindione); loss of appetite; unusual hair loss

Other side effects not listed above may also occur in some patients. If you notice any other effects, check with your doctor.

BETA-ADRENERGIC BLOCKING AGENTS Systemic

Some commonly used brand names are:

In the U.S.—

Betapace[13]	Lopressor[7]
Blocadren[14]	Normodyne[6]
Cartrol[5]	Sectral[1]
Corgard[8]	Tenormin[2]
Inderal[12]	Toprol-XL[7]
Inderal LA[12]	Trandate[6]
Kerlone[3]	Visken[11]
Levatol[10]	Zebeta[4]

In Canada—

Apo-Atenolol[2]	Blocadren[14]
Apo-Metoprolol[7]	Corgard[8]
Apo-Metoprolol (Type L)[7]	Detensol[12]
Apo-Propranolol[12]	Inderal[12]
Apo-Timol[14]	Inderal LA[12]
Betaloc[7]	Lopresor[7]
Betaloc Durules[7]	Lopresor SR[7]

In Canada (cont'd)—

Monitan[1]	Slow-Trasicor[9]
Novo-Atenol[2]	Sotacor[13]
Novometoprol[7]	Syn-Nadolol[8]
Novo-Pindol[11]	Syn-Pindolol[11]
Novo-Timol[14]	Tenormin[2]
Novopranol[12]	Trandate[6]
pms Propranolol[12]	Trasicor[9]
Sectral[1]	Visken[11]

Note: For quick reference, the following beta-adrenergic blocking agents are numbered to match the corresponding brand names.

This information applies to the following medicines:

1. Acebutolol (a-se-BYOO-toe-lole)
2. Atenolol (a-TEN-oh-lole)‡
3. Betaxolol (be-TAX-oh-lol)†
4. Bisoprolol (bis-OH-proe-lol)†
5. Carteolol (KAR-tee-oh-lole)†
6. Labetalol (la-BET-a-lole)
7. Metoprolol (me-TOE-proe-lole)§
8. Nadolol (NAY-doe-lole)§
9. Oxprenolol (ox-PREN-oh-lole)*
10. Penbutolol (pen-BYOO-toe-lole)†
11. Pindolol (PIN-doe-lole)
12. Propranolol (proe-PRAN-oh-lole)‡§
13. Sotalol (SOE-ta-lole)
14. Timolol (TIM-oh-lole)‡

*Not commercially available in the U.S.
†Not commercially available in Canada.
‡Generic name product may also be available in the U.S.
§Generic name product may also be available in Canada.

Description

This group of medicines is known as beta-adrenergic blocking agents, beta-blocking agents, or, more commonly, beta-blockers. Beta-blockers are used in the treatment of high blood pressure (hypertension). Some beta-blockers are also used to relieve angina (chest pain) and in heart attack patients to help prevent additional heart attacks. Beta-blockers are also used to correct irregular heartbeat, prevent migraine headaches, and treat tremors. They may also be used for other conditions as determined by your doctor.

Beta-blockers work by affecting the response to some nerve impulses in certain parts of the body. As a result, they decrease the heart's need for blood and oxygen by reducing its workload. They also help the heart to beat more regularly.

Beta-adrenergic blocking agents are available only with your doctor's prescription, in the following dosage forms:

Oral

Acebutolol
- Capsules (U.S.)
- Tablets (Canada)

Atenolol
- Tablets (U.S. and Canada)

Betaxolol
- Tablets (U.S.)

Bisoprolol
- Tablets (U.S.)

Carteolol
- Tablets (U.S.)

Labetalol
- Tablets (U.S. and Canada)

Metoprolol
- Tablets (U.S. and Canada)
- Extended-release tablets (U.S. and Canada)

Nadolol
- Tablets (U.S. and Canada)

Oxprenolol
- Tablets (Canada)
- Extended-release tablets (Canada)

Penbutolol
- Tablets (U.S.)

Pindolol
- Tablets (U.S. and Canada)

Propranolol
- Extended-release capsules (U.S. and Canada)
- Oral solution (U.S.)
- Tablets (U.S. and Canada)

Sotalol
- Tablets (U.S. and Canada)

Timolol
- Tablets (U.S. and Canada)

Parenteral

Atenolol
- Injection (U.S.)

Labetalol
- Injection (U.S. and Canada)

Metoprolol
- Injection (U.S. and Canada)

Propranolol
- Injection (U.S. and Canada)

Before Using This Medicine

In deciding to use a medicine, the risks of taking the medicine must be weighed against the good it will do. This is a decision you and your doctor will make. For the beta-blockers, the following should be considered:

Allergies—Tell your doctor if you have ever had any unusual or allergic reaction to the beta-blocker medicine prescribed. Also tell your health care professional if you are allergic to any other substances, such as foods, preservatives, or dyes.

Pregnancy—Use of some beta-blockers during pregnancy has been associated with low blood sugar, breathing problems, a lower heart rate, and low blood pressure in the newborn infant. Other reports have not shown unwanted effects on the newborn infant. Animal studies have shown some beta-blockers to cause problems in pregnancy when used in doses many times the usual human dose. Before taking any of these medicines, make sure your doctor knows if you are pregnant or if you may become pregnant.

Breast-feeding—It is not known whether bisoprolol, carteolol, or penbutolol passes into breast milk. All other beta-blockers pass into breast milk. Problems such as slow heartbeat, low blood pressure, and trouble in breathing have been reported in nursing babies. Mothers who are taking beta-blockers and who wish to breast-feed should discuss this with their doctor.

Children—Some of these medicines have been used in children and, in effective doses, have not been shown to cause different side effects or problems in children than they do in adults.

Older adults—Some side effects are more likely to occur in the elderly, who are usually more sensitive to the effects of beta-blockers. Also, beta-blockers may reduce tolerance to cold temperatures in elderly patients.

Other medicines—Although certain medicines should not be used together at all, in other cases two different medicines may be used together even if an interaction might occur. In these cases, your doctor may want to change the dose, or other precautions may be necessary. When you are taking or receiving a beta-blocker it is especially important that your health care professional know if you are taking any of the following:

- Allergen immunotherapy (allergy shots) or
- Allergen extracts for skin testing—Beta-blockers may increase the risk of serious allergic reaction to these medicines

- Aminophylline (e.g., Somophyllin) or
- Caffeine (e.g., NoDoz) or
- Dyphylline (e.g., Lufyllin) or
- Oxtriphylline (e.g., Choledyl) or
- Theophylline (e.g., Somophyllin-T)—The effects of both these medicines and beta-blockers may be blocked; in addition, theophylline levels in the body may be increased, especially in patients who smoke

- Antidiabetics, oral (diabetes medicine you take by mouth) or
- Insulin—There is an increased risk of hyperglycemia (high blood sugar); beta-blockers may cover up certain symptoms of hypoglycemia (low blood sugar) such as increases in pulse rate and blood pressure, and may make the hypoglycemia last longer

- Calcium channel blockers (bepridil [e.g., Bepadin], diltiazem [e.g., Cardizem], felodipine [e.g., Plendil], flunarizine [e.g., Sibelium], isradipine [e.g., DynaCirc], nicardipine [e.g., Cardene], nifedipine [e.g., Procardia], nimodipine [e.g., Nimotop], verapamil [e.g., Calan]) or

- Clonidine (e.g., Catapres) or
- Guanabenz (e.g., Wytensin)—Effects on blood pressure may be increased. In addition, unwanted effects may occur if clonidine, guanabenz, or a beta-blocker is stopped suddenly after use together. Unwanted effects on the heart may occur when beta-blockers are used with calcium channel blockers

- Cocaine—Cocaine may block the effects of beta-blockers; in addition, there is an increased risk of high blood pressure, fast heartbeat, and possibly heart problems if you use cocaine while taking a beta-blocker

- Monoamine oxidase (MAO) inhibitors (furazolidone [e.g., Furoxone], isocarboxazid [e.g., Marplan], phenelzine [e.g., Nardil], procarbazine [e.g., Matulane], selegiline [e.g., Eldepryl], tranylcypromine [e.g., Parnate])—Taking beta-blockers while you are taking or within 2 weeks of taking monoamine oxidase (MAO) inhibitors may cause severe high blood pressure

Other medical problems—The presence of other medical problems may affect the use of the beta-blockers. Make sure you tell your doctor if you have any other medical problems, especially:

- Allergy, history of (asthma, eczema, hay fever, hives), or
- Bronchitis or
- Emphysema—Severity and duration of allergic reactions to other substances may be increased; in addition, beta-blockers can increase trouble in breathing

- Bradycardia (unusually slow heartbeat) or
- Heart or blood vessel disease—There is a risk of further decreased heart function; also, if treatment is stopped suddenly, unwanted effects may occur

- Diabetes mellitus (sugar diabetes)—Beta-blockers may cause hyperglycemia (high blood sugar) and circulation problems; in addition, if your diabetes medicine causes your blood sugar to be too low, beta-blockers may cover up some of the symptoms (fast heartbeat), although they will not cover up other symptoms such as dizziness or sweating

- Kidney disease or
- Liver disease—Effects of beta-blockers may be increased because of slower removal from the body
- Mental depression (or history of)—May be increased by beta-blockers
- Myasthenia gravis or
- Psoriasis—Beta-blockers may make these conditions worse
- Overactive thyroid—Stopping beta-blockers suddenly may increase symptoms; beta-blockers may cover up fast heartbeat, which is a sign of overactive thyroid

---

Proper Use of This Medicine

For patients taking the *extended-release capsule or tablet* form of this medicine:

- Swallow the capsule or tablet whole.
- Do not crush, break (except metoprolol succinate extended-release tablets, which may be broken in half), or chew before swallowing.

For patients taking the *concentrated oral solution* form of *propranolol:*

- This medicine is to be taken by mouth even though it comes in a dropper bottle. The amount you should take is to be measured only with the specially marked dropper.
- Mix the medicine with some water, juice, or a carbonated drink. After drinking all the liquid containing the medicine, rinse the glass with a little more liquid and drink that also, to make sure you get all the medicine.

  If you prefer, you may mix this medicine with applesauce or pudding instead.

- Mix the medicine immediately before you are going to take it. Throw away any mixed medicine that you do not take immediately. Do not save medicine that has been mixed.

Ask your doctor about checking your pulse rate before and after taking beta-blocking agents. Then, while you are taking this medicine, check your pulse regularly. If it is much slower than your usual rate (or less than 50 beats per minute), check with your doctor. A pulse rate that is too slow may cause circulation problems.

To help you remember to take your medicine, try to get into the habit of taking it at the same time each day.

For patients taking this medicine *for high blood pressure:*

- In addition to the use of the medicine your doctor has prescribed, treatment for your high blood pressure may include weight control and care in the types of foods you eat, especially foods high in sodium. Your doctor will tell you which of these are most important for you. You should check with your doctor before changing your diet.

- Many patients who have high blood pressure will not notice any signs of the problem. In fact, many may feel normal. However, if high blood pressure is not treated, it can cause serious problems such as heart failure, blood vessel disease, stroke, or kidney disease.

- Remember that this medicine will not cure your high blood pressure, but it does help control it. It is very important that you *take your medicine exactly as directed*, even if you feel well. You must continue to take it as directed if you expect to lower your blood pressure and keep it down. *You may have to take high blood pressure medicine for the rest of your life.* Also, it is very important to keep your appointments with your doctor, even if you feel well.

Dosing—The dose of beta-blocker will be different for different patients. *Follow your doctor's orders or the directions on the label.* The following information includes only the average doses. *If your dose is different, do not change it* unless your doctor tells you to do so.

The number of capsules or tablets or teaspoonfuls of solution that you take depends on the strength of the medicine. Also, *the number of doses you take each day, the time allowed between doses, and the length of time you take the medicine depend on the medical problem for which you are taking the beta-blocker.*

For acebutolol

- For *oral* dosage forms (capsules and tablets):

    —For angina (chest pain) or irregular heartbeat:

    - Adults—200 milligrams (mg) two times a day. The dose may be increased up to a total of 1200 mg a day.

    - Children—Dose must be determined by your doctor.

    —For high blood pressure:

    - Adults—200 to 800 mg a day as a single dose or divided into two daily doses.

    - Children—Dose must be determined by your doctor.

For atenolol

- For *oral* dosage form (tablets):

    —For angina (chest pain):

    - Adults—50 to 100 mg once a day.

    —For high blood pressure:

    - Adults—25 to 100 mg once a day.

    - Children—Dose must be determined by your doctor.

    —For treatment after a heart attack:

    - Adults—50 mg ten minutes after the last intravenous dose, followed by another 50 mg twelve hours later. Then 100 mg once a day or 50 mg two times a day for six to nine days or until discharge from hospital.

- For *injection* dosage form:

    —For treatment of heart attacks:

• Adults—5 mg given over 5 minutes. The dose is repeated ten minutes later.

For betaxolol

• For *oral* dosage form (tablets):

—For high blood pressure:

• Adults—10 mg once a day. Your doctor may double your dose after seven to fourteen days.

• Children—Dose must be determined by your doctor.

For bisoprolol

• For *oral* dosage form (tablets):

—For high blood pressure:

• Adults—5 to 10 mg once a day.

• Children—Dose must be determined by your doctor.

For carteolol

• For *oral* dosage form (tablets):

—For high blood pressure:

• Adults—2.5 to 10 mg once a day.

• Children—Dose must be determined by your doctor.

For labetalol

• For *oral* dosage form (tablets):

—For high blood pressure:

• Adults—100 to 400 mg two times a day.

• Children—Dose must be determined by your doctor.

• For *injection* dosage form:

—For high blood pressure:

• Adults—20 mg injected slowly over two minutes with additional injections of 40 and 80 mg given every ten minutes if needed, up to a total of 300 mg; may be given instead as an infusion at a rate of 2 mg per minute to a total dose of 50 to 300 mg.

• Children—Dose must be determined by your doctor.

For metoprolol

• For *regular (short-acting) oral* dosage form (tablets):

—For high blood pressure or angina (chest pain):

• Adults—100 to 450 mg a day, taken as a single dose or in divided doses.

• Children—Dose must be determined by your doctor.

—For treatment after a heart attack:

• Adults—50 mg every six hours starting fifteen minutes after last intravenous dose. Then 100 mg two times a day for three months to 1 year.

• For *long-acting oral* dosage forms (extended-release tablets):

—For high blood pressure or angina (chest pain):

• Adults—Up to 400 mg once a day.

• Children—Dose must be determined by your doctor.

• For *injection* dosage form:

—For treatment of a heart attack:

• Adults—5 mg every two minutes for three doses.

For nadolol

• For *oral* dosage form (tablets):

—For angina (chest pain):

• Adults—40 to 240 mg once a day.

—For high blood pressure:

• Adults—40 to 320 mg once a day.

• Children—Dose must be determined by your doctor.

For oxprenolol

- For *regular (short-acting) oral* dosage form (tablets):
  - —For high blood pressure:
    - Adults—20 mg three times a day. Your doctor may increase your dose up to 480 mg a day.
    - Children—Dose must be determined by your doctor.
- For *long-acting oral* dosage form (extended-release tablets):
  - —For high blood pressure:
    - Adults—80 to 160 mg once a day.
    - Children—Dose must be determined by your doctor.

For penbutolol

- For *oral* dosage form (tablets):
  - —For high blood pressure:
    - Adults—20 mg once a day.
    - Children—Dose must be determined by your doctor.

For pindolol

- For *oral* dosage form (tablets):
  - —For high blood pressure:
    - Adults—5 mg two times a day. Your doctor may increase your dose up to 60 mg a day.
    - Children—Dose must be determined by your doctor.

For propranolol

- For *regular (short-acting) oral* dosage forms (tablets and oral solution):
  - —For angina (chest pain):
    - Adults—80 to 320 mg a day taken in two, three, or four divided doses.
  - —For irregular heartbeat:
    - Adults—10 to 30 mg three or four times a day.

  • Children—500 micrograms (0.5 mg) to 4 mg per kilogram of body weight a day taken in divided doses.

 —For high blood pressure:

  • Adults—40 mg two times a day. Your doctor may increase your dose up to 640 mg a day.

  • Children—500 micrograms (0.5 mg) to 4 mg per kilogram of body weight a day taken in divided doses.

 —For diseased heart muscle (cardiomyopathy):

  • Adults—20 to 40 mg three or four times a day.

 —For treatment after a heart attack:

  • Adults—180 to 240 mg a day taken in divided doses.

 —For treating pheochromocytoma:

  • Adults—30 to 160 mg a day taken in divided doses.

 —For preventing migraine headaches:

  • Adults—20 mg four times a day. Your doctor may increase your dose up to 240 mg a day.

 —For trembling:

  • Adults—40 mg two times a day. Your doctor may increase your dose up to 320 mg a day.

• For *long-acting oral* dosage form (extended-release capsules):

 —For high blood pressure:

  • Adults—80 to 160 mg once a day. Doses up to 640 mg once a day may be needed in some patients.

 —For angina (chest pain):

  • Adults—80 to 320 mg once a day.

 —For preventing migraine headaches:

  • Adults—80 to 240 mg once a day.

• For *injection* dosage form:

—For irregular heartbeat:

• Adults—1 to 3 mg given at a rate not greater than 1 mg per minute. Dose may be repeated after two minutes and again after four hours if needed.

• Children—10 to 100 micrograms (0.01 to 0.1 mg) per kilogram of body weight given intravenously every six to eight hours.

For sotalol

• For *oral* dosage form (tablets):

—For irregular heartbeat:

• Adults—80 mg two times a day. Your doctor may increase your dose up to 320 mg per day taken in two or three divided doses.

• Children—Dose must be determined by your doctor.

For timolol

• For *oral* dosage form (tablets):

—For high blood pressure:

• Adults—10 mg two times a day. Your doctor may increase your dose up to 60 mg per day taken as a single dose or in divided doses.

• Children—Dose must be determined by your doctor.

—For treatment after a heart attack:

• Adults—10 mg two times a day.

—For preventing migraine headaches:

• Adults—10 mg two times a day. Your doctor may increase your dose up to 30 mg once a day or in divided doses.

Missed dose—Do not miss any doses. This is especially important when you are taking only one dose per day. Some conditions may become worse if this medicine is not taken regularly.

If you do miss a dose of this medicine, take it as soon as possible. However, if it is within 4 hours of your next dose (8 hours when using atenolol, betaxolol, bisoprolol, carteolol, labetalol, nadolol, penbutolol, sotalol, or extended-release [long-acting] metoprolol, oxprenolol, or propranolol), skip the missed dose and go back to your regular dosing schedule. Do not double doses.

Storage—To store this medicine:
- Keep out of the reach of children.
- Store away from heat and direct light.
- Do not store in the bathroom, near the kitchen sink, or in other damp places. Heat or moisture may cause the medicine to break down.
- Do not keep outdated medicine or medicine no longer needed. Be sure that any discarded medicine is out of the reach of children.

Precautions While Using This Medicine

It is important that your doctor check your progress at regular visits. This is to make sure the medicine is working for you and to allow the dosage to be changed if needed.

Do not stop taking this medicine without first checking with your doctor. Your doctor may want you to reduce gradually the amount you are taking before stopping completely. Some conditions may become worse when the medicine is stopped suddenly, and the danger of heart attack is increased in some patients.

Make sure that you have enough medicine on hand to last through weekends, holidays, or vacations. You may want to carry an extra written prescription in your billfold or purse in case of an emergency. You can then have it filled if you run out of medicine while you are away from home.

Your doctor may want you to carry medical identification stating that you are taking this medicine.

Before having any kind of surgery (including dental surgery) or emergency treatment, tell the medical doctor or dentist in charge that you are taking this medicine.

For *diabetic patients:*

- *This medicine may cause your blood sugar levels to rise. Also, this medicine may cover up signs of hypoglycemia (low blood sugar),* such as change in pulse rate.

This medicine may cause some people to become dizzy, drowsy, or lightheaded. *Make sure you know how you react to this medicine before you drive, use machines, or do anything else that could be dangerous if you are dizzy or are not alert.* If the problem continues or gets worse, check with your doctor.

Beta-blockers may make you more sensitive to cold temperatures, especially if you have blood circulation problems. Beta-blockers tend to decrease blood circulation in the skin, fingers, and toes. Dress warmly during cold weather and be careful during prolonged exposure to cold, such as in winter sports.

Chest pain resulting from exercise or physical exertion is usually reduced or prevented by this medicine. This may tempt a patient to be overly active. *Make sure you discuss with your doctor a safe amount of exercise for your medical problem.*

Before you have any medical tests, tell the doctor in charge that you are taking this medicine. The results of some tests may be affected by this medicine.

Before you have any allergy shots, tell the doctor in charge that you are taking a beta-blocker. Beta-blockers may cause you to have a serious reaction to the allergy shot.

For patients with *allergies to foods, medicines, or insect stings:*

- There is a chance that this medicine will cause allergic reactions to be worse and harder to treat. If you have a severe allergic reaction while you are being treated with this medicine, check with a doctor right away so that it can be treated. Be sure to tell the doctor that you are taking a beta-blocker.

For patients taking this medicine *for high blood pressure:*

- *Do not take other medicines unless they have been discussed with your doctor.* This especially includes over-the-counter (nonprescription) medicines for appetite control, asthma, colds, cough, hay fever, or sinus problems since they may tend to increase your blood pressure.

For patients taking *labetalol by mouth:*

- *Dizziness, lightheadedness, or fainting may occur, especially when you get up from a lying or sitting position.* This is more likely to occur when you first start taking labetalol or when the dose is increased. *Getting up slowly may help.* When you get up from lying down, sit on the edge of the bed with your feet dangling for 1 to 2 minutes. Then stand up slowly. If the problem continues or gets worse, check with your doctor.
- The dizziness, lightheadedness, or fainting is also more likely to occur if you drink alcohol, stand for long periods of time, or exercise, or if the weather is hot. *While you are taking this medicine, be careful to limit the amount of alcohol you drink. Also, use extra care during exercise or hot weather or if you must stand for long periods of time.*

For patients receiving *labetalol by injection:*

- It is very important that you lie down flat while receiving labetalol and for up to 3 hours afterward. If you try to get up too soon, you may become dizzy or faint. *Do not try to sit or stand until your doctor or nurse tells you to do so.*

Side Effects of This Medicine

Along with its needed effects, a medicine may cause some unwanted effects. Although not all of these side effects may occur, if they do occur they may need medical attention.

Check with your doctor as soon as possible if any of the following side effects occur:

Less common

Breathing difficulty and/or wheezing; cold hands and feet; mental depression; shortness of breath; slow heartbeat (especially less than 50 beats per minute); swelling of ankles, feet, and/or lower legs

Rare

Back pain or joint pain; chest pain; confusion (especially in elderly); dark urine—for acebutolol, bisoprolol, or labetalol; dizziness or lightheadedness when getting up from a lying or sitting position; fever and sore throat; hallucinations (seeing, hearing, or feeling things that are not there); irregular heartbeat; red, scaling, or crusted skin; skin rash; unusual bleeding and bruising; yellow eyes or skin—for acebutolol, bisoprolol, or labetalol

Signs and symptoms of overdose (in the order in which they may occur)

Slow heartbeat; dizziness (severe) or fainting; fast or irregular heartbeat; difficulty in breathing; bluish-colored fingernails or palms of hands; convulsions (seizures)

Other side effects may occur that usually do not need medical attention. These side effects may go away during treatment as your body adjusts to the medicine. However, check with your doctor if any of the following side effects continue or are bothersome:

More common

Decreased sexual ability; dizziness or lightheadedness; drowsiness (slight); trouble in sleeping; unusual tiredness or weakness

Less common or rare

> Anxiety and/or nervousness; changes in taste—for labetalol only; constipation; diarrhea; dry, sore eyes; frequent urination—for acebutolol and carteolol only; itching of skin; nausea or vomiting; nightmares and vivid dreams; numbness and/or tingling of fingers and/or toes; numbness and/or tingling of skin, especially on scalp—for labetalol only; stomach discomfort; stuffy nose

Although not all of the side effects listed above have been reported for all of these medicines, they have been reported for at least one of them. Since all of the beta-adrenergic blocking agents are very similar, any of the above side effects may occur with any of these medicines. However, they may be more or less common with some agents than with others.

After you have been taking a beta-blocker for a while, it may cause unpleasant or even harmful effects if you stop taking it too suddenly. After you stop taking this medicine or while you are gradually reducing the amount you are taking, check with your doctor right away if any of the following occur:

> Chest pain; fast or irregular heartbeat; general feeling of discomfort or illness or weakness; headache; shortness of breath (sudden); sweating; trembling

For patients taking *labetalol:*

- You may notice a tingling feeling on your scalp when you first begin to take labetalol. This is to be expected and usually goes away after you have been taking labetalol for a while.

Other side effects not listed above may also occur in some patients. If you notice any other effects, check with your doctor.

Additional Information

Once a medicine has been approved for marketing for a certain use, experience may show that it is also useful for other medical problems. Although these uses are not included in product labeling, some beta-blockers are used in certain patients with the following medical conditions:

- Glaucoma
- Neuroleptic-induced akathisia (restlessness or the need to keep moving caused by some medicines used to treat nervousness or mental and emotional disorders)

Other than the above information, there is no additional information relating to proper use, precautions, or side effects for these uses.

BETA-ADRENERGIC BLOCKING AGENTS AND THIAZIDE DIURETICS Systemic

Some commonly used brand names are:

In the U.S.—

Corzide[4]	Tenoretic[1]
Inderide[6]	Timolide[7]
Inderide LA[6]	Ziac[2]
Lopressor HCT[3]	

In Canada—

Corzide[4]	Timolide[7]
Inderide[6]	Viskazide[5]
Tenoretic[1]	

Note: For quick reference, the following beta-adrenergic blocking agents and thiazide diuretics are numbered to match the corresponding brand names.

This information applies to the following medicines:

1. Atenolol (a-TEN-oh-lole) and Chlorthalidone (klor-THAL-i-doan)‡
2. Bisoprolol (bis-OH-proe-lol) and Hydrochlorothiazide (hye-droe-klor-oh-THYE-a-zide)†
3. Metoprolol (me-TOE-proe-lole) and Hydrochlorothiazide†
4. Nadolol (NAY-doe-lole) and Bendroflumethiazide (ben-droe-floo-meth-EYE-a-zide)
5. Pindolol (PIN-doe-lole) and Hydrochlorothiazide*
6. Propranolol (proe-PRAN-oh-lole) and Hydrochlorothiazide‡
7. Timolol (TIM-oh-lole) and Hydrochlorothiazide

*Not commercially available in the U.S.
†Not commercially available in Canada.
‡Generic name product may also be available in the U.S.

Description

Beta-adrenergic blocking agent (more commonly, beta-blockers) and thiazide diuretic combinations belong to the group of medicines known as antihypertensives (high blood pressure medicine). Both ingredients of the combination control high blood pressure, but they work in different ways. Beta-blockers (atenolol, bisoprolol, metoprolol, nadolol, pindolol, propranolol, and timolol) reduce the workload on the heart as well as having other effects. Thiazide diuretics (bendroflumethiazide, chlorthalidone, and hydrochlorothiazide) reduce the amount of fluid pressure in the body by increasing the flow of urine.

High blood pressure adds to the workload of the heart and arteries. If it continues for a long time, the heart and arteries may not function properly. This can damage the blood vessels of the brain, heart, and kidneys, resulting in a stroke, heart failure, or kidney failure. High blood pressure may also increase the risk of heart attacks. These problems may be less likely to occur if blood pressure is controlled.

Beta-blocker and thiazide diuretic combinations are available only with your doctor's prescription, in the following dosage forms:

Oral

    Atenolol and chlorthalidone
       • Tablets (U.S. and Canada)
    Bisoprolol and hydrochlorothiazide
       • Tablets (U.S.)
    Metoprolol and hydrochlorothiazide
       • Tablets (U.S.)
    Nadolol and bendroflumethiazide
       • Tablets (U.S. and Canada)
    Pindolol and hydrochlorothiazide
       • Tablets (Canada)

Propranolol and hydrochlorothiazide
  • Extended-release capsules (U.S.)
  • Tablets (U.S. and Canada)
Timolol and hydrochlorothiazide
  • Tablets (U.S. and Canada)

Before Using This Medicine

In deciding to use a medicine, the risks of taking the medicine must be weighed against the good it will do. This is a decision you and your doctor will make. For the beta-blocker and thiazide diuretic combinations, the following should be considered:

Allergies—Tell your doctor if you have ever had any unusual or allergic reaction to beta-blockers, sulfonamides (sulfa drugs), bumetanide, furosemide, acetazolamide, dichlorphenamide, methazolamide, or any of the thiazide diuretics. Also tell your health care professional if you are allergic to any other substances, such as foods, preservatives, or dyes.

Pregnancy—Use of some beta-blockers during pregnancy has been associated with low blood sugar, breathing problems, a slower heart rate, and low blood pressure in the newborn infant. Other reports have not shown unwanted effects in the newborn infant. Animal studies have shown some beta-blockers to cause problems in pregnancy when used in doses many times the usual human dose.

Studies with thiazide diuretics have not been done in pregnant women. However, use of thiazide diuretics during pregnancy may cause side effects such as jaundice, blood problems, and low potassium in the newborn infant. Animal studies have not shown thiazide diuretic medicines to cause birth defects even when used in doses several times the usual human dose.

Before taking a beta-blocker and thiazide diuretic combination, make sure your doctor knows if you are pregnant or if you may become pregnant.

Breast-feeding—Atenolol, metoprolol, nadolol, propranolol, pindolol, timolol, and thiazide diuretics pass into breast milk. It is not known whether bisoprolol passes into breast milk. Thiazide diuretics may decrease the flow of breast milk.

Children—Although there is no specific information comparing use of this combination medicine in children with use in other age groups, this medicine is not expected to cause different side effects or problems in children than it does in adults. However, extra caution may be necessary in infants with jaundice, because these medicines can make the condition worse.

Older adults—Some side effects, especially dizziness or lightheadedness and signs and symptoms of too much potassium loss, may be more likely to occur in the elderly, who are usually more sensitive to the effects of this medicine. Also, beta-blockers may reduce tolerance to cold temperatures in elderly patients.

Other medicines—Although certain medicines should not be used together at all, in other cases two different medicines may be used together even if an interaction might occur. In these cases, your doctor may want to change the dose, or other precautions may be necessary. When you are taking beta-blocker and thiazide diuretic combinations, it is especially important that your health care professional know if you are taking any of the following:

- Allergy shots or
- Allergy skin tests—The beta-blocker contained in this medicine may increase the risk of a serious allergic reaction to these medicines
- Aminophylline (e.g., Somophyllin) or
- Caffeine (e.g., NoDoz) or
- Dyphylline (e.g., Lufylline) or
- Oxtriphylline (e.g., Choledyl) or
- Theophylline (e.g., Somophyllin-T)—The effects of these medicines and beta-blockers may be blocked; in addition, theophylline levels in the body may be increased, especially in patients who smoke

- Antidiabetics, oral (diabetes medicine you take by mouth) or
- Insulin—There is an increased risk of hyperglycemia (high blood sugar); the beta-blocker contained in this medicine may also cover up certain symptoms of hypoglycemia (low blood sugar), such as increases in pulse rate and blood pressure, and may make the hypoglycemia last longer
- Calcium channel blockers (amlodipine [e.g., Norvasc], bepridil [e.g., Bepadin], diltiazem [e.g., Cardizem], felodipine [e.g., Plendil], flunarizine [e.g., Sibelium], isradipine [e.g., DynaCirc], nicardipine [e.g., Cardene], nifedipine [e.g., Procardia], nimodipine [e.g., Nimotop], verapamil [e.g., Calan]) or
- Clonidine (e.g., Catapres) or
- Guanabenz (e.g., Wytensin)—Effects on blood pressure may be increased. In addition, unwanted effects may occur if clonidine, guanabenz, or a beta-blocker is stopped suddenly after use together. Unwanted effects on the heart may occur when beta-blocker and thiazide diuretic combinations are used with calcium channel blockers
- Cocaine—Cocaine may block the effects of beta-blockers; in addition, there is an increased risk of high blood pressure, fast heartbeat, and possibly heart problems if you use cocaine while taking a beta-blocker and thiazide diuretic combination
- Digitalis glycosides (heart medicine)—Use with beta-blocker and thiazide diuretic combinations may cause high blood levels of digoxin, which may increase the chance of side effects
- Lithium—The thiazide diuretic contained in this combination may cause high blood levels of lithium, which may increase the chance of side effects
- Monoamine oxidase (MAO) inhibitors (furazolidone [e.g., Furoxone], isocarboxazid [e.g., Marplan], phenelzine [e.g., Nardil], procarbazine [e.g., Matulane], selegiline [e.g., Eldepryl], tranylcypromine [e.g., Parnate])—Taking a beta-blocker and thiazide diuretic combination while you are taking or within 2 weeks of taking monoamine oxidase (MAO) inhibitors may cause severe high blood pressure

Other medical problems—The presence of other medical problems may affect the use of the beta-blockers and thiazide diuretics. Make sure you tell your doctor if you have any other medical problems, especially:

- Allergy, history of (asthma, eczema, hay fever, hives), or
- Bronchitis or
- Emphysema—This combination medicine may make allergic reactions to other substances more severe or make the reaction last longer; in addition, the beta-blocker contained in this combination can increase trouble in breathing
- Bradycardia (unusually slow heartbeat) or
- Heart or blood vessel disease—This combination medicine may make these heart problems worse; also, if treatment is stopped suddenly, unwanted effects may occur
- Diabetes mellitus (sugar diabetes)—The beta-blocker contained in this medicine may cause hyperglycemia (high blood sugar) and circulation problems; in addition, if your diabetes medicine causes your blood sugar to be too low, beta-blockers may cover up some of the symptoms (fast heartbeat), although they will not cover up other symptoms such as dizziness or sweating; the thiazide diuretic contained in this medicine may increase the amount of sugar in the blood
- Gout (history of) or
- Lupus erythematosus (history of) or
- Pancreatitis (inflammation of the pancreas)—The thiazide diuretic contained in this medicine may make these conditions worse
- Kidney disease or
- Liver disease—Effects of this medicine may be increased because of slower removal from the body
- Mental depression (or history of) or
- Myasthenia gravis or
- Pheochromocytoma or
- Psoriasis or
- Raynaud's syndrome—The beta-blocker contained in this medicine may make these conditions worse
- Overactive thyroid—Stopping this medicine suddenly may increase symptoms of overactive thyroid; the beta-blocker contained in this medicine may cover up fast heartbeat, which is a sign of overactive thyroid

Proper Use of This Medicine

In addition to the use of the medicine your doctor has prescribed, treatment for your high blood pressure may include weight control and care in the types of foods you eat, especially foods high in sodium. Your doctor will tell you which of these are most important for you. You should check with your doctor before changing your diet.

Many patients who have high blood pressure will not notice any signs of the problem. In fact, many may feel normal. It is very important that you *take your medicine exactly as directed* and that you keep your appointments with your doctor even if you feel well.

Remember that this medicine will not cure your high blood pressure, but it does help control it. Therefore, you must continue to take it as directed if you expect to lower your blood pressure and keep it down. *You may have to take high blood pressure medicine for the rest of your life.* If high blood pressure is not treated, it can cause serious problems such as heart failure, blood vessel disease, stroke, or kidney disease.

For patients taking the *extended-release tablet* form of this medicine:

- Swallow the tablet whole.
- Do not crush, break, or chew before swallowing.

To help you remember to take your medicine, try to get into the habit of taking it at the same time each day.

Ask your doctor about checking your pulse rate before and after taking beta-blocking agents. Then, while you are taking this medicine, check your pulse regularly. If it is much slower than your usual rate (or less than 50 beats per minute), check with your doctor. A pulse rate that is too slow may cause circulation problems.

The thiazide diuretic (e.g., bendroflumethiazide, chlorthalidone, or hydrochlorothiazide) contained in this combination medicine may cause you to have an unusual feeling of tiredness when you begin to take it. You may also notice an increase in the amount of urine or in your frequency of urination. After you take the medicine for a while, these effects should lessen. To keep the increase in urine from affecting your sleep:

- If you are to take a single dose a day, take it in the morning after breakfast.

- If you are to take more than one dose a day, take the last dose no later than 6 p.m., unless otherwise directed by your doctor.

However, it is best to plan your dose or doses according to a schedule that will least affect your personal activities and sleep. Ask your health care professional to help you plan the best time to take this medicine.

Do not miss any doses. This is especially important when you are taking only one dose per day. Some conditions may become worse when this medicine is not taken regularly.

Dosing—The dose of beta-blocker and thiazide diuretic combinations will be different for different patients. *Follow your doctor's orders or the directions on the label.* The following information includes only the average doses of beta-blocker and thiazide diuretic combinations. *If your dose is different, do not change it* unless your doctor tells you to do so.

The number of capsules or tablets that you take depends on the strength of the medicine.

For atenolol and chlorthalidone combination

- For *oral* dosage form (tablets):

   —For high blood pressure:

    • Adults—1 or 2 tablets once a day.

    • Children—Dose must be determined by your doctor.

For bisoprolol and hydrochlorothiazide combination
- For *oral* dosage form (tablets):
  - —For high blood pressure:
    - Adults—1 or 2 tablets once a day.
    - Children—Dose must be determined by your doctor.

For metoprolol and hydrochlorothiazide combination
- For *oral* dosage form (tablets):
  - —For high blood pressure:
    - Adults—1 or 2 tablets a day.
    - Children—Dose must be determined by your doctor.

For nadolol and bendroflumethiazide combination
- For *oral* dosage form (tablets):
  - —For high blood pressure:
    - Adults—1 tablet once a day.
    - Children—Dose must be determined by your doctor.

For pindolol and hydrochlorothiazide combination
- For *oral* dosage form (tablets):
  - —For high blood pressure:
    - Adults—1 or 2 tablets once a day.
    - Children—Dose must be determined by your doctor.

For propranolol and hydrochlorothiazide combination
- For *regular (short-acting) oral* dosage form (tablets):
  - —For high blood pressure:
    - Adults—1 or 2 tablets two times a day.
    - Children—Dose must be determined by your doctor.
- For *long-acting oral* dosage form (capsules):
  - —For high blood pressure:
    - Adults—1 capsule a day.

- Children—Dose must be determined by your doctor.

For timolol and hydrochlorothiazide combination

- For *oral* dosage form (tablets):
  —For high blood pressure:
    - Adults—1 tablet two times a day or 2 tablets once a day.
    - Children—Dose must be determined by your doctor.

Missed dose—If you miss a dose of this medicine, take it as soon as possible. However, if it is within 4 hours of your next dose (8 hours if you are using atenolol and chlorthalidone, bisoprolol and hydrochlorothiazide, nadolol and bendroflumethiazide, or extended-release propranolol and hydrochlorothiazide), skip the missed dose and go back to your regular dosing schedule. Do not double doses.

Storage—To store this medicine:

- Keep out of the reach of children.
- Store away from heat and direct light.
- Do not store in the bathroom, near the kitchen sink, or in other damp places. Heat or moisture may cause the medicine to break down.
- Do not keep outdated medicine or medicine no longer needed. Be sure that any discarded medicine is out of the reach of children.

Precautions While Using This Medicine

It is important that your doctor check your progress at regular visits. This is to make sure the medicine is properly controlling your blood pressure and to allow the dosage to be changed if needed.

Do not stop taking this medicine without first checking with your doctor. Your doctor may want you to reduce gradually the amount you are taking before stopping completely. Some conditions may become worse when the medicine is stopped suddenly, and the risk of heart attack is increased in some patients.

Make sure that you have enough medicine on hand to last through weekends, holidays, or vacations. You may want to carry an extra written prescription in your billfold or purse in case of an emergency. You can then have it filled if you run out of medicine while you are away from home.

Your doctor may want you to carry medical identification stating that you are taking this medicine.

Do not take other medicines unless they have been discussed with your doctor. This especially includes over-the-counter (nonprescription) medicines for appetite control, asthma, colds, cough, hay fever, or sinus problems since they may increase your blood pressure.

Before having any kind of surgery (including dental surgery) or emergency treatment, tell the medical doctor or dentist in charge that you are taking this medicine.

For *diabetic patients*:

- *This medicine may increase your blood sugar levels.* Also, *this medicine may cover up signs of hypoglycemia (low blood sugar),* such as change in pulse rate. While you are taking this medicine, be especially careful in testing for sugar in your urine. If you have any questions about this, check with your doctor.

The thiazide diuretic contained in this medicine may cause a loss of potassium from your body.

- To help prevent this, your doctor may want you to:
  —eat or drink foods that have a high potassium content (for example, orange or other citrus fruit juices), or
  —take a potassium supplement, or
  —take another medicine to help prevent the loss of the potassium in the first place.

- It is very important to follow these directions. Also, it is important not to change your diet on your own. This is more important if you are already on a special diet (as for diabetes), or if you are taking a potassium supplement or a medicine to reduce potassium loss. Extra potassium may not be necessary and, in some cases, too much potassium could be harmful.

Check with your doctor if you become sick and have severe or continuing vomiting or diarrhea. These problems may cause you to lose additional water and potassium.

This medicine may cause some people to become dizzy, drowsy, lightheaded, or less alert than they are normally. *Make sure you know how you react to this medicine before you drive, use machines, or do anything else that could be dangerous if you are dizzy or are not alert.* If the problem continues or gets worse, check with your doctor.

The beta-blocker (atenolol, bisoprolol, metoprolol, nadolol, pindolol, propranolol, or timolol) contained in this medicine may make you more sensitive to cold temperatures, especially if you have blood circulation problems. Beta-blockers tend to decrease blood circulation in the skin, fingers, and toes. Dress warmly during cold weather and be careful during prolonged exposure to cold, such as in winter sports.

This medicine may cause your skin to be more sensitive to sunlight than it is normally. Exposure to sunlight, even for brief periods of time, may cause a skin rash, itching, redness or other discoloration of the skin, or a severe sunburn. When you begin taking this medicine:

- Stay out of direct sunlight, especially between the hours of 10:00 a.m. and 3:00 p.m., if possible.
- Wear protective clothing, including a hat. Also, wear sunglasses.
- Apply a sun block product that has a skin protection factor (SPF) of at least 15. Some patients may require a product with a higher SPF number, especially if

they have a fair complexion. If you have any questions about this, check with your health care professional.

• Apply a sun block lipstick that has an SPF of at least 15 to protect your lips.

• Do not use a sunlamp or tanning bed or booth.

If you have a severe reaction from the sun, check with your doctor.

Before you have any medical tests, tell the doctor in charge that you are taking this medicine. The results of some tests may be affected by this medicine.

For patients with allergies to foods, medicines, or insect stings:

• There is a chance that this medicine will make allergic reactions worse and harder to treat. If you have a severe allergic reaction while you are being treated with this medicine, check with a doctor right away so that it can be treated.

Side Effects of This Medicine

Along with its needed effects, a medicine may cause some unwanted effects. Although not all of these side effects may occur, if they do occur they may need medical attention.

Check with your doctor as soon as possible if any of the following side effects occur:

Less common

Breathing difficulty and/or wheezing; cold hands and feet; mental depression; slow heartbeat (especially less than 50 beats per minute); swelling of ankles, feet, and/or lower legs

Rare

Black, tarry stools; blood in urine or stools; chest pain; dark urine; fever, chills, cough, or sore throat; hallucinations (seeing, hearing, or feeling things that are not there); joint pain; lower back or side pain; pinpoint red spots on skin; red, scaling, or crusted skin; skin rash or hives; stomach pain (severe) with nausea and vomiting; unusual bleeding or bruising; or yellow eyes or skin

Signs and symptoms of too much potassium or sodium loss

Confusion; convulsions (seizures); dryness of mouth; increased thirst; irregular heartbeats; irritability, mood or mental changes; muscle cramps or pain; nausea or vomiting, unusual tiredness or weakness; weak pulse

Signs and symptoms of overdose (in the order in which they may occur)

Slow heartbeat; dizziness (severe) or fainting; difficulty in breathing; bluish-colored fingernails or palms of hands; convulsions (seizures)

Other side effects may occur that usually do not need medical attention. These side effects may go away during treatment as your body adjusts to the medicine. However, check with your doctor if any of the following side effects continue or are bothersome:

More common

Decreased sexual ability; dizziness or lightheadedness; drowsiness (mild); trouble in sleeping

Less common

Anxiety or nervousness; constipation; diarrhea; increased sensitivity of skin to sunlight (skin rash, itching, redness or other discoloration of skin, or severe sunburn); loss of appetite; numbness or tingling of fingers and toes; stomach discomfort or upset; stuffy nose

Rare

Changes in taste; dry, sore eyes; itching of skin; nightmares and vivid dreams

Although not all of the above side effects have been reported for all of these medicines, they have been reported for at least one of the beta-blockers or thiazide diuretics. Since all of the beta-blockers are very similar and the thiazide diuretics are also very similar, any of the above side effects may occur with any of these medicines. However, they may be more common with some combinations than with others.

After you have been taking this medicine for a while, it may cause unpleasant or even harmful effects if you stop taking it too suddenly. After you stop taking this medicine or while you are gradually reducing the amount you are taking, check with your doctor right away if any of the following occur:

> Chest pain; fast or irregular heartbeat; general feeling of discomfort, illness, or weakness; headache; shortness of breath (sudden); sweating; trembling

Other side effects not listed above may also occur in some patients. If you notice any other effects, check with your doctor.

CALCIUM CHANNEL BLOCKING AGENTS   Systemic

Some commonly used brand names are:

In the U.S.—

Adalat[7]	DynaCirc[5]
Adalat CC[7]	Isoptin[9]
Bepadin[1]	Isoptin SR[9]
Calan[9]	Nimotop[8]
Calan SR[9]	Plendil[3]
Cardene[6]	Procardia[7]
Cardizem[2]	Procardia XL[7]
Cardizem CD[2]	Vascor[1]
Cardizem SR[2]	Verelan[9]
Dilacor-XR[2]	

In Canada—

Adalat[7]	Apo-Verap[9]
Adalat FT[7]	Cardene[6]
Adalat P.A.[7]	Cardizem[2]
Apo-Diltiaz[2]	Cardizem SR[2]
Apo-Nifed[7]	Isoptin[9]

In Canada (cont'd)—

Isoptin SR[9]	Nu-Nifed[7]
Nimotop[8]	Nu-Verap[9]
Novo-Diltazem[2]	Plendil[3]
Novo-Nifedin[7]	Renedil[3]
Novo-Veramil[9]	Sibelium[4]
Nu-Diltiaz[2]	Syn-Diltiazem[2]

Note: For quick reference, the following calcium channel blocking agents are numbered to match the corresponding brand names.

This information applies to the following medicines:

1. Bepridil (BE-pri-dil)†
2. Diltiazem (dil-TYE-a-zem)‡§
3. Felodipine (fe-LOE-di-peen)
4. Flunarizine (floo-NAR-i-zeen)*
5. Isradipine (is-RA-di-peen)†
6. Nicardipine (nye-KAR-de-peen)
7. Nifedipine (nye-FED-i-peen)‡
8. Nimodipine (nye-MOE-di-peen)
9. Verapamil (ver-AP-a-mil)‡§

---

*Not commercially available in the U.S.
†Not commercially available in Canada.
‡Generic name product may also be available in the U.S.
§Generic name product may also be available in Canada.

Description

Bepridil, diltiazem, felodipine, flunarizine, isradipine, nicardipine, nifedipine, nimodipine, and verapamil belong to the group of medicines called calcium channel blockers.

Calcium channel blocking agents affect the movement of calcium into the cells of the heart and blood vessels. As a result, they relax blood vessels and increase the supply of blood and oxygen to the heart while reducing its workload.

Some of the calcium channel blocking agents are used to relieve and control angina pectoris (chest pain).

Some are also used to treat high blood pressure (hypertension). High blood pressure adds to the workload of the heart and arteries. If it continues for a long time, the heart and arteries may not function properly. This can damage the blood vessels of the brain, heart, and kidneys, resulting in a stroke, heart failure, or kidney failure. High blood pressure may also increase the risk of heart attacks. These problems may be less likely to occur if blood pressure is controlled.

Flunarizine is used to prevent migraine headaches.

Nimodipine is used to prevent and treat problems caused by a burst blood vessel in the head (also known as a ruptured aneurysm or subarachnoid hemorrhage).

Other calcium channel blocking agents may also be used for these and other conditions as determined by your doctor.

These medicines are available only with your doctor's prescription, in the following dosage forms:

Oral

Bepridil
- Tablets (U.S.)

Diltiazem
- Extended-release capsules (U.S. and Canada)
- Tablets (U.S. and Canada)

Felodipine
- Extended-release tablets (U.S. and Canada)

Flunarizine
- Capsules (Canada)

Isradipine
- Capsules (U.S.)

Nicardipine
- Capsules (U.S. and Canada)

Nifedipine
- Capsules (U.S. and Canada)
- Tablets (Canada)
- Extended-release tablets (U.S. and Canada)

Nimodipine
- Capsules (U.S. and Canada)

Verapamil
- Extended-release capsules (U.S.)
- Tablets (U.S. and Canada)
- Extended-release tablets (U.S. and Canada)

Parenteral

Diltiazem
- Injection (U.S.)

Verapamil
- Injection (U.S. and Canada)

Before Using This Medicine

In deciding to use a medicine, the risks of taking the medicine must be weighed against the good it will do. This is a decision you and your doctor will make. For the calcium channel blocking agents, the following should be considered:

Allergies—Tell your doctor if you have ever had any unusual or allergic reaction to bepridil, diltiazem, felodipine, flunarizine, isradipine, nicardipine, nifedipine, nimodipine, or verapamil. Also tell your health care professional if you are allergic to any other substances, such as foods, preservatives, or dyes.

Pregnancy—Calcium channel blockers have not been studied in pregnant women. However, studies in animals have shown that large doses of calcium channel blockers cause birth defects, prolonged pregnancy, poor bone development, and stillbirth.

Breast-feeding—Although bepridil, diltiazem, nifedipine, verapamil, and possibly other calcium channel blockers, pass into breast milk, they have not been reported to cause problems in nursing babies.

Children—Although there is no specific information comparing use of this medicine in children with use in other age groups, it is not expected to cause different side effects or problems in children than it does in adults.

Older adults—Elderly people may be especially sensitive to the effects of calcium channel blockers. This may increase the chance of side effects during treatment.

Other medicines—Although certain medicines should not be used together at all, in other cases two different medicines may be used together even if an interaction might occur. In these cases, your doctor may want to change the dose, or other precautions may be necessary. When taking calcium channel blockers it is especially important that your health care professional know if you are taking any of the following:

- Acetazolamide (e.g., Diamox) or
- Amphotericin B by injection (e.g., Fungizone) or
- Corticosteroids (cortisone-like medicine) or
- Dichlorphenamide (e.g., Daranide) or
- Diuretics (water pills) or
- Methazolamide (e.g., Naptazane)—These medicines can cause hypokalemia (low levels of potassium in the body), which can increase the unwanted effects of bepridil
- Beta-blockers (acebutolol [e.g., Sectral], atenolol [e.g., Tenormin], betaxolol [e.g., Kerlone], carteolol [e.g., Cartrol], labetalol [e.g., Normodyne], metoprolol [e.g., Lopressor], nadolol [e.g., Corgard], oxprenolol [e.g., Trasicor], penbutolol [e.g., Levatol], pindolol [e.g., Visken], propranolol [e.g., Inderal], sotalol [e.g., Sotacor], timolol [e.g., Blocadren])—Effects of both may be increased. In addition, unwanted effects may occur if a calcium channel blocker or a beta-blocker is stopped suddenly after use together
- Carbamazepine (e.g., Tegretol) or
- Cyclosporine (e.g., Sandimmune) or
- Procainamide (e.g., Pronestyl) or
- Quinidine (e.g., Quinidex)—Effects of these medicines may be increased if they are used with some calcium channel blockers
- Digitalis glycosides (heart medicine)—Effects of these medicines may be increased if they are used with some calcium channel blockers
- Disopyramide (e.g., Norpace)—Effects of some calcium channel blockers on the heart may be increased

Also, tell your health care professional if you are using any of the following medicines in the eye:

- Betaxolol (e.g., Betoptic) or
- Levobunolol (e.g., Betagan) or

- Metipranolol (e.g., OptiPranolol) or
- Timolol (e.g., Timoptic)—Effects on the heart and blood pressure may be increased

Other medical problems—The presence of other medical problems may affect the use of the calcium channel blockers. Make sure you tell your doctor if you have any other medical problems, especially:

- Heart rhythm problems (history of)—Bepridil can cause serious heart rhythm problems
- Kidney disease or
- Liver disease—Effects of the calcium channel blocker may be increased
- Mental depression (history of)—Flunarizine may cause mental depression
- Parkinson's disease or similar problems—Flunarizine can cause parkinsonian-like effects
- Other heart or blood vessel disorders—Calcium channel blockers may make some heart conditions worse

---

Proper Use of This Medicine

Take this medicine exactly as directed even if you feel well and do not notice any signs of chest pain. Do not take more of this medicine and do not take it more often than your doctor ordered. Do not miss any doses.

For patients taking *bepridil:*

- If this medicine causes upset stomach, it can be taken with meals or at bedtime.

For patients taking *diltiazem extended-release capsules:*

- Swallow the capsule whole, without crushing or chewing it.
- *Do not change to another brand without checking with your physician.* Different brands have different doses. If you refill your medicine and it looks different, check with your pharmacist.

For patients taking *nifedipine or verapamil extended-release capsules:*

- Swallow the capsule whole, without crushing or chewing it.

For patients taking *regular nifedipine or extended-release felodipine or nifedipine tablets:*

- Swallow the tablet whole, without breaking, crushing, or chewing it.
- If you are taking *Procardia XL*, you may sometimes notice what looks like a tablet in your stool. That is just the empty shell that is left after the medicine has been absorbed into your body.

For patients taking *verapamil extended-release tablets:*

- Swallow the tablet whole, without crushing or chewing it. However, if your doctor tells you to, you may break the tablet in half.
- Take the medicine with food or milk.

For patients taking this medicine *for high blood pressure:*

- In addition to the use of the medicine your doctor has prescribed, appropriate treatment for your high blood pressure may include weight control and care in the types of food you eat, especially foods high in sodium (salt). Your doctor will tell you which factors are most important for you. You should check with your doctor before changing your diet.
- Many patients who have high blood pressure will not notice any signs of the problem. In fact, many may feel normal. It is very important that you *take your medicine exactly as directed* and that you keep your appointments with your doctor even if you feel well.
- Remember that this medicine will not cure your high blood pressure but it does help control it. Therefore, you must continue to take it as directed if you expect to lower your blood pressure and keep it down. *You may have to take high blood pressure medicine for*

the rest of your life. If high blood pressure is not treated, it can cause serious problems such as heart failure, blood vessel disease, stroke, or kidney disease.

Dosing—The dose of these medicines will be different for different patients. *Follow your doctor's orders or the directions on the label.* The following information includes only the average doses of these medicines. *If your dose is different, do not change it* unless your doctor tells you to do so.

The number of capsules or tablets that you take depends on the strength of the medicine. Also, *the number of doses you take each day, the time allowed between doses, and the length of time you take the medicine depend on the medical problem for which you are taking calcium channel blocking agents.*

For bepridil

- For *oral* dosage form (tablets):

    —For angina (chest pain):

    • Adults—200 to 300 milligrams (mg) once a day.

    • Children—Use and dose must be determined by your doctor.

For diltiazem

- For *long-acting oral* dosage form (extended-release capsules):

    —For high blood pressure:

    • Adults and teenagers—

    —For *Cardizem CD* or *Dilacor-XR:* 180 to 240 milligrams (mg) once a day.

    —For *Cardizem SR:* 60 to 120 mg two times a day.

    • Children—Dose must be determined by your doctor.

- For *regular (short-acting) oral* dosage form (tablets):
  —For angina (chest pain):
  - Adults and teenagers—30 mg three or four times a day. Your doctor may gradually increase your dose as needed.
  - Children—Dose must be determined by your doctor.
- For *injection* dosage form:
  —For arrhythmias (irregular heartbeat):
  - Adults and teenagers—Dose is based on body weight and must be determined by your doctor.
  - Children—Use and dose must be determined by your doctor.

For felodipine
- For *long-acting oral* dosage form (extended-release tablets):
  —For high blood pressure:
  - Adults—5 to 10 milligrams (mg) once a day.
  - Children—Use and dose must be determined by your doctor.
  —For angina (chest pain):
  - Adults—10 mg once a day.
  - Children—Use and dose must be determined by your doctor.

For flunarizine
- For *oral* dosage form (capsules):
  —To prevent headaches:
  - Adults—10 milligrams (mg) once a day in the evening.
  - Children—Dose must be determined by your doctor.

For isradipine
- For *oral* dosage form (capsules):
  —For high blood pressure:

• Adults—2.5 milligrams (mg) two times a day. Your doctor may increase your dose as needed.

• Children—Use and dose must be determined by your doctor.

For nicardipine

• For *oral* dosage form (capsules):

—For high blood pressure or angina (chest pain):

• Adults and teenagers—20 milligrams (mg) three times a day.

• Children—Dose must be determined by your doctor.

For nifedipine

• For *regular (short-acting) oral* dosage form (capsules or tablets):

—For high blood pressure or angina (chest pain):

• Adults and teenagers—10 milligrams (mg) three times a day. Your doctor may increase your dose as needed.

• Children—Dose must be determined by your doctor.

• For *long-acting oral* dosage form (extended-release tablets):

—For high blood pressure or angina (chest pain):

• Adults and teenagers—

—For *Adalat CC* or *Procardia XL:* 30 or 60 mg once a day. Your doctor may increase your dose as needed.

—For *Adalat P.A.:* 20 mg two times a day. Your doctor may increase your dose as needed.

• Children—Dose must be determined by your doctor.

For nimodipine

• For *oral* dosage form (capsules):

—To treat a burst blood vessel in the head:

• Adults—60 milligrams (mg) every four hours.

• Children—Dose must be determined by your doctor.

For verapamil

• For *regular (short-acting) oral* dosage form (tablets):

—For angina (chest pain), arrhythmias (irregular heartbeat), or high blood pressure:

• Adults and teenagers—40 to 120 milligrams (mg) three times a day. Your doctor may increase your dose as needed.

• Children—Dose is based on body weight and must be determined by your doctor. The usual dose is 4 to 8 mg per kilogram (kg) (1.82 to 3.64 mg per pound) of body weight a day. This is divided into smaller doses.

• For *long-acting oral* dosage form (extended-release capsules):

—For high blood pressure:

• Adults and teenagers—240 to 480 mg once a day.

• Children—Dose must be determined by your doctor.

• For *long-acting oral* dosage form (extended-release tablets):

—For high blood pressure:

• Adults and teenagers—120 mg once a day to 240 mg every twelve hours.

• Children—Dose must be determined by your doctor.

• For *injection* dosage form:

—For arrhythmias (irregular heartbeat):

• Adults—5 to 10 mg slowly injected into a vein. The dose may be repeated after thirty minutes.

• Children—Dose is based on body weight and must be determined by your doctor.

—Infants up to 1 year of age: 100 to 200 micrograms (mcg) per kg (45.5 to 90.9 mcg per pound) of body weight injected slowly into a vein. The dose may be repeated after thirty minutes.

—Children 1 to 15 years of age: 100 to 300 mcg per kg (45.5 to 136.4 mcg per pound) of body weight injected slowly into a vein. The dose may be repeated after thirty minutes.

Missed dose—If you miss a dose of this medicine, take it as soon as possible. However, if it is almost time for your next dose, skip the missed dose and go back to your regular dosing schedule. Do not double doses.

Storage—To store this medicine:

- Keep out of the reach of children.
- Store away from heat and direct light.
- Do not store in the bathroom, near the kitchen sink, or in other damp places. Heat or moisture may cause the medicine to break down.
- Do not keep outdated medicine or medicine no longer needed. Be sure that any discarded medicine is out of the reach of children.

Precautions While Using This Medicine

It is important that your doctor check your progress at regular visits. This will allow your doctor to make sure the medicine is working properly and to change the dosage if needed.

If you have been using this medicine regularly for several weeks, do not suddenly stop using it. Stopping suddenly may bring on your previous problem. Check with your doctor for the best way to reduce gradually the amount you are taking before stopping completely.

Chest pain resulting from exercise or physical exertion is usually reduced or prevented by this medicine. This may tempt you to be overly active. *Make sure you discuss with your doctor a safe amount of exercise for your medical problem.*

After taking a dose of this medicine you may get a headache that lasts for a short time. This effect is more common if you are taking felodipine, isradipine, or nifedipine. This should become less noticeable after you have taken this medicine for a while. If this effect continues or if the headaches are severe, check with your doctor.

In some patients, tenderness, swelling, or bleeding of the gums may appear soon after treatment with this medicine is started. Brushing and flossing your teeth carefully and regularly and massaging your gums may help prevent this. *See your dentist regularly to have your teeth cleaned. Check with your medical doctor or dentist if you have any questions about how to take care of your teeth and gums, or if you notice any tenderness, swelling, or bleeding of your gums.*

For patients taking *bepridil, diltiazem,* or *verapamil:*

- *Ask your doctor how to count your pulse rate. Then, while you are taking this medicine, check your pulse regularly.* If it is much slower than your usual rate, or less than 50 beats per minute, check with your doctor. A pulse rate that is too slow may cause circulation problems.

For patients taking *flunarizine:*

- This medicine may cause some people to become drowsy or less alert than they are normally. This is more likely to happen when you begin to take it or when you increase the amount of medicine you are taking. *Make sure you know how you react to this medicine before you drive, use machines, or do anything else that could be dangerous if you are not alert.*

For patients taking this medicine *for high blood pressure:*

- *Do not take other medicines unless they have been discussed with your doctor.* This especially includes over-the-counter (nonprescription) medicines for appetite control, asthma, colds, cough, hay fever, or sinus problems, since they may tend to increase your blood pressure.

Side Effects of This Medicine

Along with its needed effects, a medicine may cause some unwanted effects. Although not all of these side effects may occur, if they do occur they may need medical attention.

Not all of the side effects listed below have been reported for each of these medicines, but they have been reported for at least one of them. Since many of the effects of calcium channel blockers are similar, some of these side effects may occur with any of these medicines. However, they may be more common with some of these medicines than with others.

Check with your doctor as soon as possible if any of the following side effects occur:

Less common

> Breathing difficulty, coughing, or wheezing; irregular or fast, pounding heartbeat; skin rash; slow heartbeat (less than 50 beats per minute—bepridil, diltiazem, and verapamil only); swelling of ankles, feet, or lower legs (more common with felodipine and nifedipine)

For flunarizine only—less common

> Loss of balance control; mask-like face; mental depression; shuffling walk; stiffness of arms or legs; trembling and shaking of hands and fingers; trouble in speaking or swallowing

Rare

> Bleeding, tender, or swollen gums; chest pain (may appear about 30 minutes after medicine is taken); fainting; painful, swollen joints (for nifedipine only); trouble in seeing (for nifedipine only)

For flunarizine and verapamil only—rare
    Unusual secretion of milk

Other side effects may occur that usually do not need medical attention. These side effects may go away during treatment as your body adjusts to the medicine. However, check with your doctor if any of the following side effects continue or are bothersome:

More common
    Drowsiness (for flunarizine only); increased appetite and/ or weight gain (for flunarizine only)

Less common
    Constipation; diarrhea; dizziness or lightheadedness (more common with bepridil and nifedipine); dryness of mouth (for flunarizine only); flushing and feeling of warmth (more common with nicardipine and nifedipine); headache (more common with felodipine, isradipine, and nifedipine); nausea (more common with bepridil and nifedipine); unusual tiredness or weakness

Other side effects not listed above may also occur in some patients. If you notice any other effects, check with your doctor.

Additional Information

Once a medicine has been approved for marketing for a certain use, experience may show that it is also useful for other medical problems. Although these uses are not included in product labeling, calcium channel blockers are used in certain patients with the following medical conditions:

- Hypertrophic cardiomyopathy (a heart condition) (verapamil)
- Raynaud's phenomenon (circulation problems) (nicardipine and nifedipine)

Other than the above information, there is no additional information relating to proper use, precautions, or side effects for these uses.

CHOLESTYRAMINE   Oral

Some commonly used brand names in the U.S. and Canada are Questran and Questran Light.

Description

Cholestyramine (koe-less-TEAR-a-meen) is used to lower high cholesterol levels in the blood. This may help prevent medical problems caused by cholesterol clogging the blood vessels. Cholestyramine is also used to remove substances called bile acids from your body. With some liver problems, there is too much bile acid in your body and this can cause severe itching.

Cholestyramine works by attaching to certain substances in the intestine. Since cholestyramine is not absorbed into the body, these substances also pass out of the body without being absorbed.

Cholestyramine may also be used for other conditions as determined by your doctor.

Cholestyramine is available only with your doctor's prescription, in the following dosage form:

Oral
  • Powder (U.S. and Canada)

Before Using This Medicine

In deciding to use a medicine, the risks of taking the medicine must be weighed against the good it will do. This is a decision you and your doctor will make. For cholestyramine, the following should be considered:

Allergies—Tell your doctor if you have ever had any unusual or allergic reaction to cholestyramine. Also tell your health care professional if you are allergic to any other substances, such as foods, preservatives, or dyes.

Pregnancy—Cholestyramine is not absorbed into the body and is not likely to cause problems. However, it may reduce absorption of vitamins into the body. Ask your doctor whether you need to take extra vitamins.

Breast-feeding—Cholestyramine is not absorbed into the body and is not likely to cause problems. However, the reduced absorption of vitamins by the mother may affect the nursing infant.

Children—This medicine has been tested in a limited number of children. In effective doses, the medicine has not been shown to cause different side effects or problems than it does in adults.

Older adults—Side effects may be more likely to occur in patients over 60 years of age, who are usually more sensitive to the effects of cholestyramine.

Other medicines—Although certain medicines should not be used together at all, in other cases two different medicines may be used together even if an interaction might occur. In these cases, your doctor may want to change the dose, or other precautions may be necessary. When you are taking cholestyramine it is especially important that your health care professional know if you are taking any of the following:

- Anticoagulants (blood thinners)—The effects of the anticoagulant may be changed and this may increase the chance of bleeding.
- Digitalis glycosides (heart medicine) or
- Diuretics (water pills) or
- Penicillin G, taken by mouth or
- Phenylbutazone or
- Propranolol (e.g., Inderal) or
- Tetracyclines, taken by mouth (medicine for infection) or
- Thyroid hormones or
- Vancomycin, taken by mouth—Cholestyramine may prevent these medicines from working properly

Other medical problems—The presence of other medical problems may affect the use of cholestyramine. Make sure

you tell your doctor if you have any other medical problems, especially:

- Bleeding problems or
- Constipation or
- Gallstones or
- Heart or blood vessel disease or
- Hemorrhoids or
- Stomach ulcer or other stomach problems or
- Underactive thyroid—Cholestyramine may make these conditions worse
- Kidney disease—There is an increased risk of developing electrolyte problems (problems in the blood)
- Phenylketonuria—Phenylalanine in aspartame is included in the sugar-free brand of cholestyramine and should be avoided. Aspartame can cause problems in people with phenylketonuria. Therefore, it is best if you avoid using the sugar-free product.

Proper Use of This Medicine

Take this medicine exactly as directed by your doctor. Try not to miss any doses and do not take more medicine than your doctor ordered.

This medicine should never be taken in its dry form, since it could cause you to choke. Instead, always mix as follows:

- Place the medicine in 2 ounces of any beverage and mix thoroughly. Then add an additional 2 to 4 ounces of beverage and again mix thoroughly (it will not dissolve) before drinking. After drinking all the liquid containing the medicine, rinse the glass with a little more liquid and drink that also, to make sure you get all the medicine.
- You may also mix this medicine with milk in hot or regular breakfast cereals, or in thin soups such as tomato or chicken noodle soup. Or you may add it to some pulpy fruits such as crushed pineapple, pears, peaches, or fruit cocktail.

For patients taking this medicine *for high cholesterol:*

- Importance of diet—Before prescribing medicine for your condition, your doctor will probably try to control your condition by prescribing a personal diet for you. Such a diet may be low in fats, sugars, and/or cholesterol. Many people are able to control their condition by carefully following their doctor's orders for proper diet and exercise. Medicine is prescribed only when additional help is needed. *Follow carefully the special diet your doctor gave you,* since the medicine is effective only when a schedule of diet and exercise is properly followed.

- Also, this medicine is less effective if you are greatly overweight. It may be very important for you to go on a reducing diet. However, check with your doctor before going on any diet.

- Remember that this medicine will not cure your cholesterol problem but it will help control it. Therefore, you must continue to take it as directed if you expect to lower your cholesterol level.

Dosing—The dose of cholestyramine will be different for different patients. *Follow your doctor's orders or the directions on the label.* The following information includes only the average doses of cholestyramine. *If your dose is different, do not change it* unless your doctor tells you to do so.

- For *oral* dosage form (powder for oral suspension):

  —For high cholesterol or pruritus (itching) related to biliary obstruction:

    - Adults—At first, 4 grams one or two times a day before meals. Then, your doctor may increase your dose to 8 to 24 grams a day. This is divided into two to six doses.

    - Children—At first, 4 grams a day. This is divided into two doses and taken before meals. Then, your doctor may increase your dose to 8 to 24 grams a day. This is divided into two or more doses.

Missed dose—If you miss a dose of this medicine, take it as soon as possible. Then go back to your regular dosing schedule. However, if it is almost time for your next dose, skip the missed dose and go back to your regular dosing schedule. Do not double doses.

Storage—To store this medicine:

- Keep out of the reach of children.
- Store away from heat and direct light.
- Do not store in the bathroom, near the kitchen sink, or in other damp places. Heat or moisture may cause the medicine to break down.
- Do not keep outdated medicine or medicine no longer needed. Be sure that any discarded medicine is out of the reach of children.

Precautions While Using This Medicine

It is very important that your doctor check your progress at regular visits. This will allow your doctor to see if the medicine is working properly and to decide if you should continue to take it.

Do not take any other medicine unless prescribed by your doctor since cholestyramine may change the effect of other medicines.

Do not stop taking this medicine without first checking with your doctor. When you stop taking this medicine, your blood cholesterol levels may increase again. Your doctor may want you to follow a special diet to help prevent this from happening.

Side Effects of This Medicine

In some animal studies, cholestyramine was found to cause tumors. It is not known whether cholestyramine causes tumors in humans.

Along with its needed effects, a medicine may cause some unwanted effects. Although not all of these side effects may occur, if they do occur they may need medical attention.

Check with your doctor immediately if any of the following side effects occur:

    Rare

        Black, tarry stools; stomach pain (severe) with nausea and vomiting

Check with your doctor as soon as possible if any of the following side effects occur:

    More common

        Constipation

    Rare

        Loss of weight (sudden)

Other side effects may occur that usually do not need medical attention. These side effects may go away during treatment as your body adjusts to the medicine. However, check with your doctor if any of the following side effects continue or are bothersome:

    More common

        Heartburn or indigestion; nausea or vomiting; stomach pain

    Less common

        Belching; bloating; diarrhea; dizziness; headache

Other side effects not listed above may also occur in some patients. If you notice any other effects, check with your doctor.

Additional Information

Once a medicine has been approved for marketing for a certain use, experience may show that it is also useful for other medical problems. Although these uses are not included in product labeling, cholestyramine is used in certain patients with the following medical conditions:

- Digitalis glycoside overdose
- Excess oxalate in the urine

Other than the above information, there is no additional information relating to proper use, precautions, or side effects for these uses.

CLOFIBRATE   Systemic

Some commonly used brand names are:

In the U.S.—
   Abitrate
   Atromid-S
   Generic name product may also be available.

In Canada—
   Atromid-S   Novofibrate
   Claripex

Description

Clofibrate (kloe-FYE-brate) is used to lower cholesterol and triglyceride (fat-like substances) levels in the blood. This may help prevent medical problems caused by such substances clogging the blood vessels.

Clofibrate may also be used for other conditions as determined by your doctor.

Clofibrate is available only with your doctor's prescription, in the following dosage form:

Oral

- Capsules (U.S. and Canada)

Before Using This Medicine

In addition to its helpful effects in treating your medical problem, this medicine may have some harmful effects.

You may have read or heard about a study called the World Health Organization (WHO) Study. This study compared the effects in patients who used clofibrate with effects in those who used a placebo (sugar pill). The results of this study suggested that clofibrate might increase the patient's risk of cancer, liver disease, and pancreatitis (inflammation of the pancreas), although it might also decrease the risk of heart attack. It may also increase the risk of gallstones and problems from gallbladder surgery. Other studies have not found all of these effects. Be sure you have discussed this with your doctor before taking this medicine.

In deciding to use a medicine, the risks of taking the medicine must be weighed against the good it will do. This is a decision you and your doctor will make. For clofibrate, the following should be considered:

Allergies—Tell your doctor if you have ever had any unusual or allergic reaction to clofibrate. Also tell your health care professional if you are allergic to any other substances, such as foods, preservatives, or dyes.

Diet—Before prescribing medicine for your condition, your doctor will probably try to control your condition by prescribing a personal diet for you. Such a diet may be low in fats, sugars, and/or cholesterol. Many people are able to control their condition by carefully following their doctors' orders for proper diet and exercise. *Medicine is prescribed only when additional help is needed* and is effective only when a schedule of diet and exercise is properly followed.

Also, this medicine is less effective if you are greatly overweight. It may be very important for you to go on a reducing diet. However, check with your doctor before going on any diet.

Make certain your health care professional knows if you are on a low-sodium, low-sugar, or any other special diet. Most medicines contain more than their active ingredient.

Pregnancy—Use of clofibrate is not recommended during pregnancy. Although studies have not been done in pregnant women, studies in rabbits have shown that the fetus may not be able to break down and get rid of this medicine as well as the mother. Because of this, it is possible that clofibrate may be harmful to the fetus if you take it while you are pregnant or for up to several months before you become pregnant. Be sure that you have discussed this with your doctor before taking this medicine, especially if you plan to become pregnant in the near future.

Breast-feeding—Clofibrate passes into breast milk. This medicine is not recommended during breast-feeding because it may cause unwanted effects in nursing babies.

Children—Studies on this medicine have been done only in adult patients, and there is no specific information comparing use of clofibrate in children with use in other age groups. However, use is not recommended in children under 2 years of age since cholesterol is needed for normal development.

Older adults—Many medicines have not been studied specifically in older people. Therefore, it may not be known whether they work exactly the same way they do in younger adults. Although there is no specific information comparing use of clofibrate in the elderly with use in other age groups, this medicine is not expected to cause different side effects or problems in older people than it does in younger adults.

Other medicines—Although certain medicines should not be used together at all, in other cases two different medicines may be used together even if an interaction might occur. In these cases, your doctor may want to change the dose, or other precautions may be necessary. When you are taking clofibrate, it is especially important that your health care professional knows if you are taking the following:

- Anticoagulants (blood thinners)—Use with clofibrate may increase the effects of the anticoagulant

Other medical problems—The presence of other medical problems may affect the use of clofibrate. Make sure you tell your doctor if you have any other medical problems, especially:

- Gallstones or
- Stomach or intestinal ulcer—May make these conditions worse

- Heart disease or
- Kidney disease or
- Liver disease—Higher blood levels may result and increase the risk of side effects

- Underactive thyroid—Clofibrate may cause or make muscle disease worse

---

Proper Use of This Medicine

Use this medicine only as directed by your doctor. Do not use more or less of it, and do not use it more often or for a longer time than your doctor ordered.

Follow carefully the special diet your doctor gave you. This is the most important part of controlling your condition and is necessary if the medicine is to work properly.

Stomach upset may occur but usually lessens after a few doses. Take this medicine with food or immediately after meals to lessen possible stomach upset.

Dosing—The dose of clofibrate will be different for different patients. *Follow your doctor's orders or the directions on the label.* The following information includes only the average doses of clofibrate. *If your dose is different, do not change it* unless your doctor tells you to do so.

The number of capsules that you take depends on the strength of the medicine.

- For *oral* dosage form (capsules):
    —For high cholesterol:

- Adults—1.5 to 2 grams a day. This is divided into two to four doses.
- Children—Dose must be determined by your doctor.

Missed dose—If you miss a dose of this medicine, take it as soon as possible. However, if it is almost time for your next dose, skip the missed dose and go back to your regular dosing schedule. Do not double doses.

Storage—To store this medicine:
- Keep out of the reach of children.
- Store away from heat and direct light.
- Do not store in the bathroom, near the kitchen sink, or in other damp places. Heat or moisture may cause the medicine to break down.
- Do not keep outdated medicine or medicine no longer needed. Be sure that any discarded medicine is out of the reach of children.

Precautions While Using This Medicine

It is very important that your doctor check your progress at regular visits. This will allow your doctor to see if the medicine is working properly to lower your cholesterol and triglyceride levels and to decide if you should continue to take it.

Do not stop taking this medicine without first checking with your doctor. When you stop taking this medicine, your blood fat levels may increase again. Your doctor may want you to follow a special diet to help prevent that.

Side Effects of This Medicine

Along with its needed effects, a medicine may cause some unwanted effects. Although not all of these side effects

may occur, if they do occur they may need medical attention.

Check with your doctor immediately if you think you have taken an overdose or if any of the following side effects occur:

Rare

> Chest pain; irregular heartbeat; shortness of breath; stomach pain (severe) with nausea and vomiting

Check with your doctor as soon as possible if any of the following side effects occur:

Rare

> Blood in urine; cough or hoarseness; decrease in urination; fever or chills; lower back or side pain; painful or difficult urination; swelling of feet or lower legs

Other side effects may occur that usually do not need medical attention. These side effects may go away during treatment as your body adjusts to the medicine. However, check with your doctor if any of the following side effects continue or are bothersome:

More common

> Diarrhea; nausea

Less common or rare

> Decreased sexual ability; headache; increased appetite or weight gain (slight); muscle aches or cramps; sores in mouth and on lips; stomach pain, gas, or heartburn; unusual tiredness or weakness; vomiting

Other side effects not listed above may also occur in some patients. If you notice any other effects, check with your doctor.

Additional Information

Once a medicine has been approved for marketing for a certain use, experience may show that it is also useful for other medical problems. Although this use is not included in product labeling, clofibrate is used in certain patients with the following medical condition:

• Certain types of diabetes insipidus (water diabetes)

Other than the above information, there is no additional information relating to proper use, precautions, or side effects for this use.

CLONIDINE Systemic

Some commonly used brand names are:

In the U.S.—
  Catapres
  Catapres-TTS
  Generic name product may also be available.

In Canada—
  Catapres
  Dixarit

Description

Clonidine (KLOE-ni-deen) belongs to the general class of medicines called antihypertensives. It is used to treat high blood pressure (hypertension).

High blood pressure adds to the workload of the heart and arteries. If it continues for a long time, the heart and arteries may not function properly. This can damage the blood vessels of the brain, heart, and kidneys, resulting in a stroke, heart failure, or kidney failure. Hypertension may also increase the risk of heart attacks. These problems may be less likely to occur if blood pressure is controlled.

Clonidine works by controlling nerve impulses along certain nerve pathways. As a result, it relaxes blood vessels so that blood passes through them more easily. This helps to lower blood pressure.

Clonidine may also be used for other conditions as determined by your doctor.

Clonidine is available only with your doctor's prescription, in the following dosage forms:

Oral
- Tablets (U.S. and Canada)

Transdermal
- Skin patch (U.S.)

Before Using This Medicine

In deciding to use a medicine, the risks of taking the medicine must be weighed against the good it will do. This is a decision you and your doctor will make. For clonidine, the following should be considered:

Allergies—Tell your doctor if you have ever had any unusual or allergic reaction to clonidine. Also tell your health care professional if you are allergic to any other substance, such as foods, preservatives, or dyes.

Pregnancy—Clonidine has not been studied in pregnant women. However, studies in animals have shown that clonidine causes harmful effects in the fetus, but not birth defects.

Breast-feeding—Although clonidine passes into breast milk, it has not been reported to cause problems in nursing babies.

Children—Children may be more sensitive than adults to clonidine. Clonidine overdose has been reported when children accidentally took this medicine.

Older adults—Dizziness or faintness may be more likely to occur in the elderly, who are more sensitive than younger adults to the effects of clonidine.

Other medicines—Although certain medicines should not be used together at all, in other cases two different medicines may be used together even if an interaction might occur. In these cases, your doctor may want to change the dose, or other precautions may be necessary. When you are taking clonidine, it is especially important that your health care professional know if you are taking any of the following:

- Beta-blockers (acebutolol [e.g., Sectral], atenolol [e.g., Tenormin], betaxolol [e.g., Kerlone], carteolol [e.g., Cartrol], labetalol [e.g., Normodyne], metoprolol [e.g., Lopressor], nadolol [e.g., Corgard], oxprenolol [e.g., Trasicor], penbutolol [e.g., Levatol], pindolol [e.g., Visken], propranolol [e.g., Inderal], sotalol [e.g., Sotacor], timolol [e.g., Blocadren])—These medicines may increase the risk of harmful effects when clonidine treatment is stopped suddenly
- Tricyclic antidepressants (amitriptyline [e.g., Elavil], amoxapine [e.g., Asendin], clomipramine [e.g., Anafranil], desipramine [e.g., Pertofrane], doxepin [e.g., Sinequan], imipramine [e.g., Tofranil], nortriptyline [e.g., Aventyl], protriptyline [e.g., Vivactil], trimipramine [e.g., Surmontil])—These medicines may decrease clonidine's effects on blood pressure

Other medical problems—The presence of other medical problems may affect the use of clonidine. Make sure you tell your doctor if you have any other medical problems, especially:

- Heart or blood vessel disease—Clonidine may make these conditions worse
- Irritated or scraped skin (with transdermal system [skin patch] only)—The effects of clonidine may be increased if the skin patch is placed on an area of scraped or irritated skin because more medicine is absorbed into the body
- Kidney disease—Effects of clonidine may be increased because of slower removal of clonidine from the body
- Mental depression (history of) or
- Raynaud's syndrome—Clonidine may make these conditions worse
- Polyarteritis nodosa or
- Scleroderma or
- Systemic lupus erythematosus (SLE)—with transdermal system (skin patch) only—Effects of clonidine may be decreased because absorption of this medicine into the body is blocked

Proper Use of This Medicine

For patients taking this medicine *for high blood pressure:*

• In addition to the use of the medicine your doctor has prescribed, treatment for your high blood pressure may include weight control and care in the types of foods you eat, especially foods high in sodium. Your doctor will tell you which of these are most important for you. You should check with your doctor before changing your diet.

• Many patients who have high blood pressure will not notice any signs of the problem. In fact, many may feel normal. It is very important that you *take your medicine exactly as directed* and that you keep your appointments with your doctor even if you feel well.

• Remember that this medicine will not cure your high blood pressure, but it does help control it. Therefore, you must continue to use it as directed if you expect to lower your blood pressure and keep it down. *You may have to take high blood pressure medicine for the rest of your life.* If high blood pressure is not treated, it can cause serious problems such as heart failure, blood vessel disease, stroke, or kidney disease.

For patients using the *transdermal system (skin patch):*

• *Use this medicine exactly as directed by your doctor. It will work only if applied correctly. This medicine usually comes with patient instructions. Read them carefully before using.*

• Do not try to trim or cut the adhesive patch to adjust the dosage. Check with your doctor if you think the medicine is not working as it should.

• Apply the patch to a clean, dry area of skin on your upper arm or chest. Choose an area with little or no hair and free of scars, cuts, or irritation.

• The system should stay in place even during show-

ering, bathing, or swimming. If the patch becomes
loose, cover it with the extra adhesive overlay provided. Apply a new patch if the first one becomes
too loose or falls off.

• Each dose is best applied to a different area of skin
to prevent skin problems or other irritation.

• After removing a used patch, fold the patch in half
with the sticky sides together. Make sure to dispose
of it out of the reach of children.

To help you remember to use your medicine, try to get
into the habit of using it at regular times. If you are taking
the tablets, take them at the same time each day. If you are
using the transdermal system (skin patch), try to change it
at the same time and day of the week.

Dosing—The dose of clonidine will be different for different patients. *Follow your doctor's orders or the directions
on the label.* The following information includes only the
average doses of clonidine used for the treatment of high
blood pressure. *If your dose is different, do not change it*
unless your doctor tells you to do so:

• For *oral* dosage form (tablets):

—For high blood pressure:

• Adults—100 mcg (0.1 mg) two times a day.
Your doctor may increase your dose up to
200 mcg (0.2 mg) to 600 mcg (0.6 mg) a day
taken in divided doses.

• Children—Use and dose must be determined by
your doctor.

• For *transdermal* dosage form (skin patch):

—For high blood pressure:

• Adults—One transdermal dosage system (skin
patch) applied once a week.

• Children—Use and dose must be determined by
your doctor.

Missed dose—If you miss a dose of this medicine, take
it or use it as soon as possible. Then go back to your

regular dosing schedule. *If you miss 2 or more doses of the tablets in a row or if you miss changing the transdermal patch for 3 or more days, check with your doctor right away.* If your body goes without this medicine for too long, your blood pressure may go up to a dangerously high level and some unpleasant effects may occur.

Storage—To store this medicine:
- Keep out of the reach of children.
- Store away from heat and direct light.
- Do not store in the bathroom, near the kitchen sink, or in other damp places. Heat or moisture may cause the medicine to break down.
- Do not keep outdated medicine or medicine no longer needed. Be sure that any discarded medicine is out of the reach of children.

Precautions While Using This Medicine

It is important that your doctor check your progress at regular visits to make sure that this medicine is working properly.

Check with your doctor before you stop using this medicine. Your doctor may want you to reduce gradually the amount you are using before stopping completely.

Make sure that you have enough clonidine on hand to last through weekends, holidays, or vacations. You should not miss any doses. You may want to ask your doctor for another written prescription for clonidine to carry in your wallet or purse. You can then have it filled if you run out of medicine when you are away from home.

For patients taking this medicine *for high blood pressure:*
- *Do not take other medicines unless they have been discussed with your doctor.* This especially includes over-the-counter (nonprescription) medicines for ap-

petite control, asthma, colds, cough, hay fever, or sinus problems, since they may tend to increase your blood pressure.

Clonidine will add to the effects of alcohol and other CNS depressants (medicines that slow down the nervous system, possibly causing drowsiness). Some examples of CNS depressants are antihistamines or medicine for hay fever, other allergies, or colds; sedatives, tranquilizers, or sleeping medicine; prescription pain medicine or narcotics; barbiturates; medicine for seizures; muscle relaxants; or anesthetics, including some dental anesthetics. *Check with your doctor before taking any of the above while you are using this medicine.*

Clonidine may cause some people to become drowsy or less alert than they are normally. This is more likely to happen when you begin to take it or when you increase the amount of medicine you are taking. *Make sure you know how you react to this medicine before you drive, use machines, or do anything else that could be dangerous if you are not alert.*

Before having any kind of surgery (including dental surgery) or emergency treatment, *tell the medical doctor or dentist in charge that you are using this medicine.*

Dizziness, lightheadedness, or fainting may occur after you take this medicine, especially when you get up from a lying or sitting position. Getting up slowly may help, but if the problem continues or gets worse, check with your doctor.

The dizziness, lightheadedness, or fainting is also more likely to occur if you drink alcohol, stand for long periods of time, exercise, or if the weather is hot. While you are taking clonidine, be careful to limit the amount of alcohol you drink. Also, use extra care during exercise or hot weather or if you must stand for a long time.

Clonidine may cause dryness of the mouth. For temporary relief, use sugarless candy or gum, melt bits of ice in your mouth, or use a saliva substitute. However, if your mouth continues to feel dry for more than 2 weeks, check with your medical doctor or dentist. Continuing dryness of the mouth may increase the chance of dental disease, including tooth decay, gum disease, and fungus infections.

Side Effects of This Medicine

Along with its needed effects, a medicine may cause some unwanted effects. Although not all of these side effects may occur, if they do occur they may need medical attention.

Check with your doctor immediately if any of the following side effects occur:

Signs and symptoms of overdose

Difficulty in breathing; dizziness (extreme) or faintness; pinpoint pupils of eyes; slow heartbeat; unusual tiredness or weakness (extreme)

Check with your doctor as soon as possible if any of the following side effects occur:

More common—with transdermal system (skin patch) only

Itching or redness of skin

Less common

Mental depression; swelling of feet and lower legs

Rare

Paleness or cold feeling in fingertips and toes; vivid dreams or nightmares

Other side effects may occur that usually do not need medical attention. These side effects may go away during treatment as your body adjusts to the medicine. However, check with your doctor if any of the following side effects continue or are bothersome:

More common

Constipation; dizziness; drowsiness; dryness of mouth; unusual tiredness or weakness

Less common

Darkening of skin—with transdermal system (skin patch) only; decreased sexual ability; dizziness, lightheadedness, or fainting, especially when getting up from a lying or sitting position; dry, itching, or burning eyes; loss of appetite; nausea or vomiting; nervousness

After you have been using this medicine for a while, it may cause unpleasant or even harmful effects if you stop taking it too suddenly. After you stop taking this medicine, *check with your doctor immediately* if any of the following occur:

Anxiety or tenseness; chest pain; fast or pounding heartbeat; headache; increased salivation; nausea; nervousness; restlessness; shaking or trembling of hands and fingers; stomach cramps; sweating; trouble in sleeping; vomiting

Other side effects not listed above may also occur in some patients. If you notice any other effects, check with your doctor.

Additional Information

Once a medicine has been approved for marketing for a certain use, experience may show that it is also useful for other medical problems. Although these uses are not included in product labeling, clonidine is used in certain patients with the following medical conditions:

- Migraine headache
- Symptoms associated with menopause or menstrual discomfort
- Symptoms of withdrawal associated with alcohol, nicotine, or narcotics
- Gilles de la Tourette's syndrome

Other than the above information, there is no additional information relating to proper use, precautions, or side effects for these uses.

CLONIDINE AND CHLORTHALIDONE   Systemic

A commonly used brand name in the U.S. and Canada is Combipres. Generic name product may also be available in the U.S.

Description

Clonidine (KLOE-ni-deen) and chlorthalidone (klor-THAL-i-done) combinations are used in the treatment of high blood pressure (hypertension).

High blood pressure adds to the workload of the heart and arteries. If it continues for a long time, the heart and arteries may not function properly. This can damage the blood vessels of the brain, heart, and kidneys, resulting in a stroke, heart failure, or kidney failure. Hypertension may also increase the risk of heart attacks. These problems may be less likely to occur if blood pressure is controlled.

Clonidine works by controlling nerve impulses along certain body nerve pathways. As a result, it relaxes blood vessels so that blood passes through them more easily. The chlorthalidone in this combination is a diuretic (water pill) that helps reduce the amount of water in the body by increasing the flow of urine.

Clonidine and chlorthalidone combination is available only with your doctor's prescription, in the following dosage form:

Oral
  • Tablets (U.S. and Canada)

Before Using This Medicine

In deciding to use a medicine, the risks of taking the medicine must be weighed against the good it will do. This is a decision you and your doctor will make. For clonidine and chlorthalidone, the following should be considered:

Allergies—Tell your doctor if you have ever had any unusual or allergic reaction to clonidine, chlorthalidone, sulfonamides (sulfa drugs), or other thiazide diuretics (water pills). Also tell your health care professional if you are allergic to any other substance, such as foods, preservatives, or dyes.

Pregnancy—Clonidine has not been studied in pregnant women. However, studies in animals have shown that clonidine does not cause birth defects but does cause other harmful effects in the fetus. When chlorthalidone is used during pregnancy, it may cause side effects including jaundice, blood problems, and low potassium in the newborn infant. Be sure you have discussed this with your doctor before taking this medicine.

Breast-feeding—Both clonidine and chlorthalidone pass into breast milk. Chlorthalidone may decrease the flow of breast milk. Therefore, you should avoid use of clonidine and chlorthalidone combination during the first month of breast-feeding.

Children—Studies on this medicine have been done only in adult patients, and there is no specific information comparing use of clonidine and chlorthalidone combination in children with use in other age groups. However, children may be more sensitive than adults to clonidine. Clonidine overdose has been reported when children accidentally took this medicine.

Older adults—Dizziness or lightheadedness and signs of too much potassium loss may be more likely to occur in the elderly, who are more sensitive to the effects of clonidine and chlorthalidone.

Other medicines—Although certain medicines should not be used together at all, in other cases two different medicines may be used together even if an interaction might occur. In these cases, your doctor may want to change the dose, or other precautions may be necessary. When you are taking clonidine and chlorthalidone, it is especially important that your health care professional know if you are taking any of the following:

- Beta-blockers (acebutolol [e.g., Sectral], atenolol [e.g., Tenormin], betaxolol [Kerlone], bisoprolol [Zebeta], carteolol [e.g., Cartrol], labetalol [e.g., Normodyne], metoprolol [e.g., Lopressor], nadolol [e.g., Corgard], oxprenolol [e.g., Trasicor], penbutolol [e.g., Levatol], pindolol [e.g., Visken], propranolol [e.g., Inderal], sotalol [e.g., Sotacor], timolol [e.g., Blocadren])—These medicines may increase the risk of harmful effects when clonidine and chlorthalidone combination treatment is stopped suddenly

- Cholestyramine or
- Colestipol—Use with clonidine and chlorthalidone combination may prevent the chlorthalidone portion of the medicine from working properly; take clonidine and chlorthalidone combination at least 1 hour before or 4 hours after cholestyramine or colestipol

- Digitalis glycosides (heart medicine)—This medicine may cause low potassium in the blood, which may increase the chance of side effects of digitalis glycosides

- Lithium (e.g., Lithane)—Use with clonidine and chlorthalidone combination may cause high blood levels of lithium, which may increase the chance of side effects

- Tricyclic antidepressants (amitriptyline [e.g., Elavil], amoxapine [e.g., Asendin], clomipramine [e.g., Anafranil], desipramine [e.g., Pertofrane], doxepin [e.g., Sinequan], imipramine [e.g., Tofranil], nortriptyline [e.g., Aventyl], protriptyline [e.g., Vivactil], trimipramine [e.g., Surmontil])—These medicines may decrease the effects of clonidine and chlorthalidone combination on blood pressure

Other medical problems—The presence of other medical problems may affect the use of clonidine and chlorthalidone. Make sure you tell your doctor if you have any other medical problems, especially:

- Diabetes mellitus (sugar diabetes)—This medicine may change the amount of diabetes medicine needed

- Gout—This medicine may increase the amount of uric acid in the blood, which can lead to gout

- Heart or blood vessel disease or
- Lupus erythematosus (history of) or
- Mental depression (history of) or
- Pancreatitis (inflammation of the pancreas) or
- Raynaud's syndrome—This medicine may make these conditions worse

- Kidney disease—Effects of this medicine may be increased because of slower removal from the body. If severe, the chlorthalidone portion of this medicine may not work

- Liver disease—If this medicine causes loss of too much water from the body, liver disease can become much worse

---

Proper Use of This Medicine

This medicine may cause you to have an unusual feeling of tiredness when you begin to take it. You may also notice an increase in the amount of urine or in your frequency of urination. After taking the medicine for a while, these effects should lessen. It is best to plan your doses according to a schedule that will least affect your personal activities and sleep. Ask your health care professional to help you plan the best time to take this medicine.

In addition to the use of the medicine your doctor has prescribed, appropriate treatment for your high blood pressure may include weight control and care in the types of foods you eat, especially foods high in sodium. Your doctor will tell you which factors are most important for you. You should check with your doctor before changing your diet.

Many patients who have high blood pressure will not notice any signs of the problem. In fact, many may feel normal. It is very important that you *take your medicine exactly as directed* and that you keep your appointments with your doctor even if you feel well.

Remember that this medicine will not cure your high blood pressure but it does help control it. Therefore, you must continue to take it as directed if you expect to lower your blood pressure and keep it down. *You may have to take high blood pressure medicine for the rest of your life.* If high blood pressure is not treated, it can cause serious problems such as heart failure, blood vessel disease, stroke, or kidney disease.

To help you remember to take your medicine, try to get into the habit of taking it at the same time each day.

Dosing—The dose of clonidine and chlorthalidone combination will be different for different patients. *Follow your doctor's orders or the directions on the label.* The following information includes only the average doses of clonidine and chlorthalidone combination. *If your dose is different, do not change it* unless your doctor tells you to do so.

The number of tablets that you take depends on the strength of the medicine.

- For *oral* dosage form (tablets):
  —For high blood pressure:
    - Adults—1 or 2 tablets two to four times a day.
    - Children—Dose must be determined by your doctor.

Missed dose—If you miss a dose of this medicine, take it as soon as possible. Then go back to your regular dosing schedule. *If you miss two or more doses in a row, check with your doctor right away.* If your body goes without this medicine for too long, your blood pressure may go up to a dangerously high level and some unpleasant effects may occur.

Storage—To store this medicine:

- Keep out of the reach of children.
- Store away from heat and direct light.
- Do not store in the bathroom, near the kitchen sink,

or in other damp places. Heat or moisture may cause
the medicine to break down.

- Do not keep outdated medicine or medicine no longer
  needed. Be sure that any discarded medicine is out
  of the reach of children.

Precautions While Using This Medicine

It is important that your doctor check your progress at
regular visits to make sure that this medicine is working
properly.

*Check with your doctor before you stop taking this medi-
cine.* Your doctor may want you to reduce gradually the
amount you are taking before stopping completely.

*Make sure that you have enough medicine on hand to last
through weekends, holidays, or vacations.* You should not
miss taking any doses. You may want to ask your doctor
for another written prescription to carry in your wallet or
purse. You can then have it filled if you run out of medicine when you are away from home.

Before having any kind of surgery (including dental surgery) or emergency treatment, *make sure the medical doctor or dentist in charge knows that you are taking this
medicine.*

*Do not take other medicines unless they have been dis-
cussed with your doctor.* This especially includes over-the-
counter (nonprescription) medicines for appetite control,
asthma, colds, cough, hay fever, or sinus problems, since
they may tend to increase your blood pressure.

This medicine will add to the effects of alcohol and other
CNS depressants (medicines that slow down the nervous
system, possibly causing drowsiness). Some examples of
CNS depressants are antihistamines or medicine for hay
fever, other allergies, or colds; sedatives, tranquilizers, or
sleeping medicine; prescription pain medicine or narcotics;

barbiturates; medicine for seizures; muscle relaxants; or anesthetics, including some dental anesthetics. *Check with your doctor before taking any of the above while you are using this medicine.*

This medicine may cause some people to become drowsy or less alert than they are normally. This is more likely to happen when you begin to take it or when you increase the amount of medicine you are taking. *Make sure you know how you react to this medicine before you drive, use machines, or do anything else that could be dangerous if you are not alert.*

Dizziness, lightheadedness, or fainting may occur, especially when you get up from a lying or sitting position. Getting up slowly may help, but if the problem continues or gets worse, check with your doctor.

The dizziness, lightheadedness, or fainting is also more likely to occur if you drink alcohol, stand for long periods of time, exercise, or if the weather is hot. Drinking alcoholic beverages may also make the drowsiness worse. While you are taking this medicine, be careful to limit the amount of alcohol you drink. Also, use extra care during exercise or hot weather or if you must stand for long periods of time.

This medicine may cause a loss of potassium from your body.

- To help prevent this, your doctor may want you to:
  —eat or drink foods that have a high potassium content (for example, orange or other citrus fruit juices), or
  —take a potassium supplement, or
  —take another medicine to help prevent the loss of the potassium in the first place.
- It is very important to follow these directions. Also, it is important not to change your diet on your own. This is more important if you are already on a special

diet (as for diabetes), or if you are taking a potassium supplement or a medicine to reduce potassium loss. Extra potassium may not be necessary and, in some cases, too much potassium could be harmful.

Check with your doctor if you become sick and have severe or continuing vomiting or diarrhea. These problems may cause you to lose additional water and potassium.

For *diabetic patients:*

• The chlorthalidone contained in this medicine may raise blood sugar levels. While you are using this medicine, be especially careful in testing for sugar in your urine.

This medicine may cause your skin to be more sensitive to sunlight than it is normally. Exposure to sunlight, even for brief periods of time, may cause a skin rash, itching, redness or other discoloration of the skin, or a severe sunburn. When you begin taking this medicine:

• Stay out of direct sunlight, especially between the hours of 10:00 a.m. and 3:00 p.m., if possible.

• Wear protective clothing, including a hat. Also, wear sunglasses.

• Apply a sun block product that has a skin protection factor (SPF) of at least 15. Some patients may require a product with a higher SPF number, especially if they have a fair complexion. If you have any questions about this, check with your health care professional.

• Apply a sun block lipstick that has an SPF of at least 15 to protect your lips.

• Do not use a sunlamp or tanning bed or booth.

If you have a severe reaction from the sun, check with your doctor.

This medicine may cause dryness of the mouth. For temporary relief, use sugarless candy or gum, melt bits of ice in your mouth, or use a saliva substitute. However, if your mouth continues to feel dry for more than 2 weeks, check with your medical doctor or dentist. Continuing dryness of the mouth may increase the chance of dental disease, including tooth decay, gum disease, and fungus infections.

Side Effects of This Medicine

Along with its needed effects, a medicine may cause some unwanted effects. Although not all of these side effects may occur, if they do occur they may need medical attention.

Check with your doctor immediately if any of the following side effects occur:

Signs and symptoms of overdose

Difficulty in breathing; dizziness (extreme) or faintness; feeling cold; pinpoint pupils of eyes; slow heartbeat; unusual tiredness or weakness (extreme)

Check with your doctor as soon as possible if any of the following side effects occur:

Signs and symptoms of too much potassium loss

Dryness of mouth; increased thirst; irregular heartbeat; mood or mental changes; muscle cramps or pain; nausea or vomiting; weak pulse

Signs and symptoms of too much sodium loss

Confusion; convulsions (seizures); decreased mental activity; irritability; muscle cramps; unusual tiredness or weakness

Less common

Mental depression; swelling of feet and lower legs

Rare

Black, tarry stools; blood in urine or stools; cough or hoarseness; fever or chills; joint pain; lower back or side pain; paleness or cold feeling in fingertips and toes; pinpoint red spots on skin; skin rash or hives; stomach pain (severe) with nausea and vomiting; unusual bleeding or bruising; vivid dreams or nightmares; yellow eyes or skin

Other side effects may occur that usually do not need medical attention. These side effects may go away during treatment as your body adjusts to the medicine. However, check with your doctor if any of the following side effects continue or are bothersome:

More common

Constipation; dizziness; drowsiness; dryness of mouth; unusual tiredness or weakness

Less common

Decreased sexual ability; diarrhea; dizziness or lightheadedness when getting up from a lying or sitting position; dry, itching, or burning eyes; increased sensitivity of skin to sunlight; loss of appetite; nausea or vomiting; nervousness; upset stomach

After you have been using this medicine for a while, it may cause unpleasant or even harmful effects if you stop taking it too suddenly. After you stop taking this medicine, check with your doctor if any of the following occur:

Anxiety or tenseness; chest pain; fast or irregular heartbeat; headache; increased salivation; nausea; nervousness; restlessness; shaking or trembling of hands and fingers; stomach cramps; sweating; trouble in sleeping; vomiting

Other side effects not listed above may also occur in some patients. If you notice any other effects, check with your doctor.

COLESTIPOL Oral

A commonly used brand name is:

In the U.S.—
Colestid

In Canada—
Colestid

Description

Colestipol (koe-LES-ti-pole) is used to lower high cholesterol levels in the blood. This may help prevent medical problems caused by cholesterol clogging the blood vessels.

Colestipol works by attaching to certain substances in the intestine. Since colestipol is not absorbed into the body, these substances also pass out of the body without being absorbed.

Colestipol may also be used for other conditions as determined by your doctor.

Colestipol is available only with your doctor's prescription, in the following dosage form:

Oral
- Powder (U.S. and Canada)

Before Using This Medicine

In deciding to use a medicine, the risks of taking the medicine must be weighed against the good it will do. This is a decision you and your doctor will make. For colestipol, the following should be considered:

Allergies—Tell your doctor if you have ever had any unusual or allergic reaction to colestipol. Also tell your health care professional if you are allergic to any substances, such as foods, preservatives, or dyes.

Diet—Before prescribing medicine for your condition, your doctor will probably try to control your condition by prescribing a personal diet for you. Such a diet may be low in fats, sugars, and/or cholesterol. Many people are able to control their condition by carefully following their doctor's orders for proper diet and exercise. Medicine is prescribed only when additional help is needed and is effective only when a schedule of diet and exercise is properly followed.

Also, this medicine is less effective if you are greatly overweight. It may be very important for you to go on a reducing diet. However, check with your doctor before going on any diet.

Make certain your health care professional knows if you are on a low-sodium, low-sugar, or any other special diet.

Pregnancy—Colestipol is not absorbed into the body and is not likely to cause problems. However, it may reduce absorption of vitamins into the body. Ask your doctor whether you need to take extra vitamins.

Breast-feeding—Colestipol is not absorbed into the body and is not likely to cause problems.

Children—There is no specific information comparing use of colestipol in children with use in other age groups. However, use is not recommended in children under 2 years of age since cholesterol is needed for normal development.

Older adults—Side effects may be more likely to occur in patients over 60 years of age, who are usually more sensitive to the effects of colestipol.

Other medicines—Although certain medicines should not be used together at all, in other cases two different medicines may be used together even if an interaction might occur. In these cases, your doctor may want to change the dose, or other precautions may be necessary. When you are taking colestipol it is especially important that your health care professional knows if you are taking any of the following:

* Anticoagulants (blood thinners)—The effects of the anticoagulant may be altered
* Digitalis glycosides (heart medicine) or
* Diuretics (water pills) or
* Penicillin G, taken by mouth, or

- Propranolol, taken by mouth, or
- Tetracyclines (medicine for infection), taken by mouth, or
- Thyroid hormones or
- Vancomycin, taken by mouth—Colestipol may cause these medicines to be less effective; these medicines should be taken 4 to 5 hours apart from colestipol

Other medical problems—The presence of other medical problems may affect the use of colestipol. Make sure you tell your doctor if you have any other medical problems, especially:

- Bleeding problems or
- Constipation or
- Gallstones or
- Heart or blood vessel disease or
- Hemorrhoids or
- Stomach ulcer or other stomach problems or
- Underactive thyroid—Colestipol may make these conditions worse
- Kidney disease—There is an increased risk of developing electrolyte problems
- Liver disease—Cholesterol levels may be raised

Proper Use of This Medicine

Take this medicine exactly as directed by your doctor. Try not to miss any doses and do not take more medicine than your doctor ordered.

Follow carefully the special diet your doctor gave you. This is the most important part of controlling your condition and is necessary if the medicine is to work properly.

This medicine should never be taken in its dry form, since it could cause you to choke. Instead, always mix as follows:

- Add this medicine to 3 ounces or more of water, milk, flavored drink, or your favorite juice or carbonated drink. If you use a carbonated drink, slowly mix in the powder in a large glass to prevent too much foaming. Stir until it is completely mixed (it will *not* dissolve) before drinking. After drinking all the liquid containing the medicine, rinse the glass with a little more liquid and drink that also, to make sure you get all the medicine.

- You may also mix this medicine with milk in hot or regular breakfast cereals, or in thin soups such as tomato or chicken noodle soup. Or you may add it to some pulpy fruits such as crushed pineapple, pears, peaches, or fruit cocktail.

Dosing—The dose of colestipol will be different for different patients. *Follow your doctor's orders or the directions on the label.* The following information includes only the average doses of colestipol. *If your dose is different, do not change it* unless your doctor tells you to do so.

- For *oral* dosage form (powder for oral suspension):
  —For high cholesterol:
    - Adults—15 to 30 grams a day. This is divided into two to four doses and taken before meals.
    - Children—Use and dose must be determined by your doctor.

Missed dose—If you miss a dose of this medicine, take it as soon as possible. Then go back to your regular dosing schedule. However, if it is almost time for your next dose, skip the missed dose and go back to your regular dosing schedule. Do not double doses.

Storage—To store this medicine:

- Keep out of the reach of children.
- Store away from heat and direct light.
- Do not store in the bathroom, near the kitchen sink or in other damp places. Heat or moisture may cause the medicine to break down.
- Do not keep outdated medicine or medicine no longer needed. Be sure that any discarded medicine is out of the reach of children.

Precautions While Using This Medicine

It is very important that your doctor check your progress at regular visits. This will allow your doctor to see if the medicine is working properly to lower your cholesterol levels and to decide if you should continue to take it.

Do not stop taking this medicine without first checking with your doctor. When you stop taking this medicine, your blood cholesterol levels may increase again. Your doctor may want you to follow a special diet to help prevent this from happening.

Do not take any other medicine unless prescribed by your doctor since colestipol may interfere with other medicines.

Side Effects of This Medicine

Along with its needed effects, a medicine may cause some unwanted effects. Although not all of these side effects may occur, if they do occur they may need medical attention.

Check with your doctor immediately if either of the following side effects occurs:

Rare
   Black, tarry stools; stomach pain (severe) with nausea and vomiting

Check with your doctor as soon as possible if either of the following side effects occurs:

More common
   Constipation
Rare
   Loss of weight (sudden)

Other side effects may occur that usually do not need medical attention. These side effects may go away during treatment as your body adjusts to the medicine. However,

check with your doctor if any of the following side effects continue or are bothersome:

Less common

> Belching; bloating; diarrhea; dizziness; headache; nausea or vomiting; stomach pain

Other side effects not listed above may also occur in some patients. If you notice any other effects, check with your doctor.

Additional Information

Once a medicine has been approved for marketing for a certain use, experience may show that it is also useful for other medical problems. Although these uses are not included in product labeling, colestipol is used in certain patients with the following medical conditions:

- Diarrhea caused by bile acids
- Digitalis glycoside overdose
- Excess oxalate in the urine
- Itching (pruritus) associated with partial biliary obstruction

Other than the above information, there is no additional information relating to proper use, precautions, or side effects for these uses.

CYCLANDELATE   Systemic

A commonly used brand name is Cyclospasmol.

Generic name product may also be available in the U.S.

Description

Cyclandelate (sye-KLAN-de-late) belongs to the group of medicines commonly called vasodilators. These medicines increase the size of blood vessels. Cyclandelate is used to treat problems resulting from poor blood circulation.

In the U.S., cyclandelate is available only with your doctor's prescription. It is available in the following dosage forms:

Oral

- Capsules (U.S.)
- Tablets (Canada)

Before Using This Medicine

In deciding to use a medicine, the risks of taking the medicine must be weighed against the good it will do. This is a decision you and your doctor will make. For cyclandelate, the following should be considered:

Allergies—Tell your doctor if you have ever had any unusual or allergic reaction to cyclandelate. Also tell your health care professional if you are allergic to any other substances, such as foods, preservatives, or dyes.

Pregnancy—Studies on effects in pregnancy have not been done in either humans or animals.

Breast-feeding—It is not known whether cyclandelate passes into breast milk. However, cyclandelate has not been reported to cause problems in nursing babies.

Children—Studies on this medicine have been done only in adult patients, and there is no specific information comparing use of cyclandelate in children with use in other age groups.

Older adults—Many medicines have not been studied specifically in older people. Therefore, it may not be known whether they work exactly the same way they do in younger adults. Although there is no specific information comparing use of cyclandelate in the elderly with use in other age groups, this medicine is not expected to cause different side effects or problems in older people than in younger adults.

Other medicines—Although certain medicines should not be used together at all, in other cases two different medicines may be used together even if an interaction might occur. In these cases, your doctor may want to change the dose, or other precautions may be necessary. Tell your health care professional if you are taking any other prescription or nonprescription (over-the-counter [OTC]) medicine, or if you smoke.

Other medical problems—The presence of other medical problems may affect the use of cyclandelate. Make sure you tell your doctor if you have any other medical problems, especially:

- Angina (chest pain) or
- Bleeding problems or
- Glaucoma or
- Hardening of the arteries or
- Heart attack (recent) or
- Stroke (recent)—The chance of unwanted effects may be increased

---

Proper Use of This Medicine

If this medicine upsets your stomach, it may be taken with meals, milk, or antacids.

Dosing—The dose of cyclandelate will be different for different patients. *Follow your doctor's orders or the directions on the label.* The following information includes only the average doses of cyclandelate. *If your dose is different, do not change it* unless your doctor tells you to do so.

The number of capsules or tablets that you take depends on the strength of the medicine.

- For *oral* dosage form (capsules or tablets):
    - —For treating poor circulation:
        - Adults—At first, 1.2 to 1.6 grams a day. This is taken in divided doses before meals and at bed-

time. Then, your doctor will gradually lower your dose to 400 to 800 milligrams (mg) a day. This is divided into two to four doses.

• Children—Use and dose must be determined by your doctor.

Missed dose—If you miss a dose of this medicine, take it as soon as you remember. Then go back to your regular dosing schedule. However, if it is almost time for your next dose, skip the missed dose and go back to your regular dosing schedule. Do not double doses.

Storage—To store this medicine:

• Keep out of the reach of children.

• Store away from heat and direct light.

• Do not store in the bathroom, near the kitchen sink, or in other damp places. Heat or moisture may cause the medicine to break down.

• Do not keep outdated medicine or medicine no longer needed. Be sure that any discarded medicine is out of the reach of children.

Precautions While Using This Medicine

It may take some time for this medicine to work. If you feel that the medicine is not working, do not stop taking it on your own. Instead, check with your doctor.

The helpful effects of this medicine may be decreased if you smoke.

Dizziness may occur, especially when you get up from a lying or sitting position or climb stairs. Getting up slowly may help. If this problem continues or gets worse, check with your doctor.

Side Effects of This Medicine

Along with its needed effects, a medicine may cause some unwanted effects. The following side effects may go away during treatment as your body adjusts to the medicine. However, check with your doctor if any of these effects continue or are bothersome:

Less common

Belching, heartburn, nausea, or stomach pain; dizziness; fast heartbeat; flushing of face; headache; sweating; tingling sensation in face, fingers, or toes; weakness

Other side effects not listed above may also occur in some patients. If you notice any other effects, check with your doctor.

DEXTROTHYROXINE   Systemic

Some commonly used brand names are:

In the U.S.—
  Choloxin

In Canada—
  Choloxin

Other—

Biotirmone	Dynothel
Debetrol	Eulipos
Dethyrona	Lisolipin
Dethyrone	Nadrothyron-D

Description

Dextrothyroxine (dex-troe-thye-ROX-een) is used to lower high cholesterol levels in the blood. However, it has generally been replaced by safer medicines for the treatment of high cholesterol.

Dextrothyroxine is available only with your doctor's prescription, in the following dosage form:

Oral

  • Tablets (U.S. and Canada)

Before Using This Medicine

In deciding to use a medicine, the risks of taking the medicine must be weighed against the good it will do. This is a decision you and your doctor will make. For dextrothyroxine, the following should be considered:

Allergies—Tell your doctor if you have ever had any unusual or allergic reaction to dextrothyroxine. Also tell your health care professional if you are allergic to any other substances, such as foods, preservatives, or dyes.

Diet—Before prescribing medicine for your condition, your doctor will probably try to control your condition by prescribing a personal diet for you. Such a diet may be low in fats, sugars, and/or cholesterol. Many people are able to control their condition by carefully following their doctor's orders for proper diet and exercise. *Medicine is prescribed only when additional help is needed* and is effective only when a schedule of diet and exercise is properly followed.

Also, this medicine is less effective if you are greatly overweight. It may be very important for you to go on a reducing diet. However, check with your doctor before going on any diet.

Make certain your health care professional knows if you are on any special diet, such as a low-sodium or low-sugar diet.

Pregnancy—Dextrothyroxine has not been studied in pregnant women. However, studies in animals have not shown that dextrothyroxine causes birth defects or other problems. Before taking this medicine, make sure your doctor knows if you are pregnant or if you may become pregnant.

Breast-feeding—It is not known whether dextrothyroxine passes into breast milk. Although most medicines pass into breast milk in small amounts, many of them may be used safely while breast-feeding. Mothers who are taking this medicine and who wish to breast-feed should discuss this with their doctor.

Children—There is no specific information comparing use of dextrothyroxine in children to use in other age groups. However, use is not recommended in children under 2 years of age since cholesterol is needed for normal development.

Older adults—Side effects are more likely to occur in the elderly, who are usually more sensitive to the effects of dextrothyroxine.

Other medicines—Although certain medicines should not be used together at all, in other cases two different medicines may be used together even if an interaction might occur. In these cases, your doctor may want to change the dose, or other precautions may be necessary. When you are taking dextrothyroxine, it is especially important that your health care professional know if you are taking any of the following:

- Anticoagulants (blood thinners)—The effects of the anticoagulant may be altered; a change in dosage of the anticoagulant may be necessary
- Cholestyramine (e.g., Questran) or
- Colestipol (e.g., Colestid)—The effects of dextrothyroxine may decrease; these two medicines should be taken at least 4 to 5 hours before or after dextrothyroxine

Other medical problems—The presence of other medical problems may affect the use of dextrothyroxine. Make sure you tell your doctor if you have any other medical problems, especially:

- Diabetes mellitus (sugar diabetes)—Blood sugar levels may be increased
- Heart or blood vessel disease or
- High blood pressure or
- Overactive thyroid—Dextrothyroxine may make these conditions worse

- Kidney disease—Higher blood levels of dextrothyroxine may result and increase the chance of side effects
- Liver disease—May lead to an increase in cholesterol blood levels
- Underactive thyroid—There may be an increased sensitivity to the effects of dextrothyroxine

---

Proper Use of This Medicine

Take this medicine exactly as directed by your doctor. Try not to miss any doses and do not take more medicine than your doctor ordered.

Remember that this medicine will not cure your cholesterol problem, but it does help control it. Therefore, you must continue to take it as directed if you expect to lower your cholesterol level.

Follow carefully the special diet your doctor gave you. This is the most important part of controlling your condition, and is necessary if the medicine is to work properly.

Dosing—The dose of dextrothyroxine will be different for different patients. *Follow your doctor's orders or the directions on the label.* The following information includes only the average doses of dextrothyroxine. *If your dose is different, do not change it* unless your doctor tells you to do so.

The number of tablets that you take depends on the strength of the medicine.

- For *tablets* dosage form:
  —For treatment of high cholesterol:
    - Adults—1 to 8 milligrams (mg) a day.
    - Children up to two years of age—Use is not recommended.
    - Children two years of age and older—50 to 100 micrograms (0.05 to 0.1 mg) per kilogram of body weight a day.

Missed dose—If you miss a dose of this medicine, take it as soon as possible. However, if it is almost time for your next dose, skip the missed dose and go back to your regular dosing schedule. Do not double doses.

Storage—To store this medicine:

- Keep out of the reach of children.
- Store away from heat and direct light.
- Do not store in the bathroom, near the kitchen sink, or in other damp places. Heat or moisture may cause the medicine to break down.
- Do not keep outdated medicine or medicine no longer needed. Be sure that any discarded medicine is out of the reach of children.

Precautions While Using This Medicine

It is very important that your doctor check your progress at regular visits. This will allow your doctor to see if the medicine is working properly to lower your cholesterol levels and if you should continue to take it.

Do not stop taking this medicine without first checking with your doctor. When you stop taking this medicine, your blood cholesterol levels may increase again. Your doctor may want you to follow a special diet to help prevent this from happening.

Before having any kind of surgery (including dental surgery) or emergency treatment, *tell the medical doctor or dentist in charge that you are taking this medicine.*

Side Effects of This Medicine

Along with its needed effects, a medicine may cause some unwanted effects. Although not all of these side effects may occur, if they do occur they may need medical attention.

Check with your doctor immediately if any of the following side effects occur:

> *Rare*
>
>> Chest pain; fast or irregular heartbeat; stomach pain (severe) with nausea and vomiting

Check with your doctor as soon as possible if the following side effects occur, since they may indicate too much medicine is being taken:

> *Rare*
>
>> Changes in appetite; changes in menstrual periods; diarrhea; fast or irregular heartbeat; fever; hand tremors; headache; increase in urination; irritability, nervousness, or trouble in sleeping; leg cramps; shortness of breath; skin rash or itching; sweating, flushing, or increased sensitivity to heat; unusual weight loss; vomiting

Other side effects not listed above may also occur in some patients. If you notice any other effects, check with your doctor.

DIGITALIS MEDICINES Systemic

Some commonly used brand names are:

In the U.S.—
Crystodigin[1]   Lanoxin[2]
Lanoxicaps[2]

In Canada—
Digitaline[1]   Novodigoxin[2]
Lanoxin[2]

Note: For quick reference, the following digitalis medicines are numbered to match the corresponding brand names.

This information applies to the following medicines:

1. Digitoxin (di-ji-TOX-in)‡
2. Digoxin (di-JOX-in)‡

---

‡Generic name product may also be available in the U.S.

Description

Digitalis medicines are used to improve the strength and efficiency of the heart, or to control the rate and rhythm of the heartbeat. This leads to better blood circulation and reduced swelling of hands and ankles in patients with heart problems.

Although digitalis has been prescribed to help some patients lose weight, it should *never* be used in this way. When used improperly, digitalis can cause serious problems.

Digitalis medicines are available only with your doctor's prescription, in the following dosage forms:

Oral

Digitoxin
- Tablets (U.S. and Canada)

Digoxin
- Capsules (U.S.)
- Elixir (U.S. and Canada)
- Tablets (U.S. and Canada)

Parenteral

Digoxin
- Injection (U.S. and Canada)

Before Using This Medicine

In deciding to use a medicine, the risks of taking the medicine must be weighed against the good it will do. This is a decision you and your doctor will make. For digitalis medicines, the following should be considered:

Allergies—Tell your doctor if you have ever had any unusual or allergic reaction to digitalis medicines. Also tell your health care professional if you are allergic to any other substances, such as foods, preservatives, or dyes.

Pregnancy—Digitalis medicines pass from the mother to the fetus. However, studies on effects in pregnancy have not been done in either humans or animals. Make sure your doctor knows if you are pregnant or if you may become pregnant before taking digitalis medicines.

Breast-feeding—Although small amounts of digitalis medicines pass into breast milk, they have not been reported to cause problems in nursing babies.

Children—This medicine has been tested in children and, in effective doses, has not been shown to cause different side effects or problems than it does in adults. However, the dose is very different for babies and children, and it is important to follow your doctor's instructions exactly.

Older adults—Signs and symptoms of overdose may be especially likely to occur in elderly patients, who are usually more sensitive than younger adults to the effects of digitalis medicines.

Other medicines—Although certain medicines should not be used together at all, in other cases two different medicines may be used together even if an interaction might occur. In these cases, your doctor may want to change the dose, or other precautions may be necessary. When you are taking or receiving digitalis medicines it is especially important that your health care professional know if you are taking any of the following:

- Amiodarone (e.g., Cordarone)—May cause levels of digitalis medicines in the body to be higher than usual, which could lead to signs or symptoms of overdose
- Amphetamines or
- Appetite suppressants (diet pills) or
- Digitalis medicines (other) or other heart medicine or
- Medicine for asthma or other breathing problems or
- Medicine for colds, sinus problems, or hay fever or other allergies (including nose drops or sprays)—May increase the risk of heart rhythm problems
- Calcium channel blocking agents (bepridil [e.g., Bepadin, Vascor], diltiazem [e.g., Cardizem, Cardizem CD, Cardizem SR],

felodipine [e.g., Plendil], flunarizine [e.g., Sibelium], israd-
ipine [e.g., DynaCirc], nicardipine [e.g., Cardene], nifedi-
pine [e.g., Adalat, Procardia, Procardia XL], nimodipine
[e.g., Nimotop], verapamil [e.g., Calan, Calan SR, Isoptin,
Isoptin SR, Verelan]) or
- Propafenone—May cause levels of digitalis medicines in
  the body to be higher than usual, which could lead to signs
  or symptoms of overdose
- Cholestyramine (e.g., Questran) or
- Colestipol (e.g., Colestid) or
- Diarrhea medicine or
- Sucralfate or
- If your diet contains large amounts of fiber, such as bran—
  May decrease effects of digitalis medicines by keeping
  them from being absorbed into the body; digitalis medi-
  cines should be taken several hours apart from these
- Diuretics (water pills) or
- Other medicines that decrease the amount of potassium in
  the body (corticosteroids [cortisone-like medicines], alco-
  hol, capreomycin, corticotropin, insulin, laxatives, salicylates [aspirin], vitamin B;i1;i2, vitamin D [high doses])—
  These medicines can cause hypokalemia (low levels of
  potassium in the body), which can increase the unwanted
  effects of digitalis medicines
- Potassium-containing medicines or supplements—If levels
  of potassium in the body become too high, there is a serious risk of heart rhythm problems being caused by digitalis medicines
- Quinidine (e.g., Quinidex)—May cause levels of digitalis
  medicines in the body to be higher than usual, which could
  lead to signs or symptoms of overdose

Other medical problems—The presence of other medical
problems may affect the use of digitalis medicines. Make
sure you tell your doctor if you have any other medical
problems, especially:
- Heart disease or
- Lung disease (severe)—The heart may be more sensitive to
  the effects of digitalis medicines
- Heart rhythm problems—Digitalis glycosides may make
  certain heart rhythm problems worse

- Kidney disease or
- Liver disease—Effects may be increased because of slower removal of digitalis medicines from the body
- Thyroid disease—Patients with low or high thyroid gland activity may be more or less sensitive to the effects of digitalis glycosides

---

Proper Use of This Medicine

To keep your heart working properly, *take this medicine exactly as directed even though you may feel well*. Do not take more of it than your doctor ordered and do not miss any doses.

For patients taking the *liquid form of digoxin:*
- This medicine is to be taken by mouth even if it comes in a dropper bottle. The amount you should take is to be measured only with the specially marked dropper.

To help you remember to take your dose of medicine, try to take it at the same time every day.

Ask your doctor about checking your pulse rate. Then, while you are taking this medicine, check your pulse regularly. If it is much slower, or faster, than your usual rate (or less than 60 beats per minute), or if it changes in rhythm or force, check with your doctor. Such changes may mean that side effects are developing.

Dosing—When you are taking digitalis medicines, it is very important that you get the exact amount of medicine that you need. The dose of digitalis medicine will be different for different patients. Your doctor will determine the proper dose of digitalis medicine for you. *Follow your doctor's orders or the directions on the label.*

After you begin taking digitalis medicines, your doctor may sometimes check your blood level of digitalis medicine to find out if your dose needs to be changed. *Do not change your dose of digitalis medicine* unless your doctor tells you to do so.

The number of capsules or tablets or teaspoonfuls of solution that you take depends on the strength of the medicine.

Missed dose—If you miss a dose of this medicine, and you remember it within 12 hours, take it as soon as you remember. However, if you do not remember until later, do not take the missed dose at all and do not double the next one. Instead, go back to your regular dosing schedule. If you have any questions about this or if you miss doses for 2 or more days in a row, check with your doctor.

Storage—To store this medicine:

- Keep out of the reach of children.
- Store away from heat and direct light.
- Do not store in the bathroom, near the kitchen sink, or in other damp places. Heat or moisture may cause the medicine to break down.
- Keep the oral liquid form of this medicine from freezing.
- Do not keep outdated medicine or medicine no longer needed. Be sure that any discarded medicine is out of the reach of children.

Precautions While Using This Medicine

It is important that your doctor check your progress at regular visits to make sure the medicine is working properly. This will allow your doctor to make any changes in directions for taking it, if necessary.

Do not stop taking this medicine without first checking with your doctor. Stopping suddenly may cause a serious change in heart function.

Keep this medicine out of the reach of children. Digitalis medicines are a major cause of accidental poisoning in children.

Watch for signs and symptoms of overdose while you are taking digitalis medicine. Follow your doctor's directions carefully. The amount of this medicine needed to help most people is very close to the amount that could cause serious problems from overdose. Some early warning signs of overdose are loss of appetite, nausea, vomiting, diarrhea, or extremely slow heartbeat. In infants and small children, the earliest signs of overdose are changes in the rate and rhythm of the heartbeat. Children may not show the other symptoms as soon as adults.

Before having any kind of surgery (including dental surgery) or emergency treatment, tell the medical doctor or dentist in charge that you are using this medicine.

Your doctor may want you to carry a medical identification card or bracelet stating that you are taking this medicine.

Do not take any other medicine unless ordered by your doctor. Many over-the-counter (OTC) or nonprescription medicines contain ingredients that interfere with digitalis medicines or that may make your condition worse. These medicines include antacids; laxatives; asthma remedies; cold, cough, or sinus preparations; medicine for diarrhea; and reducing or diet medicines.

For patients taking the *tablet or capsule* form of this medicine:

- This medicine may look like other tablets or capsules you now take. It is very important that you do not get the medicines mixed up since this may have serious results. Ask your pharmacist for ways to avoid mix-ups with medicines that look alike.

Side Effects of This Medicine

Along with its needed effects, a medicine may cause some unwanted effects. Although not all of these side effects

may occur, if they do occur they may need medical attention.

Check with your doctor as soon as possible if any of the following side effects or symptoms of overdose occur:

Rare

Skin rash or hives

Signs and symptoms of overdose (in the order in which they may occur)

Loss of appetite; nausea or vomiting; lower stomach pain; diarrhea; unusual tiredness or weakness (extreme); slow or irregular heartbeat (may be fast heartbeat in children); blurred vision or ''yellow, green, or white vision'' (yellow, green, or white halo seen around objects); drowsiness; confusion or mental depression; headache; fainting

Note: Overdose symptoms in infants and small children may occur at first only as changes in the heartbeat rate or rhythm, while in adults and older children the first symptoms may be mostly stomach upset, stomach pain, loss of appetite, or unusually slow heartbeat.

Other side effects not listed above may also occur in some patients. If you notice any other effects, check with your doctor.

DIPYRIDAMOLE—Diagnostic
Systemic

Some commonly used brand names are:

In the U.S.—

Dipridacot   Persantine
I.V. Persantine

Generic name product may also be available.

In Canada—

Apo-Dipyridamole   Persantine
Novodipiradol

Description

Dipyridamole (dye-peer-ID-a-mole) is used as part of a medical test that shows how well blood is flowing to your heart. The test can show your doctor whether any of the blood vessels that bring blood to the heart are blocked or in danger of becoming blocked. Your doctor can then decide on the best treatment for you. Exercise (for example, walking on a treadmill) is usually used to give your doctor this information. Dipyridamole is used instead of exercise for people who are not able to exercise at all, or cannot exercise hard enough.

The dose of dipyridamole that is used to test how well blood is flowing to your heart will be different for different patients and depends on your body weight.

For information on other uses of dipyridamole, see Dipyridamole—Therapeutic (Systemic).

Dipyridamole is available only with your doctor's prescription, in the following dosage forms:

Oral
- Tablets (U.S. and Canada)

Parenteral
- Injection (U.S. and Canada)

Before Having This Test

In deciding to use a diagnostic test, any risks of the test must be weighed against the good it will do. This is a decision you and your doctor will make. Also, test results may be affected by other things. For dipyridamole, the following should be considered:

Allergies—Tell your doctor if you have ever had any unusual or allergic reaction to dipyridamole. Also tell your

health care professional if you are allergic to any other substances, such as foods, preservatives, or dyes.

Pregnancy—Although studies have not been done in pregnant women, dipyridamole has not been reported to cause birth defects or other problems. Also, dipyridamole has not been shown to cause birth defects or other problems in mice, rats, or rabbits given many times the maximum human dose.

Breast-feeding—Although dipyridamole passes into breast milk, it has not been reported to cause problems in nursing babies.

Children—This medicine has been tested only in adults, and there is no specific information comparing use of dipyridamole in children with use in other age groups.

Older adults—Dipyridamole for diagnostic use has been tested in older people. It has not been shown to cause different side effects or problems in older people than it does in younger adults.

Other medicines—Although certain medicines should not be used together at all, in other cases two different medicines may be used together even if an interaction might occur. In these cases, your doctor may want to change the dose, or other precautions may be necessary. Before you receive dipyridamole, it is especially important that your doctor knows if you are taking any of the following:

- Aminophylline (e.g., Somophyllin) or
- Caffeine (e.g., NoDoz) or
- Dyphylline (e.g., Lufyllin) or
- Oxtriphylline (e.g., Choledyl) or
- Theophylline (e.g., Somophyllin-T)—These medicines will interfere with the results of this test. Caffeine should not be taken for 8 to 12 hours before the test. It is present in many medicines (for example, stay-awake products, pain relievers, and medicines for relieving migraine headaches) and foods or beverages (for example, coffee, tea, colas or other soft drinks, cocoa, and chocolate). If you are not sure whether any medicine you are taking contains caffeine, check with your pharmacist

The other medicines listed here are used to treat asthma or other lung or breathing problems. They should not be taken for about 36 hours before the test. However, *do not stop taking the medicine on your own.* Instead, at least 3 or 4 days before the test, tell the doctor in charge of giving the test that you are taking the medicine. He or she can call the doctor who ordered the medicine for you, and together they will decide whether you should stop taking the medicine for a while

- Anticoagulants (blood thinners) or
- Aspirin or
- Carbenicillin by injection (e.g., Geopen) or
- Cefamandole (e.g., Mandol) or
- Cefoperazone (e.g., Cefobid) or
- Cefotetan (e.g., Cefotan) or
- Divalproex (e.g., Depakote) or
- Heparin or
- Inflammation or pain medicine, except narcotics, or
- Pentoxifylline (e.g., Trental) or
- Plicamycin (e.g., Mithracin) or
- Sulfinpyrazone (e.g., Anturane) or
- Ticarcillin (e.g., Ticar) or
- Ticlopidine (e.g., Ticlid) or
- Valproic acid (e.g., Depakene)—The chance of bleeding may be increased

Other medical problems—The presence of other medical problems may affect the use of dipyridamole. Make sure you tell your doctor if you have any other medical problems, especially:

- Asthma or history of or
- Chest pain—The chance of side effects may be increased
- Low blood pressure—Large amounts of dipyridamole can make your condition worse

---

Side Effects of This Medicine

Along with its needed effects, a medicine may cause some unwanted effects. Although not all of these side effects

may occur, if they do occur they may need medical attention.

While you are receiving dipyridamole, and for a while after you have received it, your doctor will closely follow its effects. If necessary, your doctor can give you a medicine that will stop any unwanted effects. *Tell your doctor right away if you notice any of the following side effects:*

More common

Chest pain

Less common or rare

Headache (severe and throbbing); shortness of breath, troubled breathing, tightness in chest, or wheezing

Other side effects may occur that usually do not need medical attention. These side effects may go away in a little while. However, check with your doctor if they continue or are bothersome:

More common

Dizziness or lightheadedness; headache

Less common

Flushing; nausea or vomiting

Other side effects not listed above may also occur in some patients. If you notice any other effects, check with your doctor.

DIPYRIDAMOLE—Therapeutic
Systemic

Some commonly used brand names are:

In the U.S.—

Dipridacot   Persantine

Generic name product may also be available.

In Canada—

Apo-Dipyridamole   Persantine
Novodipiradol

Description

Dipyridamole (dye-peer-ID-a-mole) is used to lessen the chance of stroke or other serious medical problems that may occur when a blood vessel is blocked by blood clots. It is given only when there is a larger-than-usual chance that these problems may occur. For example, it is given to people who have had diseased heart valves replaced by mechanical valves, because dangerous blood clots are especially likely to occur in these patients. Dipyridamole works by helping to prevent dangerous blood clots from forming.

Dipyridamole may also be used for other heart and blood conditions as determined by your doctor.

Dipyridamole is also sometimes used as part of a medical test that shows how well blood is flowing to your heart. For information on this use of dipyridamole, see Dipyridamole—Diagnostic (Systemic).

Dipyridamole is available only with your doctor's prescription, in the following dosage forms:

Oral
  • Tablets (U.S. and Canada)

Parenteral
  • Injection (Canada)

Before Using This Medicine

In deciding to use a medicine, the risks of taking the medicine must be weighed against the good it will do. This is a decision you and your doctor will make. For dipyridamole, the following should be considered:

Allergies—Tell your doctor if you have ever had any unusual or allergic reaction to dipyridamole. Also tell your

health care professional if you are allergic to any other substances, such as foods, preservatives, or dyes.

Pregnancy—Although studies have not been done in pregnant women, dipyridamole has not been reported to cause birth defects or other problems. Also, dipyridamole has not been shown to cause birth defects or other problems in mice, rats, or rabbits given many times the maximum human dose.

Breast-feeding—Although dipyridamole passes into breast milk, it has not been reported to cause problems in nursing babies.

Children—This medicine has been tested only in adults, and there is no specific information comparing use of dipyridamole in children with use in other age groups.

Older adults—Dipyridamole has not been studied specifically in older people taking the medicine regularly to prevent blood clots from forming. Although there is no specific information comparing this use of dipyridamole in the elderly with use in other age groups, it is not expected to cause different side effects or problems in older people than it does in younger adults.

Other medicines—Although certain medicines should not be used together at all, in other cases two different medicines may be used together even if an interaction might occur. In these cases, your doctor may want to change the dose, or other precautions may be necessary. When you are taking dipyridamole, it is especially important that your health care professional know if you are taking any of the following:

- Anticoagulants (blood thinners) or
- Aspirin or
- Carbenicillin by injection (e.g., Geopen) or
- Cefamandole (e.g., Mandol) or
- Cefoperazone (e.g., Cefobid) or
- Cefotetan (e.g., Cefotan) or
- Divalproex (e.g., Depakote) or

- Heparin or
- Inflammation or pain medicine, except narcotics, or
- Pentoxifylline (e.g., Trental) or
- Plicamycin (e.g., Mithracin) or
- Sulfinpyrazone (e.g., Anturane) or
- Ticarcillin (e.g., Ticar) or
- Ticlopidine (e.g., Ticlid) or
- Valproic acid (e.g., Depakene)—The chance of bleeding may be increased

Other medical problems—The presence of other medical problems may affect the use of dipyridamole. Make sure you tell your doctor if you have any other medical problems, especially:

- Chest pain—The chance of side effects may be increased
- Low blood pressure—Large amounts of dipyridamole can make your condition worse

---

Proper Use of This Medicine

This medicine works best when there is a constant amount in the blood. To help keep the amount constant, *dipyridamole must be taken in regularly spaced doses,* as ordered by your doctor.

This medicine works best when taken with a full glass (8 ounces) of water at least 1 hour before or 2 hours after meals. However, to lessen stomach upset, your doctor may want you to take the medicine with food or milk.

Dosing—The dose of dipyridamole will be different for different patients. *Follow your doctor's orders or the directions on the label.* The following information includes only the average doses of dipyridamole. *If your dose is different, do not change it* unless your doctor tells you to do so.

- For preventing blood clots:
  —For *oral* dosage form (tablets):
  - Adults—The usual dose is 75 to 100 milligrams

(mg) four times a day taken together with an anti-coagulant (blood-thinning) medicine.

- Children—Use and dose must be determined by your doctor.

Missed dose—If you miss a dose of this medicine, take it as soon as possble. However, if it is within 4 hours of your next scheduled dose, skip the missed dose and go back to your regular dosing schedule. Do not double doses.

Storage—To store this medicine:

- Keep out of the reach of children.
- Store away from heat and direct light.
- Do not store in the bathroom, near the kitchen sink, or in other damp places. Heat or moisture may cause the medicine to break down.
- Do not keep outdated medicine or medicine no longer needed. Be sure that any discarded medicine is out of the reach of children.

Precautions While Using This Medicine

Dipyridamole is sometimes used together with an anticoagulant (blood thinner) or aspirin. The combination of medicines may provide better protection against the formation of blood clots than any of the medicines used alone. However, the risk of bleeding may also be increased. To reduce the risk of bleeding:

- *Do not take aspirin, or any combination medicine containing aspirin, unless the same doctor who directed you to take dipyridamole also directs you to take aspirin.* This is especially important if you are taking an anticoagulant together with dipyridamole.
- If you have been directed to take aspirin together with dipyridamole, *take only the amount of aspirin ordered by your doctor.* If you need a medicine to relieve pain or a fever, your doctor may not want

you to take extra aspirin. It is a good idea to discuss this with your doctor, so that you will know ahead of time what medicine to take.

• Your doctor should check your progress at regular visits.

Tell all medical doctors and dentists you go to that you are taking dipyridamole, and whether or not you are taking an anticoagulant (blood thinner) or aspirin together with it.

Dizziness, lightheadedness, or fainting may occur, especially when you get up from a lying or sitting position. Getting up slowly may help. If this problem continues or gets worse, check with your doctor.

Side Effects of This Medicine

Along with its needed effects, a medicine may cause some unwanted effects. Although not all of these side effects may occur, if they do occur they may need medical attention.

Check with your doctor as soon as possible if the following side effect occurs shortly after you start taking this medicine:

Less common
    Skin rash or itching
Rare
    Chest pain or tightness in chest

Other side effects may occur that usually do not need medical attention. These side effects may go away during treatment as your body adjusts to the medicine. However, check with your doctor if they continue or are bothersome:

More common
    Dizziness
Less common
    Flushing; headache; nausea or vomiting; stomach cramping; weakness

Other side effects not listed above may also occur in some patients. If you notice any other effects, check with your doctor.

DISOPYRAMIDE Systemic

Some commonly used brand names are:

In the U.S.—
Norpace
Norpace CR

Generic name product may also be available.

In Canada—
Norpace   Rythmodan
Norpace CR   Rythmodan-LA

Description

Disopyramide (dye-soe-PEER-a-mide) is used to correct irregular heartbeats to a normal rhythm and to slow an overactive heart. This allows the heart to work more efficiently.

Disopyramide is available only with your doctor's prescription, in the following dosage forms:

Oral

- Capsules (U.S. and Canada)
- Extended-release capsules (U.S.)
- Extended-release tablets (Canada)

Parenteral

- Injection (Canada)

Before Using This Medicine

In deciding to use a medicine, the risks of taking the medicine must be weighed against the good it will do. This is a decision you and your doctor will make. For disopyramide, the following should be considered:

Allergies—Tell your doctor if you have ever had any unusual or allergic reaction to disopyramide. Also tell your health care professional if you are allergic to any other substance, such as foods, preservatives, or dyes.

Pregnancy—Disopyramide has not been studied in pregnant women. However, use of disopyramide in a small number of pregnant women seems to show that this medicine may cause contractions of the uterus. Studies in animals have shown that disopyramide increases the risk of miscarriages. Before taking this medicine, make sure your doctor knows if you are pregnant or if you may become pregnant.

Breast-feeding—Disopyramide passes into breast milk.

Children—This medicine has been tested in children and has not been shown to cause different side effects or problems than it does in adults.

Older adults—Some side effects, such as difficult urination and dry mouth, may be especially likely to occur in elderly patients, who are usually more sensitive than younger adults to the effects of disopyramide.

Other medicines—Although certain medicines should not be used together at all, in other cases two different medicines may be used together even if an interaction might occur. In these cases, your doctor may want to change the dose, or other precautions may be necessary. When you are taking disopyramide, it is especially important that your health care professional know if you are taking any of the following:

- Other heart medicine—Effects on the heart may be increased
- Pimozide (e.g., Orap)—Risk of heart rhythm problems may be increased

Other medical problems—The presence of other medical problems may affect the use of disopyramide. Make sure

you tell your doctor if you have any other medical problems, especially:

- Diabetes mellitus (sugar diabetes)—Disopyramide may cause low blood sugar
- Difficult urination or
- Enlarged prostate—Disopyramide may cause difficult urination
- Glaucoma (history of) or
- Myasthenia gravis—Disopyramide may make these conditions worse
- Kidney disease or
- Liver disease—Effects may be increased because of slower removal of disopyramide from the body

---

Proper Use of This Medicine

Take disopyramide exactly as directed by your doctor even though you may feel well. Do not take more medicine than ordered.

For patients taking the *extended-release capsules:*
- Swallow the capsule whole without breaking, crushing, or chewing.

For patients taking the *extended-release tablets:*
- Do not crush or chew the tablet.

This medicine works best when there is a constant amount in the blood. *To help keep the amount constant, do not miss any doses. Also, it is best to take the doses at evenly spaced times day and night.* For example, if you are to take 4 doses a day, the doses should be spaced about 6 hours apart. If this interferes with your sleep or other daily activities, or if you need help in planning the best times to take your medicine, check with your health care professional.

Dosing—The dose of disopyramide will be different for different patients. *Follow your doctor's orders or the di-*

rections on the label. The following information includes only the average doses of disopyramide. *If your dose is different, do not change it* unless your doctor tells you to do so.

The number of tablets or capsules that you take depends on the strength of the medicine.

- For *treatment* of arrhythmias:

    —For *short-acting oral* dosage forms (capsules):

    - Adults—300 milligrams (mg) for the first dose. Then 100 to 150 mg taken every six to eight hours.

    - Children—Dose is based on body weight and age. It must be determined by your doctor. The dose is usually 6 to 30 mg per kilogram (kg) of body weight (2.73 to 13.64 mg per pound) per day. This dose is evenly divided and taken every six hours.

    —For *long-acting oral* dosage forms (extended-release capsules or tablets):

    - Adults—200 or 300 mg every twelve hours.

    - Children—Use is not recommended.

    —For *injection* dosage form:

    - Adults—

        —*First few doses:* Dose is based on body weight and must be determined by your doctor. It is usually 2 mg per kg of body weight (0.91 mg per pound) injected in three divided doses, or, 2 mg per kg of body weight (0.91 mg per pound) infused over fifteen minutes.

        —*Dose following first few doses:* Dose is based on body weight and must be determined by your doctor. It is usually 0.4 mg per kg of body weight (0.18 mg per pound) per hour given for up to twenty-four hours.

    - Children—Use is not recommended.

Missed dose—*If you miss a dose of this medicine, take it as soon as possible unless the next scheduled dose is in less than 4 hours.* If you do not remember until later, skip the missed dose and go back to your regular dosing schedule. Do not double doses.

Storage—To store this medicine:

- Keep out of the reach of children.
- Store away from heat and direct light.
- Do not store in the bathroom, near the kitchen sink, or in other damp places. Heat or moisture may cause the medicine to break down.
- Do not keep outdated medicine or medicine no longer needed. Be sure that any discarded medicine is out of the reach of children.

Precautions While Using This Medicine

Your doctor should check your progress at regular visits to make sure the medicine is working properly.

Do not stop taking this medicine without first checking with your doctor. Stopping suddenly may cause a serious change in heart function.

Dizziness, lightheadedness, or fainting may occur, especially when you get up from a lying or sitting position. This is due to lowered blood pressure. Getting up slowly may help. This effect does not occur often at doses of disopyramide usually used; however, *make sure you know how you react to this medicine before you drive, use machines, or do anything else that could be dangerous if you are not alert.* If the problem continues or gets worse, check with your doctor.

Avoid alcoholic beverages until you have discussed their use with your doctor. Alcohol may make the low blood sugar effect worse and/or increase the possibility of dizziness or fainting.

Disopyramide may cause hypoglycemia (low blood sugar) in some people. Patients with congestive heart disease or diabetes especially should be aware of the signs of hypoglycemia. (See Side Effects of This Medicine.) If these signs appear, eat or drink a food containing sugar and call your doctor right away.

This medicine may cause blurred vision or other vision problems. If any of these occur, *do not drive, use machines, or do anything else that could be dangerous if you are not able to see well.*

Disopyramide may cause dryness of the mouth, nose, and throat. For temporary relief of mouth dryness, use sugarless candy or gum, melt bits of ice in your mouth, or use a saliva substitute. However, if dry mouth continues for more than 2 weeks, check with your medical doctor or dentist. Continuing dryness of the mouth may increase the chance of dental disease, including tooth decay, gum disease, and fungus infections.

This medicine will often make you sweat less, allowing your body temperature to increase. *Use extra care not to become overheated during exercise or hot weather while you are taking this medicine,* since overheating could possibly result in heat stroke.

Side Effects of This Medicine

Along with its needed effects, a medicine may cause some unwanted effects. Although not all of these side effects may occur, if they do occur they may need medical attention.

Check with your doctor as soon as possible if any of the following side effects occur:

More common
   Difficult urination

Less common

Chest pains; dizziness, lightheadedness, or fainting; fast or slow heartbeat; muscle weakness; shortness of breath (unexplained); swelling of feet or lower legs; weight gain (rapid)

Rare

Eye pain; mental depression; sore throat and fever; yellow eyes or skin

Signs and symptoms of hypoglycemia (low blood sugar)

Anxious feeling; chills; cold sweats; confusion; cool, pale skin; drowsiness; fast heartbeat; headache; hunger (excessive); nausea; nervousness; shakiness; unsteady walk; unusual tiredness or weakness

Other side effects may occur that usually do not need medical attention. These side effects may go away during treatment as your body adjusts to the medicine. However, check with your health care professional if any of the following side effects continue or are bothersome:

More common

Dryness of mouth and throat

Less common

Bloating or stomach pain; blurred vision; constipation; decreased sexual ability; dry eyes and nose; frequent urge to urinate; loss of appetite

Other side effects not listed above may also occur in some patients. If you notice any other effects, check with your doctor.

DIURETICS, LOOP   Systemic

Some commonly used brand names are:

In the U.S.—

Bumex[1]	Lasix[3]
Edecrin[2]	Myrosemide[3]

In Canada—

Apo-Furosemide[3]	Edecrin[2]

In Canada (cont'd)—
Furoside[3]   Novosemide[3]
Lasix[3]   Uritol[3]
Lasix Special[3]

Note: For quick reference, the following loop diuretics are numbered to match the corresponding brand names.

This information applies to the following medicines:

1. Bumetanide (byoo-MET-a-nide)[†][‡]
2. Ethacrynic Acid (eth-a-KRIN-ik AS-id)
3. Furosemide (fur-OH-se-mide)[‡][§]

[†]Not commercially available in Canada.
[‡]Generic name product may also be available in the U.S.
[§]Generic name product may also be available in Canada.

Description

Loop diuretics are given to help reduce the amount of water in the body. They work by acting on the kidneys to increase the flow of urine.

Furosemide is also used to treat high blood pressure (hypertension) in those patients who are not helped by other medicines or in those patients who have kidney problems.

High blood pressure adds to the workload of the heart and arteries. If it continues for a long time, the heart and arteries may not function properly. This can damage the blood vessels of the brain, heart, and kidneys, resulting in a stroke, heart failure, or kidney failure. High blood pressure may also increase the risk of heart attacks. These problems may be less likely to occur if blood pressure is controlled.

Loop diuretics may also be used for other conditions as determined by your doctor.

This medicine is available only with your doctor's prescription, in the following dosage forms:

Oral

Bumetanide
• Tablets (U.S.)

Ethacrynic Acid
- Oral solution (U.S. and Canada)
- Tablets (U.S. and Canada)

Furosemide
- Oral solution (U.S. and Canada)
- Tablets (U.S. and Canada)

Parenteral

Bumetanide
- Injection (U.S.)

Ethacrynic Acid
- Injection (U.S. and Canada)

Furosemide
- Injection (U.S. and Canada)

Before Using This Medicine

In deciding to use a medicine, the risks of taking the medicine must be weighed against the good it will do. This is a decision you and your doctor will make. For loop diuretics, the following should be considered:

Allergies—Tell your doctor if you have ever had any unusual or allergic reaction to bumetanide, ethacrynic acid, furosemide, sulfonamides (sulfa drugs), or thiazide diuretics (water pills). Also tell your health care professional if you are allergic to any other substances, such as foods, preservatives, or dyes.

Pregnancy—Studies have not been done in pregnant women. However, studies in animals have shown this medicine to cause harmful effects.

In general, diuretics are not useful for normal swelling of feet and hands that occurs during pregnancy. Diuretics should not be taken during pregnancy unless recommended by your doctor.

Breast-feeding—These medicines have not been reported to cause problems in nursing babies. Furosemide passes into breast milk; it is not known whether bumetanide or ethacrynic acid passes into breast milk.

Children—Although there is no specific information comparing the use of loop diuretics in children with use in any other age group, these medicines are not expected to cause different side effects in children than they do in adults.

Older adults—Dizziness, lightheadedness, or signs of too much potassium loss may be more likely to occur in the elderly, who are more sensitive to the effects of this medicine. Elderly patients may also be more likely to develop blood clots.

Other medicines—Although certain medicines should not be used together at all, in other cases two different medicines may be used together even if an interaction might occur. In these cases, your doctor may want to change the dose, or other precautions may be necessary. When you are taking loop diuretics, it is especially important that your health care professional know if you are taking *any* other medicines.

Other medical problems—The presence of other medical problems may affect the use of loop diuretics. Make sure you tell your doctor if you have any other medical problems, especially:

- Diabetes mellitus (sugar diabetes)—Loop diuretics may increase the amount of sugar in the blood
- Gout or
- Hearing problems or
- Pancreatitis (inflammation of the pancreas)—Loop diuretics may make these conditions worse
- Heart attack, recent—Use of loop diuretics after a recent heart attack may increase the chance of side effects
- Kidney disease (severe) or
- Liver disease—Higher blood levels of the loop diuretic may occur, which may increase the chance of side effects
- Lupus erythematosus (history of)—Ethacrynic acid and furosemide may make this condition worse

Proper Use of This Medicine

This medicine may cause you to have an unusual feeling of tiredness when you begin to take it. You may also notice an increase in the amount of urine or in your frequency of urination. After you have taken the medicine for a while, these effects should lessen. In general, to keep the increase in urine from affecting your sleep:

- If you are to take a single dose a day, take it in the morning after breakfast.
- If you are to take more than one dose a day, take the last dose no later than 6 p.m., unless otherwise directed by your doctor.

However, it is best to plan your dose or doses according to a schedule that will least affect your personal activities and sleep. Ask your health care professional to help you plan the best time to take this medicine.

To help you remember to take your medicine, try to get into the habit of taking it at the same time each day.

For patients taking the *oral liquid form* of furosemide:

- This medicine is to be taken by mouth even if it comes in a dropper bottle. If this medicine does not come in a dropper bottle, use a specially marked measuring spoon or other device to measure each dose accurately, since the average household teaspoon may not hold the right amount of liquid.

For patients taking this medicine for *high blood pressure:*

- In addition to the use of the medicine your doctor has prescribed, appropriate treatment for your high blood pressure may include weight control and care in the types of foods you eat, especially foods high in sodium. Your doctor will tell you which factors are most important for you. You should check with your doctor before changing your diet.
- Many patients who have high blood pressure will not

notice any signs of the problem. In fact, many may feel normal. It is very important that you *take your medicine exactly as directed* and that you keep your appointments with your doctor even if you feel well.

• Remember that this medicine will not cure your high blood pressure, but it does help control it. Therefore, you must continue to take it as directed if you expect to lower your blood pressure and keep it down. *You may have to take high blood pressure medicine for the rest of your life.* If high blood pressure is not treated, it can cause serious problems such as heart failure, blood vessel disease, stroke, or kidney disease.

If this medicine upsets your stomach, it may be taken with meals or milk. If stomach upset (nausea, vomiting, or stomach pain) continues or gets worse, or if you suddenly get severe diarrhea, check with your doctor.

Dosing—The dose of loop diuretics will be different for different patients. *Follow your doctor's orders or the directions on the label.* The following information includes only the average doses of loop diuretics. *If your dose is different, do not change it* unless your doctor tells you to do so.

The number of tablets or teaspoonfuls of solution that you take depends on the strength of the medicine. Also, *the number of doses you take each day, the time allowed between doses, and the length of time you take the medicine depend on the medical problem for which you are taking loop diuretics.*

For bumetanide

• For *oral* dosage form (tablets):

—To lower the amount of water in the body:

• Adults—0.5 to 2 milligrams (mg) once a day. Your doctor may increase your dose if needed.

• Children—Dose must be determined by your doctor.

- For *injection* dosage form:

  —To lower the amount of water in the body:

    - Adults—0.5 to 1 mg injected into a muscle or a vein every two to three hours as needed.

    - Children—Dose must be determined by your doctor.

For ethacrynic acid

- For *oral* dosage form (oral solution or tablets):

  —To lower the amount of water in the body:

    - Adults—50 to 200 milligrams (mg) a day. This may be taken as a single dose or divided into smaller doses.

    - Children—At first, 25 mg a day. Your doctor may increase your dose as needed.

- For *injection* dosage form:

  —To lower the amount of water in the body:

    - Adults—50 mg injected into a vein every two to six hours as needed.

    - Children—Dose is based on body weight and must be determined by your doctor. The usual dose is 1 mg per kilogram (kg) (0.45 mg per pound) of body weight injected into a vein.

For furosemide

- For *oral* dosage form (oral solution or tablets):

  —To lower the amount of water in the body:

    - Adults—At first, 20 to 80 milligrams (mg) once a day. Then, your doctor may increase your dose as needed. Your doctor may tell you to take a dose once a day, two or three times a day, or every other day.

    - Children—Dose is based on body weight and must be determined by your doctor. The usual dose is 2 mg per kilogram (kg) (0.91 mg per pound) of body weight for one dose. Then, your doctor may increase your dose every six to eight hours as needed.

—For high blood pressure:

- Adults—40 mg two times a day. Your doctor may increase your dose.

- For *injection* dosage form:

—To lower the amount of water in the body:

- Adults—At first, 20 to 40 mg injected into a muscle or a vein for one dose. Then, your doctor may increase your dose every two hours as needed. Once the medicine is working, the dose is injected into a muscle or a vein one or two times a day.

- Children—Dose is based on body weight and must be determined by your doctor. The usual dose is 1 mg per kg (0.45 mg per pound) of body weight injected into a muscle or a vein for one dose. Your doctor may increase your dose every two hours as needed.

—For very high blood pressure:

- Adults—40 to 200 mg injected into a vein.

Missed dose—If you miss a dose of this medicine, take it as soon as possible. However, if it is almost time for your next dose, skip the missed dose and go back to your regular dosing schedule. Do not double doses.

Storage—To store this medicine:

- Keep out of the reach of children.

- Store away from heat and direct light.

- Do not store in the bathroom, near the kitchen sink, or in other damp places. Heat or moisture may cause the medicine to break down.

- Keep the oral liquid form of this medicine from freezing.

- Do not keep outdated medicine or medicine no longer

needed. Be sure that any discarded medicine is out of the reach of children.

Precautions While Using This Medicine

It is important that your doctor check your progress at regular visits to make sure that this medicine is working properly.

This medicine may cause a loss of potassium from your body:

- To help prevent this, your doctor may want you to:

  —eat or drink foods that have a high potassium content (for example, orange or other citrus fruit juices), or

  —take a potassium supplement, or

  —take another medicine to help prevent the loss of the potassium in the first place.

- It is very important to follow these directions. Also, it is important not to change your diet on your own. This is more important if you are already on a special diet (as for diabetes), or if you are taking a potassium supplement or a medicine to reduce potassium loss. Extra potassium may not be necessary and, in some cases, too much potassium could be harmful.

To prevent the loss of too much water and potassium, tell your doctor if you become sick, especially with severe or continuing nausea and vomiting or diarrhea.

Before having any kind of surgery (including dental surgery) or emergency treatment, make sure the medical doctor or dentist in charge knows that you are taking this medicine.

Dizziness, lightheadedness, or fainting may occur, especially when you get up from a lying or sitting position. This is more likely to occur in the morning. Getting up

slowly may help. When you get up from lying down, sit on the edge of the bed with your feet dangling for 1 or 2 minutes. Then stand up slowly. If the problem continues or gets worse, check with your doctor.

The dizziness, lightheadedness, or fainting is also more likely to occur if you drink alcohol, stand for long periods of time, exercise, or if the weather is hot. *While you are taking this medicine, be careful to limit the amount of alcohol you drink. Also, use extra care during exercise or hot weather or if you must stand for long periods of time.*

For *diabetic patients:*
• This medicine may affect blood sugar levels. While you are using this medicine, be especially careful in testing for sugar in your blood or urine.

For patients taking this medicine for *high blood pressure:*
• *Do not take other medicines unless they have been discussed with your doctor.* This especially includes over-the-counter (nonprescription) medicines for appetite control, asthma, colds, cough, hay fever, or sinus problems, since they may tend to increase your blood pressure.

For patients taking *furosemide:*
• Furosemide may cause your skin to be more sensitive to sunlight than it is normally. Exposure to sunlight, even for brief periods of time, may cause a skin rash, itching, redness or other discoloration of the skin, or a severe sunburn. When you begin taking this medicine:

—Stay out of direct sunlight, especially between the hours of 10:00 a.m. and 3:00 p.m., if possible.

—Wear protective clothing, including a hat. Also, wear sunglasses.

—Apply a sun block product that has a skin protection factor (SPF) of at least 15. Some patients may require a product with a higher SPF number, especially if they have a fair complexion. If you have any questions about this, check with your health care professional.

—Apply a sun block lipstick that has an SPF of at least 15 to protect your lips.

—Do not use a sunlamp or tanning bed or booth.

If you have a severe reaction from the sun, check with your doctor.

Side Effects of This Medicine

Along with its needed effects, a medicine may cause some unwanted effects. Although not all of these side effects may occur, if they do occur they may need medical attention.

Check with your doctor as soon as possible if any of the following side effects occur:

Rare

Black, tarry stools; blood in urine or stools; cough or hoarseness; fever or chills; joint pain; lower back or side pain; painful or difficult urination; pinpoint red spots on skin; ringing or buzzing in ears or any loss of hearing—more common with ethacrynic acid; skin rash or hives; stomach pain (severe) with nausea and vomiting; unusual bleeding or bruising; yellow eyes or skin; yellow vision—for furosemide only

Signs and symptoms of too much potassium loss

Dryness of mouth; increased thirst; irregular heartbeat; mood or mental changes; muscle cramps or pain; nausea or vomiting; unusual tiredness or weakness; weak pulse

Other side effects may occur that usually do not need medical attention. These side effects may go away during treatment as your body adjusts to the medicine. However, check with your doctor if any of the following side effects continue or are bothersome:

More common

Dizziness or lightheadedness when getting up from a lying or sitting position

Less common or rare

Blurred vision; chest pain—with bumetanide only; confusion—with ethacrynic acid only; diarrhea—more common with ethacrynic acid; headache; increased sensitivity of skin to sunlight—with furosemide only; loss of appetite—more common with ethacrynic acid; nervousness—with ethacrynic acid only; premature ejaculation or difficulty in keeping an erection—with bumetanide only; redness or pain at place of injection; stomach cramps or pain

Other side effects not listed above may also occur in some patients. If you notice any other effects, check with your doctor.

Additional Information

Once a medicine has been approved for marketing for a certain use, experience may show that it is also useful for other medical problems. Although these uses are not included in product labeling, loop diuretics are used in certain patients with the following medical conditions:

- Hypercalcemia (too much calcium in the blood)
- Diagnostic aid for kidney disease

Other than the above information, there is no additional information relating to proper use, precautions, or side effects for these uses.

DIURETICS, POTASSIUM-SPARING   Systemic

Some commonly used brand names are:

In the U.S.—
Aldactone[2]   Midamor[1]
Dyrenium[3]

In Canada—
Aldactone[2]   Midamor[1]
Dyrenium[3]   Novospiroton[2]

Note: For quick reference, the following potassium-sparing diuretics are
      numbered to match the corresponding brand names.

This information applies to the following medicines:

1. Amiloride (a-MILL-oh-ride)‡
2. Spironolactone (speer-on-oh-LAK-tone)‡
3. Triamterene (trye-AM-ter-een)

---

‡Generic name product may also be available in the U.S.

Description

Potassium-sparing diuretics are commonly used to help
reduce the amount of water in the body. Unlike some
other diuretics, these medicines do not cause your body to
lose potassium.

Amiloride and spironolactone are also used to treat high
blood pressure (hypertension). High blood pressure adds
to the workload of the heart and arteries. If the condition
continues for a long time, the heart and arteries may not
function properly. This can damage the blood vessels of
the brain, heart, and kidneys, resulting in a stroke, heart
failure, or kidney failure. High blood pressure may also
increase the risk of heart attacks. These problems may be
less likely to occur if blood pressure is controlled.

Spironolactone is also used to help increase the amount of
potassium in the body when it is getting too low.

Potassium-sparing diuretics help to reduce the amount of
water in the body by acting on the kidneys to increase the
flow of urine. This also helps to lower blood pressure.

These medicines can also be used for other conditions as determined by your doctor.

Potassium-sparing diuretics are available only with your doctor's prescription, in the following dosage forms:

   Oral

   Amiloride
      • Tablets (U.S. and Canada)
   Spironolactone
      • Tablets (U.S. and Canada)
   Triamterene
      • Capsules (U.S.)
      • Tablets (Canada)

Before Using This Medicine

In deciding to use a medicine, the risks of taking the medicine must be weighed against the good it will do. This is a decision you and your doctor will make. For potassium-sparing diuretics, the following should be considered:

Allergies—Tell your doctor if you have ever had any unusual or allergic reaction to amiloride, spironolactone, or triamterene. Also tell your health care professional if you are allergic to any other substances, such as foods, preservatives, or dyes.

Pregnancy—Studies have not been done in pregnant women. However, this medicine has not been shown to cause birth defects or other problems in animals.

In general, diuretics are not useful for the normal swelling of feet and hands that occurs during pregnancy. Diuretics should not be taken during pregnancy unless recommended by your doctor.

Breast-feeding—Although amiloride, spironolactone, and triamterene may pass into breast milk, these medicines have not been reported to cause problems in nursing babies.

Children—This medicine has been tested in children and, in effective doses, has not been shown to cause different side effects or problems in children than it does in adults.

Older adults—Signs and symptoms of too much potassium are more likely to occur in the elderly, who are more sensitive than younger adults to the effects of this medicine.

Other medicines—Although certain medicines should not be used together at all, in other cases two different medicines may be used together even if an interaction might occur. In these cases, your doctor may want to change the dose, or other precautions may be necessary. When you are taking potassium-sparing diuretics, it is especially important that your health care professional know if you are taking any of the following:

- Angiotensin-converting enzyme (ACE) inhibitors (benazepril [e.g., Lotensin], captopril [e.g., Capoten], enalapril [e.g., Vasotec], fosinopril [e.g., Monopril], lisinopril [e.g., Prinivil, Zestril], quinapril [e.g., Accupril], ramipril [e.g., Altace]) or
- Cyclosporine (e.g., Sandimmune) or
- Potassium-containing medicines or supplements—Use with potassium-sparing diuretics may cause high blood levels of potassium, which may increase the chance of side effects
- Digoxin—Use with spironolactone may cause high blood levels of digoxin, which may increase the chance of side effects
- Lithium (e.g., Lithane)—Use with potassium-sparing diuretics may cause high blood levels of lithium, which may increase the chance of side effects

Other medical problems—The presence of other medical problems may affect the use of potassium-sparing diuretics. Make sure you tell your doctor if you have any other medical problems, especially:

- Diabetes mellitus (sugar diabetes) or

- Kidney disease or
- Liver disease—Higher blood levels of potassium may occur, which may increase the chance of side effects

- Gout or
- Kidney stones (history of)—Triamterene may make these conditions worse

- Menstrual problems or breast enlargement—Spironolactone may make these conditions worse

---

Proper Use of This Medicine

This medicine may cause you to have an unusual feeling of tiredness when you begin to take it. You may also notice an increase in the amount of urine or in your frequency of urination. After you have taken the medicine for a while, these effects should lessen. In general, to keep the increase in urine from affecting your sleep:

- If you are to take a single dose a day, take it in the morning after breakfast.
- If you are to take more than one dose a day, take the last dose no later than 6 p.m., unless otherwise directed by your doctor.

However, it is best to plan your dose or doses according to a schedule that will least affect your personal activities and sleep. Ask your health care professional to help you plan the best time to take this medicine.

To help you remember to take your medicine, try to get into the habit of taking it at the same time each day.

If this medicine upsets your stomach, it may be taken with meals or milk. If stomach upset (nausea, vomiting, stomach pain or cramps) continues, check with your doctor.

For patients taking this medicine for *high blood pressure:*

- In addition to the use of the medicine your doctor has prescribed, treatment for your high blood pressure may include weight control and care in the types of foods you eat, especially foods high in sodium. Your doctor will tell you which of these are most important for you. You should check with your doctor before changing your diet.

- Many patients who have high blood pressure will not notice any signs of the problem. In fact, many may feel normal. It is very important that you *take your medicine exactly as directed* and that you keep your appointments with your doctor even if you feel well.

- Remember that this medicine will not cure your high blood pressure, but it does help control it. Therefore, you must continue to take it as directed if you expect to lower your blood pressure and keep it down. *You may have to take high blood pressure medicine for the rest of your life.* If high blood pressure is not treated, it can cause serious problems such as heart failure, blood vessel disease, stroke, or kidney disease.

Dosing—The dose of potassium-sparing diuretics will be different for different patients. *Follow your doctor's orders or the directions on the label.* The following information includes only the average doses of potassium-sparing diuretics. *If your dose is different, do not change it* unless your doctor tells you to do so.

The number of capsules or tablets that you take depends on the strength of the medicine. Also, *the number of doses you take each day, the time allowed between doses, and the length of time you take the medicine depend on the medical problem for which you are taking potassium-sparing diuretics.*

For amiloride

- For *oral* dosage form (tablets):

  —For high blood pressure or to lower the amount of water in the body:

  - Adults—5 to 10 milligrams (mg) once a day.

  - Children—Dose must be determined by your doctor.

For spironolactone
- For *oral* dosage form (tablets):
  - —To lower the amount of water in the body:
    - Adults—At first, 25 to 200 milligrams (mg) a day. This is divided into two to four doses. Your doctor may increase your dose to 75 to 400 mg a day.
    - Children—Dose is based on body weight and must be determined by your doctor. The usual dose is 1 to 3 mg per kilogram (kg) (0.45 to 1.36 mg per pound) of body weight a day. The dose may be taken as a single dose or divided into two to four doses. Your doctor may increase your dose as needed.
  - —For high blood pressure:
    - Adults—At first, 50 to 100 milligrams (mg) a day. This may be taken as a single dose or divided into two to four doses. Your doctor may gradually increase your dose up to 200 mg a day.
    - Children—Dose is based on body weight and must be determined by your doctor. The usual dose is 1 to 3 mg per kg (0.45 to 1.36 mg per pound) of body weight a day. The dose may be taken as a single dose or divided into two to four doses. Your doctor may increase your dose as needed.
  - —To treat high aldosterone levels in the body:
    - Adults—100 to 400 mg a day. This is divided into two to four doses and taken until you have surgery. If you are not having surgery, your doses may be smaller.
  - —For detecting high aldosterone levels in the body:
    - Adults—400 mg a day, taken in two to four divided doses. Your doctor may want you to take this dose for as little as four days or as long as three to four weeks. Follow your doctor's instructions.

—To treat low potassium levels in the blood:

  • Adults—25 to 100 mg a day. This may be taken as a single dose or divided into two to four doses.

For triamterene

  • For *oral* dosage form (capsules or tablets):

    —To lower the amount of water in the body:

      • Adults—25 to 100 milligrams (mg) a day. Your doctor may gradually increase your dose.

      • Children—Dose is based on body weight and must be determined by your doctor. To start, the usual dose is 2 to 4 mg per kilogram (kg) (0.9 to 1.82 mg per pound) of body weight a day or every other day. This is divided into smaller doses. Your doctor may increase your dose as needed.

Missed dose—If you miss a dose of this medicine, take it as soon as possible. However, if it is almost time for your next dose, skip the missed dose and go back to your regular dosing schedule. Do not double doses.

Storage—To store this medicine:

  • Keep out of the reach of children.

  • Store away from heat and direct light.

  • Do not store in the bathroom, near the kitchen sink, or in other damp places. Heat or moisture may cause the medicine to break down.

  • Do not keep outdated medicine or medicine no longer needed. Be sure that any discarded medicine is out of the reach of children.

Precautions While Using This Medicine

It is important that your doctor check your progress at regular visits to make sure that this medicine is working properly.

This medicine does not cause a loss of potassium from your body as some other diuretics (water pills) do. Therefore, it is not necessary for you to get extra potassium in your diet, and too much potassium could even be harmful. Since salt substitutes and low-sodium milk may contain potassium, do not use them unless told to do so by your doctor.

Check with your doctor if you become sick and have severe or continuing nausea, vomiting, or diarrhea. These problems may cause you to lose additional water, which could be harmful, or to lose potassium, which could lessen the medicine's helpful effects.

Before having any kind of surgery (including dental surgery) or emergency treatment, tell the medical doctor or dentist in charge that you are taking this medicine.

Before you have any medical tests, tell the doctor in charge that you are taking this medicine. The results of some tests may be affected by this medicine.

For patients taking this medicine for *high blood pressure:*

• *Do not take other medicines unless they have been discussed with your doctor.* This especially includes over-the-counter (nonprescription) medicines for appetite control, asthma, colds, cough, hay fever, or sinus problems, since these medicines may tend to increase your blood pressure.

For patients taking *triamterene:*

• This medicine may cause your skin to be more sensitive to sunlight than it is normally. Exposure to sunlight, even for brief periods of time, may cause a skin rash, itching, redness or other discoloration of the skin, or a severe sunburn. When you begin taking this medicine:

—Stay out of direct sunlight, especially between the hours of 10:00 a.m. and 3:00 p.m., if possible.

—Wear protective clothing, including a hat. Also, wear sunglasses.

—Apply a sun block product that has a skin protection factor (SPF) of at least 15. Some patients may require a product with a higher SPF number, especially if they have a fair complexion. If you have any questions about this, check with your health care professional.

—Apply a sun block lipstick that has an SPF of at least 15 to protect your lips.

—Do not use a sunlamp or tanning bed or booth.

—If you have a severe reaction from the sun, check with your doctor.

Side Effects of This Medicine

In rats, spironolactone has been found to increase the risk of tumors. It is not known if spironolactone increases the chance of tumors in humans.

Along with its needed effects, a medicine may cause some unwanted effects. Although not all of these side effects may occur, if they do occur they may need medical attention.

Check with your doctor as soon as possible if any of the following side effects occur:

Rare

For amiloride, spironolactone, and triamterene

Skin rash or itching; shortness of breath

For spironolactone and triamterene only (in addition to effects listed above)

Cough or hoarseness; fever or chills; lower back or side pain; painful or difficult urination

For triamterene only (in addition to effects listed above)

Black, tarry stools; blood in urine or stools; bright red

tongue; burning, inflamed feeling in tongue; cracked corners of mouth; lower back pain (severe); pinpoint red spots on skin; unusual bleeding or bruising; weakness

Signs and symptoms of too much potassium

Confusion; irregular heartbeat; nervousness; numbness or tingling in hands, feet, or lips; shortness of breath or difficult breathing; unusual tiredness or weakness; weakness or heaviness of legs

Other side effects may occur that usually do not need medical attention. These side effects may go away during treatment as your body adjusts to the medicine. However, check with your doctor if any of the following side effects continue or are bothersome:

More common (less common with amiloride and triamterene)

Nausea and vomiting; stomach cramps and diarrhea

Less common

For amiloride, spironolactone, and triamterene

Dizziness; headache

For amiloride and spironolactone only (in addition to effects listed above)

Decreased sexual ability

For amiloride only (in addition to effects listed above)

Constipation; muscle cramps

For spironolactone only (in addition to effects listed above for spironolactone)

Breast tenderness in females; clumsiness; deepening of voice in females; enlargement of breasts in males; inability to have or keep an erection; increased hair growth in females; irregular menstrual periods; sweating

For triamterene only (in addition to effects listed above for triamterene)

Increased sensitivity of skin to sunlight

Signs and symptoms of too little sodium

Drowsiness; dryness of mouth; increased thirst; lack of energy

For *male patients:*

- Spironolactone sometimes causes enlarged breasts in males, especially when they take large doses of it for a long time. Breasts usually decrease in size gradually over several months after this medicine is stopped. If you have any questions about this, check with your doctor.

Other side effects not listed above may also occur in some patients. If you notice any other effects, check with your doctor.

Additional Information

Once a medicine has been approved for marketing for a certain use, experience may show that it is also useful for other medical problems. Although these uses are not included in product labeling, spironolactone is used in certain patients with the following medical conditions:

- Polycystic ovary syndrome
- Hirsutism, female (increased hair growth)

Other than the above information, there is no additional information relating to proper use, precautions, or side effects for these uses.

DIURETICS, POTASSIUM-SPARING, AND HYDROCHLOROTHIAZIDE Systemic

Some commonly used brand names are:

In the U.S.—

Aldactazide[2]	Moduretic[1]
Dyazide[3]	Spirozide[2]
Maxzide[3]	

Generic name product may also be available.

In Canada—

Aldactazide[2]   Moduret[1]
Apo-Triazide[3]   Novo-Spirozine[2]
Dyazide[3]   Novo-Triamzide[3]

Note: For quick reference, the following medicines are numbered to match the corresponding brand names.

This information applies to the following medicines:

1. Amiloride (a-MILL-oh-ride) and Hydrochlorothiazide (hye-droe-klor-oh-THYE-a-zide)‡
2. Spironolactone (speer-on-oh-LAK-tone) and Hydrochlorothiazide‡
3. Triamterene (trye-AM-ter-een) and Hydrochlorothiazide‡

---

‡Generic name product may also be available in the U.S.

Description

This medicine is a combination of two diuretics (water pills). It is commonly used to help reduce the amount of water in the body.

This combination is also used to treat high blood pressure (hypertension). High blood pressure adds to the workload of the heart and arteries. If it continues for a long time, the heart and arteries may not function properly. This can damage the blood vessels of the brain, heart, and kidneys, resulting in a stroke, heart failure, or kidney failure. High blood pressure may also increase the risk of heart attacks. These problems may be less likely to occur if blood pressure is controlled.

Diuretics help to reduce the amount of water in the body by acting on the kidneys to increase the flow of urine. This also helps to lower blood pressure.

This combination is also used to treat problems caused by too little potassium in the body.

This medicine is available only with your doctor's prescription, in the following dosage forms:

Oral

Amiloride and Hydrochlorothiazide
• Tablets (U.S. and Canada)

Spironolactone and Hydrochlorothiazide
* Tablets (U.S. and Canada)
Triamterene and Hydrochlorothiazide
* Capsules (U.S.)
* Tablets (U.S. and Canada)

Before Using This Medicine

In deciding to use a medicine, the risks of taking the medicine must be weighed against the good it will do. This is a decision you and your doctor will make. For potassium-sparing diuretics and hydrochlorothiazide, the following should be considered:

Allergies—Tell your doctor if you have ever had any unusual or allergic reaction to amiloride, spironolactone, triamterene, sulfonamides (sulfa drugs), bumetanide, furosemide, acetazolamide, dichlorphenamide, methazolamide, or to hydrochlorothiazide or any of the other thiazide diuretics. Also tell your health care professional if you are allergic to any other substances, such as foods, preservatives, or dyes.

Pregnancy—In general, diuretics are not useful for normal swelling of feet and hands that occurs during pregnancy. They should not be taken during pregnancy unless recommended by your doctor.

Breast-feeding—Hydrochlorothiazide and spironolactone pass into breast milk. It is not known whether amiloride or triamterene passes into breast milk. Hydrochlorothiazide may also decrease the flow of breast milk. Therefore, you should avoid use of potassium-sparing diuretic and hydrochlorothiazide combinations during the first month of breast-feeding.

Children—Studies on this combination medicine have been done only in adult patients, and there is no specific information comparing use of potassium-sparing diuretic and hydrochlorothiazide combinations in children with use in other age groups.

Older adults—Dizziness or lightheadedness and signs and symptoms of too much potassium in the body or too little potassium in the body may be more likely to occur in the elderly, who are more sensitive than younger adults to the effects of this medicine.

Other medicines—Although certain medicines should not be used together at all, in other cases two different medicines may be used together even if an interaction might occur. In these cases, your doctor may want to change the dose, or other precautions may be necessary. When you are taking potassium-sparing diuretics and hydrochlorothiazide, it is especially important that your health care professional know if you are taking any of the following:

- Angiotensin-converting enzyme (ACE) inhibitors (benazepril [e.g., Lotensin], captopril [e.g., Capoten], enalapril [e.g., Vasotec], fosinopril [e.g., Monopril], lisinopril [e.g., Prinivil, Zestril], quinapril [e.g., Accupril], ramipril [e.g., Altace]) or
- Cyclosporine (e.g., Sandimmune) or
- Potassium-containing medicines or supplements—Use with potassium-sparing diuretic and hydrochlorothiazide combinations may cause high blood levels of potassium, which may increase the chance of side effects
- Cholestyramine or
- Colestipol—Use with potassium-sparing diuretic and hydrochlorothiazide combinations may prevent the diuretic from working properly; take the diuretic at least 1 hour before or 4 hours after cholestyramine or colestipol
- Digitalis glycosides (heart medicine)—Use with diuretics may cause high blood levels of digoxin, which may increase the chance of side effects
- Lithium (e.g., Lithane)—Use with diuretics may cause high blood levels of lithium, which may increase the chance of side effects

Other medical problems—The presence of other medical problems may affect the use of potassium-sparing diuretics and hydrochlorothiazide. Make sure you tell your doctor if you have any other medical problems, especially:

- Diabetes mellitus (sugar diabetes) or
- Kidney disease or
- Liver disease—Higher blood levels of potassium may occur, which may increase the chance of side effects

- Gout (history of) or
- Kidney stones (history of)—Triamterene and hydrochlorothiazide combination may make these conditions worse

- Heart or blood vessel disease—These medicines may cause high cholesterol levels or high triglyceride levels

- Lupus erythematosus (history of) or
- Pancreatitis (inflammation of pancreas)—Potassium-sparing diuretic and hydrochlorothiazide combinations may make these conditions worse

- Menstrual problems in women or breast enlargement in men—Spironolactone and hydrochlorothiazide combination may make these conditions worse

---

Proper Use of This Medicine

This medicine may cause you to have an unusual feeling of tiredness when you begin to take it. You may also notice an increase in the amount of urine or in your frequency of urination. After you have taken the medicine for a while, these effects should lessen. In general, to keep the increase in urine from affecting your sleep:

- If you are to take a single dose a day, take it in the morning after breakfast.

- If you are to take more than one dose a day, take the last dose no later than 6 p.m., unless otherwise directed by your doctor.

However, it is best to plan your dose or doses according to a schedule that will least affect your personal activities and sleep. Ask your health care professional to help you plan the best time to take this medicine.

To help you remember to take your medicine, try to get into the habit of taking it at the same time each day.

If this medicine upsets your stomach, it may be taken with meals or milk. If stomach upset (nausea, vomiting, stomach pain, or cramps) continues, check with your doctor.

For patients taking this medicine for *high blood pressure:*

- In addition to the use of the medicine your doctor has prescribed, treatment for your high blood pressure may include weight control and care in the types of foods you eat, especially foods high in sodium. Your doctor will tell you which of these are most important for you. You should check with your doctor before changing your diet.

- Many patients who have high blood pressure will not notice any signs of the problem. In fact, many may feel normal. It is very important that you *take your medicine exactly as directed* and that you keep your appointments with your doctor even if you feel well.

- Remember that this medicine will not cure your high blood pressure, but it does help control it. Therefore, you must continue to take it as directed if you expect to lower your blood pressure and keep it down. *You may have to take high blood pressure medicine for the rest of your life.* If high blood pressure is not treated, it can cause serious problems such as heart failure, blood vessel disease, stroke, or kidney disease.

Dosing—The dose of potassium-sparing diuretic and hydrochlorothiazide combinations will be different for different patients. *Follow your doctor's orders or the directions on the label.* The following information includes only the average doses of potassium-sparing diuretic and hydrochlorothiazide combinations. *If your dose is different, do not change it* unless your doctor tells you to do so.

The number of capsules or tablets that you take depends on the strength of the medicine. Also, *the number of doses you take each day depends on the strength of the medicine*

*and the medical problem for which you are taking po-
tassium-sparing diuretic and hydrochlorothiazide combinations.*

For amiloride and hydrochlorothiazide combination

- For *oral* dosage form (tablets):

  —For high blood pressure or lowering the amount
  of water in the body:

  - Adults—1 or 2 tablets a day.
  - Children—Dose must be determined by your
    doctor.

For spironolactone and hydrochlorothiazide combination

- For *oral* dosage form (tablets):

  —For high blood pressure or lowering the amount
  of water in the body:

  - Adults—1 to 4 tablets a day.
  - Children—Dose is based on body weight and
    must be determined by your doctor.

For triamterene and hydrochlorothiazide combination

- For *oral* dosage form (capsules):

  —For high blood pressure or lowering the amount
  of water in the body:

  - Adults—1 or 2 capsules once a day.
  - Children—Dose must be determined by your
    doctor.

- For *oral* dosage form (tablets):

  —For high blood pressure or lowering the amount
  of water in the body:

  - Adults—1 to 4 tablets a day, depending on the
    strength of your tablet.
  - Children—Dose must be determined by your
    doctor.

Missed dose—If you miss a dose of this medicine, take
it as soon as possible. However, if it is almost time for
your next dose, skip the missed dose and go back to your
regular dosing schedule. Do not double doses.

Storage—To store this medicine:
- Keep out of the reach of children.
- Store away from heat and direct light.
- Do not store in the bathroom, near the kitchen sink, or in other damp places. Heat or moisture may cause the medicine to break down.
- Do not keep outdated medicine or medicine no longer needed. Be sure that any discarded medicine is out of the reach of children.

Precautions While Using This Medicine

It is important that your doctor check your progress at regular visits to make sure that this medicine is working properly.

This medicine may cause a loss or increase of potassium in your body. Your doctor may have special instructions about whether or not you need to eat or drink foods or beverages that have a high potassium content (for example, orange or other citrus fruit juices), take a potassium supplement, or use salt substitutes. Since too much potassium can be harmful, it is important not to change your diet on your own. Tell your doctor if you are already on a special diet (as for diabetes). Since salt substitutes and low-sodium milk may contain potassium, do not use them unless told to do so by your doctor. Check with your health care professional if you need a list of foods that are high in potassium or if you have any questions.

Check with your doctor if you become sick and have severe or continuing vomiting or diarrhea. These problems may cause you to lose additional water and potassium and lead to low blood pressure.

For *diabetic patients:*
- Hydrochlorothiazide (contained in this combination medicine) may raise blood sugar levels. While you

are taking this medicine, be especially careful in testing for sugar in your blood or urine.

Potassium-sparing diuretics and hydrochlorothiazide may cause your skin to be more sensitive to sunlight than it is normally. Exposure to sunlight, even for brief periods of time, may cause a skin rash, itching, redness or other discoloration of the skin, or a severe sunburn. When you begin taking this medicine:

- Stay out of direct sunlight, especially between the hours of 10:00 a.m. and 3:00 p.m., if possible.
- Wear protective clothing, including a hat. Also, wear sunglasses.
- Apply a sun block product that has a skin protection factor (SPF) of at least 15. Some patients may require a product with a higher SPF number, especially if they have a fair complexion. If you have any questions about this, check with your health care professional.
- Apply a sun block lipstick that has an SPF of at least 15 to protect your lips.
- Do not use a sunlamp or tanning bed or booth.

If you have a severe reaction from the sun, check with your doctor.

Before having any kind of surgery (including dental surgery) or emergency treatment, tell the medical doctor or dentist in charge that you are taking this medicine.

For patients taking *triamterene and hydrochlorothiazide combination:*

- Do not change brands of triamterene and hydrochlorothiazide without first checking with your doctor. Different products may not work the same way. If you refill your medicine and it looks different, check with your pharmacist.

For patients taking this medicine for *high blood pressure:*

- *Do not take other medicines unless they have been discussed with your doctor.* This especially includes over-the-counter (nonprescription) medicines for appetite control, asthma, colds, cough, hay fever, or sinus problems, since they may tend to increase your blood pressure.

Tell the doctor in charge that you are taking this medicine before you have any medical tests. The results of some tests may be affected by this medicine.

Side Effects of This Medicine

In rats, spironolactone has been found to increase the risk of development of tumors. However, the doses given were many times the dose of spironolactone given to humans. It is not known whether spironolactone causes tumors in humans.

Along with its needed effects, a medicine may cause some unwanted effects. Although not all of these side effects may occur, if they do occur they may need medical attention.

Check with your doctor as soon as possible if any of the following side effects occur:

Rare

Black, tarry stools; blood in urine or stools; cough or hoarseness; fever or chills; joint pain; lower back or side pain; painful or difficult urination; pinpoint red spots on skin; skin rash or hives; stomach pain (severe) with nausea and vomiting; unusual bleeding or bruising; yellow eyes or skin

Signs and symptoms of changes in potassium

Confusion; dryness of mouth; increased thirst; irregular heartbeat; mood or mental changes; muscle cramps or pain; numbness or tingling in hands, feet, or lips; shortness of breath or difficulty breathing; unusual tiredness or weakness; weak pulse; weakness or heaviness of legs

Reported for triamterene only (rare)

Bright red tongue; burning, inflamed feeling in tongue; cracked corners of mouth

Other side effects may occur that usually do not need medical attention. These side effects may go away during treatment as your body adjusts to the medicine. However, check with your doctor if any of the following side effects continue or are bothersome:

More common (less common with triamterene)

Loss of appetite; nausea and vomiting; stomach cramps and diarrhea; upset stomach

Less common

Decreased sexual ability; dizziness or lightheadedness when getting up from a lying or sitting position; headache; increased sensitivity of skin to sunlight

Reported for amiloride only (less common)

Constipation

Reported for spironolactone only (less common)

Breast tenderness in females; deepening of voice in females; enlargement of breasts in males; increased hair growth in females; irregular menstrual periods; sweating

Spironolactone sometimes causes enlarged breasts in males, especially when they take large doses of it for a long time. Breasts usually decrease in size gradually over several months after this medicine is stopped. If you have any questions about this, check with your doctor.

Other side effects not listed above may also occur in some patients. If you notice any other effects, check with your doctor.

DIURETICS, THIAZIDE   Systemic

Some commonly used brand names are:

In the U.S.—

Anhydron[5]	Diuril[3]
Aquatensen[8]	Enduron[8]
Diucardin[7]	Esidrix[6]
Diulo[9]	Exna[2]

In the U.S. (cont'd)—

Hydrex[2]
Hydro-chlor[6]
Hydro-D[6]
HydroDIURIL[6]
Hydromox[11]
Hygroton[4]
Metahydrin[12]
Mykrox[9]

Naqua[12]
Naturetin[1]
Oretic[6]
Renese[10]
Saluron[7]
Thalitone[4]
Trichlorex[12]
Zaroxolyn[9]

In Canada—

Apo-Chlorthalidone[4]
Apo-Hydro[6]
Diuchlor H[6]
Duretic[8]
HydroDIURIL[6]
Hygroton[4]
Naturetin[1]

Neo-Codema[6]
Novo-Hydrazide[6]
Novo-Thalidone[4]
Uridon[4]
Urozide[6]
Zaroxolyn[9]

Note: For quick reference, the following thiazide diuretics are numbered to match the corresponding brand names.

This information applies to the following medicines:

1. Bendroflumethiazide (ben-droe-floo-meth-EYE-a-zide)
2. Benzthiazide (benz-THYE-a-zide)†‡
3. Chlorothiazide (klor-oh-THYE-a-zide)†‡
4. Chlorthalidone (klor-THAL-i-doan)‡§
5. Cyclothiazide (sye-kloe-THYE-a-zide)†
6. Hydrochlorothiazide (hye-droe-klor-oh-THYE-a-zide)‡§
7. Hydroflumethiazide (hye-droe-floo-meth-EYE-a-zide)†‡
8. Methyclothiazide (meth-ee-kloe-THYE-a-zide)‡
9. Metolazone (me-TOLE-a-zone)
10. Polythiazide (pol-i-THYE-a-zide)†
11. Quinethazone (kwin-ETH-a-zone)†
12. Trichlormethiazide (trye-klor-meth-EYE-a-zide)†‡

---

†Not commercially available in Canada.
‡Generic name product may also be available in the U.S.
§Generic name product may also be available in Canada.

Description

Thiazide or thiazide-like diuretics are commonly used to treat high blood pressure (hypertension). High blood pressure adds to the workload of the heart and arteries. If it continues for a long time, the heart and arteries may not function properly. This can damage the blood vessels of the brain, heart, and kidneys, resulting in a stroke, heart failure, or kidney failure. High blood pressure may also increase the risk of heart attacks. These problems may be less likely to occur if blood pressure is controlled.

Thiazide diuretics are also used to help reduce the amount of water in the body by increasing the flow of urine. They may also be used for other conditions as determined by your doctor.

Thiazide diuretics are available only with your doctor's prescription, in the following dosage forms:

Oral

Bendroflumethiazide
- Tablets (U.S. and Canada)

Benzthiazide
- Tablets (U.S.)

Chlorothiazide
- Oral suspension (U.S.)
- Tablets (U.S.)

Chlorthalidone
- Tablets (U.S. and Canada)

Cyclothiazide
- Tablets (U.S.)

Hydrochlorothiazide
- Oral solution (U.S.)
- Tablets (U.S. and Canada)

Hydroflumethiazide
- Tablets (U.S.)

Methyclothiazide
- Tablets (U.S. and Canada)

Metolazone
- Tablets (U.S. and Canada)

Polythiazide
- Tablets (U.S.)

Quinethazone
- Tablets (U.S.)

Trichlormethiazide
- Tablets (U.S.)

Parenteral

Chlorothiazide
- Injection (U.S.)

Before Using This Medicine

In deciding to use a medicine, the risks of taking the medicine must be weighed against the good it will do. This is a decision you and your doctor will make. For thiazide diuretics, the following should be considered:

Allergies—Tell your doctor if you have ever had any unusual or allergic reaction to sulfonamides (sulfa drugs), bumetanide, furosemide, acetazolamide, dichlorphenamide, methazolamide, or to any of the thiazide diuretics. Also tell your health care professional if you are allergic to any other substances, such as foods, preservatives, or dyes.

Pregnancy—When this medicine is used during pregnancy, it may cause side effects including jaundice, blood problems, and low potassium in the newborn infant. In addition, although this medicine has not been shown to cause birth defects or other problems in animals, studies have not been done in humans.

In general, diuretics are not useful for normal swelling of feet and hands that occurs during pregnancy. They should not be taken during pregnancy unless recommended by your doctor.

Breast-feeding—Thiazide diuretics pass into breast milk. These medicines may also decrease the flow of breast milk. Therefore, you should avoid use of thiazide diuretics during the first month of breast-feeding.

Children—Although there is no specific information comparing the use of thiazide diuretics in children with use in other age groups, these medicines are not expected to cause different side effects or problems in children than they do in adults. However, extra caution may be necessary in infants with jaundice, because these medicines can make the condition worse.

Older adults—Dizziness or lightheadedness and signs of too much potassium loss may be more likely to occur in the elderly, who are more sensitive than younger adults to the effects of thiazide diuretics.

Other medicines—Although certain medicines should not be used together at all, in other cases two different medicines may be used together even if an interaction might occur. In these cases, your doctor may want to change the dose, or other precautions may be necessary. When you are taking thiazide diuretics, it is especially important that your health care professional know if you are taking any of the following:

- Cholestyramine or
- Colestipol—Use with thiazide diuretics may prevent the diuretic from working properly; take the diuretic at least 1 hour before or 4 hours after cholestyramine or colestipol
- Digitalis glycosides (heart medicine)—Use with thiazide diuretics may cause high blood levels of digoxin, which may increase the chance of side effects
- Lithium (e.g., Lithane)—Use with thiazide diuretics may cause high blood levels of lithium, which may increase the chance of side effects

Other medical problems—The presence of other medical problems may affect the use of thiazide diuretics. Make sure you tell your doctor if you have any other medical problems, especially:

- Diabetes mellitus (sugar diabetes)—Thiazide diuretics may increase the amount of sugar in the blood
- Gout (history of) or
- Lupus erythematosus (history of) or
- Pancreatitis (inflammation of the pancreas)—Thiazide diuretics may make these conditions worse
- Heart or blood vessel disease—Thiazide diuretics may cause high cholesterol levels or high triglyceride levels
- Liver disease or
- Kidney disease (severe)—Higher blood levels of the thiazide diuretic may occur, which may prevent the thiazide diuretic from working properly

Proper Use of This Medicine

This medicine may cause you to have an unusual feeling of tiredness when you begin to take it. You may also notice an increase in the amount of urine or in your frequency of urination. After you have taken the medicine for a while, these effects should lessen. In general, to keep the increase in urine from affecting your sleep:

- If you are to take a single dose a day, take it in the morning after breakfast.

- If you are to take more than one dose a day, take the last dose no later than 6 p.m., unless otherwise directed by your doctor.

However, it is best to plan your dose or doses according to a schedule that will least affect your personal activities and sleep. Ask your health care professional to help you plan the best time to take this medicine.

To help you remember to take your medicine, try to get into the habit of taking it at the same time each day.

For patients taking this medicine for *high blood pressure:*

- In addition to the use of the medicine your doctor has prescribed, appropriate treatment for your high blood pressure may include weight control and care in the types of foods you eat, especially foods high in sodium. Your doctor will tell you which factors are most important for you. You should check with your doctor before changing your diet.

- Many patients who have high blood pressure will not notice any signs of the problem. In fact, many may feel normal. It is very important that you *take your medicine exactly as directed* and that you keep your appointments with your doctor even if you feel well.

- Remember that this medicine will not cure your high blood pressure but it does help control it. Therefore, you must continue to take it as directed if you expect to lower your blood pressure and keep it down. *You*

*may have to take high blood pressure medicine for
the rest of your life.* If high blood pressure is not
treated, it can cause serious problems such as heart
failure, blood vessel disease, stroke, or kidney
disease.

For patients taking the *oral liquid form of hydrochlorothiazide,* which comes in a dropper bottle:

- This medicine is to be taken by mouth. The amount
  you should take is to be measured only with the specially marked dropper.

Dosing—The dose of these medicines will be different
for different patients. *Follow your doctor's orders or the
directions on the label.* The following information includes
only the average doses of these medicines. *If your dose is
different, do not change it* unless your doctor tells you to
do so.

The number of tablets or teaspoonfuls of solution or suspension that you take depends on the strength of the medicine. Also, *the number of doses you take each day, the
time allowed between doses, and the length of time you
take the medicine depend on the medical problem for
which you are taking thiazide diuretics.*

For bendroflumethiazide

- For *oral* dosage form (tablets):

  —To lower the amount of water in the body:

    - Adults—At first, 2.5 to 10 milligrams (mg) one
      or two times a day. Then, your doctor may lower
      your dose to 2.5 to 5 mg once a day. Or, your
      doctor may want you to take this dose once every
      other day or once a day for only three to five
      days out of the week.

    - Children—Dose is based on body weight and
      must be determined by your doctor. The usual
      dose is 50 to 100 micrograms (mcg) per kilogram
      (kg) (22.7 to 45.4 mcg per pound) of body weight
      once a day.

—For high blood pressure:

  • Adults—2.5 to 20 mg a day. This may be taken as a single dose or divided into two doses.

  • Children—Dose is based on body weight and must be determined by your doctor. The usual dose is 50 to 400 mcg per kg (22.7 to 181.8 mcg per pound) of body weight a day. This may be taken as a single dose or divided into two doses.

For benzthiazide

  • For *oral* dosage form (tablets):

    —To lower the amount of water in the body:

      • Adults—25 to 100 milligrams (mg) two times a day. Or, your doctor may want you to take this dose once every other day or once a day for only three to five days out of the week.

      • Children—Dose is based on body weight and must be determined by your doctor.

    —For high blood pressure:

      • Adults—50 to 100 mg a day. This may be taken as a single dose or divided into two doses.

      • Children—Dose is based on body weight and must be determined by your doctor.

For chlorothiazide

  • For *oral* dosage forms (oral suspension or tablets):

    —To lower the amount of water in the body:

      • Adults—250 milligrams (mg) every six to twelve hours.

      • Children—Dose is based on body weight and must be determined by your doctor.

    —For high blood pressure:

      • Adults—250 to 1000 mg a day. This may be taken as a single dose or divided into smaller doses.

      • Children—Dose is based on body weight and must be determined by your doctor.

- For *injection* dosage form:
    - —To lower the amount of water in the body:
        - Adults—250 mg injected into a vein every six to twelve hours.
        - Children—Use and dose must be determined by your doctor.
    - —For high blood pressure:
        - Adults—500 to 1000 mg a day, injected into a vein. This dose may be given as a single dose or divided into two doses.
        - Children—Use and dose must be determined by your doctor.

For chlorthalidone
- For *oral* dosage form (tablets):
    - —To lower the amount of water in the body:
        - Adults—25 to 100 milligrams (mg) once a day. Or, 100 to 200 mg taken once every other day or once a day for three days out of the week.
        - Children—Dose is based on body weight and must be determined by your doctor.
    - —For high blood pressure:
        - Adults—25 to 100 mg once a day.
        - Children—Dose is based on body weight and must be determined by your doctor.

For cyclothiazide
- For *oral* dosage form (tablets):
    - —To lower the amount of water in the body:
        - Adults—1 to 2 milligrams (mg) once a day. Or, your doctor may want you to take this dose once every other day or once a day for only two or three days out of the week.
        - Children—Dose is based on body weight and must be determined by your doctor.
    - —For high blood pressure:
        - Adults—2 mg once a day.

• Children—Dose is based on body weight and must be determined by your doctor.

For hydrochlorothiazide

• For *oral* dosage forms (oral solution or tablets):

—To lower the amount of water in the body:

• Adults—25 to 100 milligrams (mg) one or two times a day. Or, your doctor may want you to take this dose once every other day or once a day for three to five days out of the week.

• Children—Dose is based on body weight and must be determined by your doctor.

—For high blood pressure:

• Adults—25 to 100 mg a day. This may be taken as a single dose or divided into two doses.

• Children—Dose is based on body weight and must be determined by your doctor.

For hydroflumethiazide

• For *oral* dosage form (tablets):

—To lower the amount of water in the body:

• Adults—25 to 100 milligrams (mg) one or two times a day. Or, your doctor may want you to take this dose once every other day or once a day for three to five days out of the week.

• Children—Dose is based on body weight and must be determined by your doctor.

—For high blood pressure:

• Adults—50 to 100 mg a day. This may be taken as a single dose or divided into two doses.

• Children—Dose is based on body weight and must be determined by your doctor.

For methyclothiazide

• For *oral* dosage form (tablets):

—To lower the amount of water in the body:

• Adults—2.5 to 10 milligrams (mg) once a day. Or, your doctor may want you to take this dose once every other day or once a day for three to five days out of the week.

• Children—Dose is based on body weight and must be determined by your doctor.

—For high blood pressure:

• Adults—2.5 to 5 mg once a day.

• Children—Dose is based on body weight and must be determined by your doctor.

For metolazone

• For *oral* dosage form (*extended* metolazone tablets):

—To lower the amount of water in the body:

• Adults—5 to 20 milligrams (mg) once a day.

• Children—Dose must be determined by your doctor.

—For high blood pressure:

• Adults—2.5 to 5 mg once a day.

• Children—Dose must be determined by your doctor.

• For *oral* dosage form (*prompt* metolazone tablets):

—For high blood pressure:

• Adults—At first, 500 micrograms (mcg) once a day. Then, 500 to 1000 mcg once a day.

• Children—Dose must be determined by your doctor.

For polythiazide

• For *oral* dosage form (tablets):

—To lower the amount of water in the body:

• Adults—1 to 4 milligrams (mg) once a day. Or, your doctor may want you to take this dose once every other day or once a day for three to five days out of the week.

• Children—Dose is based on body weight and must be determined by your doctor.

—For high blood pressure:

- Adults—2 to 4 mg once a day.
- Children—Dose is based on body weight and must be determined by your doctor.

For quinethazone

- For *oral* dosage form (tablets):

  —To lower the amount of water in the body or for high blood pressure:

  - Adults—50 to 200 milligrams (mg) a day. This may be taken as a single dose or divided into two doses.
  - Children—Dose must be determined by your doctor.

For trichlormethiazide

- For *oral* dosage form (tablets):

  —To lower the amount of water in the body:

  - Adults—1 to 4 milligrams (mg) once a day. Or, your doctor may want you to take this dose once every other day or once a day for three to five days out of the week.
  - Children—Dose is based on body weight and must be determined by your doctor.

  —For high blood pressure:

  - Adults—2 to 4 mg once a day.
  - Children—Dose is based on body weight and must be determined by your doctor.

Missed dose—If you miss a dose of this medicine, take it as soon as possible. However, if it is almost time for your next dose, skip the missed dose and go back to your regular dosing schedule. Do not double doses.

Storage—To store this medicine:

- Keep out of the reach of children.
- Store away from heat and direct light.
- Do not store in the bathroom, near the kitchen sink, or in other damp places. Heat or moisture may cause the medicine to break down.

- Keep the oral liquid form of this medicine from freezing.
- Do not keep outdated medicine or medicine no longer needed. Be sure that any discarded medicine is out of the reach of children.

Precautions While Using This Medicine

It is important that your doctor check your progress at regular visits to make sure that this medicine is working properly.

This medicine may cause a loss of potassium from your body:

- To help prevent this, your doctor may want you to:

  —eat or drink foods that have a high potassium content (for example, orange or other citrus fruit juices), or

  —take a potassium supplement, or

  —take another medicine to help prevent the loss of the potassium in the first place.

- It is very important to follow these directions. Also, it is important not to change your diet on your own. This is more important if you are already on a special diet (as for diabetes), or if you are taking a potassium supplement or a medicine to reduce potassium loss. Extra potassium may not be necessary and, in some cases, too much potassium could be harmful.

Check with your doctor if you become sick and have severe or continuing vomiting or diarrhea. These problems may cause you to lose additional water and potassium.

For *diabetic patients:*

- Thiazide diuretics may raise blood sugar levels. While you are using this medicine, be especially careful in testing for sugar in your blood or urine.

Thiazide diuretics may cause your skin to be more sensitive to sunlight than it is normally. Exposure to sunlight, even for brief periods of time, may cause a skin rash, itching, redness or other discoloration of the skin, or a severe sunburn. When you begin taking this medicine:

- Stay out of direct sunlight, especially between the hours of 10:00 a.m. and 3:00 p.m., if possible.
- Wear protective clothing, including a hat. Also, wear sunglasses.
- Apply a sun block product that has a skin protection factor (SPF) of at least 15. Some patients may require a product with a higher SPF number, especially if they have a fair complexion. If you have any questions about this, check with your health care professional.
- Apply a sun block lipstick that has an SPF of at least 15 to protect your lips.
- Do not use a sunlamp or tanning bed or booth.

If you have a severe reaction from the sun, check with your doctor.

For patients taking this medicine for *high blood pressure:*

- *Do not take other medicines unless they have been discussed with your doctor.* This especially includes over-the-counter (nonprescription) medicines for appetite control, asthma, colds, cough, hay fever, or sinus problems, since they may tend to increase your blood pressure.

Side Effects of This Medicine

Along with its needed effects, a medicine may cause some unwanted effects. Although not all of these side effects may occur, if they do occur they may need medical attention.

Check with your doctor as soon as possible if any of the following side effects occur:

Rare

> Black, tarry stools; blood in urine or stools; cough or
> hoarseness; fever or chills; joint pain; lower back or
> side pain; painful or difficult urination; pinpoint red
> spots on skin; skin rash or hives; stomach pain (severe)
> with nausea and vomiting; unusual bleeding or bruis-
> ing; yellow eyes or skin

Signs and symptoms of too much potassium loss

> Dryness of mouth; increased thirst; irregular heartbeat;
> mood or mental changes; muscle cramps or pain; nau-
> sea or vomiting; unusual tiredness or weakness; weak
> pulse

Signs and symptoms of too much sodium loss

> Confusion; convulsions; decreased mental activity; irrita-
> bility; muscle cramps; unusual tiredness or weakness

Other side effects may occur that usually do not need
medical attention. These side effects may go away during
treatment as your body adjusts to the medicine. However,
check with your doctor if any of the following side effects
continue or are bothersome:

Less common

> Decreased sexual ability; diarrhea; dizziness or lighthead-
> edness when getting up from a lying or sitting position;
> increased sensitivity of skin to sunlight; loss of appe-
> tite; upset stomach

Other side effects not listed above may also occur in some
patients. If you notice any other effects, check with your
doctor.

Additional Information

Once a medicine has been approved for marketing for a
certain use, experience may show that it is also useful
for other medical problems. Although these uses are not
specifically included in product labeling, thiazide diuretics
are used in certain patients with the following medical
conditions:

- Diabetes insipidus (water diabetes)
- Kidney stones (calcium-containing)

For patients taking this medicine for *diabetes insipidus (water diabetes):*

- Some thiazide diuretics are used in the treatment of diabetes insipidus (water diabetes). In patients with water diabetes, this medicine causes a decrease in the flow of urine and helps the body hold water. Thus, the information given above about increased urine flow will not apply to you.

Other than the above information, there is no additional information relating to proper use, precautions, or side effects for these uses.

DOXAZOSIN   Systemic

A commonly used brand name in the U.S. and Canada is Cardura.

Description

Doxazosin (dox-AY-zoe-sin) belongs to the general class of medicines called antihypertensives. It is used to treat high blood pressure (hypertension).

High blood pressure adds to the workload of the heart and arteries. If it continues for a long time, the heart and arteries may not function properly. This can damage the blood vessels of the brain, heart, and kidneys, resulting in a stroke, heart failure, or kidney failure. High blood pressure may also increase the risk of heart attacks. These problems may be less likely to occur if blood pressure is controlled.

Doxazosin works by relaxing blood vessels so that blood passes through them more easily. This helps to lower blood pressure.

Doxazosin is also used to treat benign (noncancerous) enlargement of the prostate (benign prostatic hyperplasia

[BPH]). Benign enlargement of the prostate is a problem that can occur in men as they get older. The prostate gland is located below the bladder. As the prostate gland enlarges, certain muscles in the gland may become tight and get in the way of the tube that drains urine from the bladder. This can cause problems in urinating, such as a need to urinate often, a weak stream when urinating, or a feeling of not being able to empty the bladder completely.

Doxazosin helps relax the muscles in the prostate and the opening of the bladder. This may help increase the flow of urine and/or decrease the symptoms. However, doxazosin will not shrink the prostate. The prostate may continue to get larger. This may cause the symptoms to become worse over time. Therefore, even though doxazosin may lessen the problems caused by enlarged prostate now, surgery still may be needed in the future.

Doxazosin is available only with your doctor's prescription, in the following dosage form:
Oral
- Tablets (U.S. and Canada)

Before Using This Medicine

In deciding to use a medicine, the risks of taking the medicine must be weighed against the good it will do. This is a decision you and your doctor will make. For doxazosin, the following should be considered:

Allergies—Tell your doctor if you have ever had any unusual or allergic reaction to doxazosin, prazosin, or terazosin. Also tell your health care professional if you are allergic to any other substances, such as foods, preservatives, or dyes.

Pregnancy—Doxazosin has not been studied in pregnant women. However, studies in rabbits have shown that doxazosin given at very high doses may cause death of the fetus. Before taking this medicine, make sure your doctor knows if you are pregnant or if you may become pregnant.

Breast-feeding—It is not known whether doxazosin passes into breast milk. However, doxazosin passes into the milk of rats. Although most medicines pass into breast milk in small amounts, many of them may be used safely while breast-feeding. Mothers who are taking this medicine and who wish to breast-feed should discuss this with their doctor.

Children—Studies on this medicine have been done only in adult patients, and there is no specific information comparing use of doxazosin in children with use in other age groups.

Older adults—Dizziness, lightheadedness, or fainting may be especially likely to occur in elderly patients with high blood pressure, because these patients are usually more sensitive than younger adults to the effects of doxazosin.

Other medicines—Although certain medicines should not be used together at all, in other cases two different medicines may be used together even if an interaction might occur. In these cases, your doctor may want to change the dose, or other precautions may be necessary. Tell your health care professional if you are using any other prescription or nonprescription (over-the-counter [OTC]) medicine.

Other medical problems—The presence of other medical problems may affect the use of doxazosin. Make sure you tell your doctor if you have any other medical problems, especially:

- Kidney disease—Possible increased sensitivity to the effects of doxazosin
- Liver disease—The effects of doxazosin may be increased, which may increase the chance of side effects

Proper Use of This Medicine

For patients *taking this medicine for high blood pressure:*
- In addition to the use of the medicine your doctor

has prescribed, treatment for your high blood pressure may include weight control and care in the types of foods you eat, especially foods high in sodium. Your doctor will tell you which of these are most important for you. You should check with your doctor before changing your diet.

- Many patients who have high blood pressure will not notice any signs of the problem. In fact, many may feel normal. It is very important that you *take your medicine exactly as directed* and that you keep your appointments with your doctor even if you feel well.

- Remember that doxazosin will not cure your high blood pressure, but it does help control it. Therefore, you must continue to take it as directed if you expect to lower your blood pressure and keep it down. *You may have to take high blood pressure medicine for the rest of your life.* If high blood pressure is not treated, it can cause serious problems such as heart failure, blood vessel disease, stroke, or kidney disease.

For patients *taking this medicine for benign enlargement of the prostate:*

- Remember that doxazosin will not shrink the size of your prostate, but it does help to relieve the symptoms of this condition. You may still need to have surgery later.

- It may take up to 2 weeks before your symptoms improve.

To help you remember to take your medicine, try to get into the habit of taking it at the same time each day.

Dosing—The dose of doxazosin will be different for different patients. *Follow your doctor's orders or the directions on the label.* The following information includes only the average doses of doxazosin. *If your dose is different, do not change it* unless your doctor tells you to do so.

The number of tablets that you take depends on the strength of the medicine.

- For *oral* dosage form (tablets):
  —For benign enlargement of the prostate:
    - Adults—At first, 1 milligram (mg) taken at bedtime. Your doctor may increase your dose up to 8 mg once a day.
  —For high blood pressure:
    - Adults—1 mg once a day to start. Your doctor may increase your dose slowly to as much as 16 mg once a day.
    - Children—Use and dose must be determined by your doctor.

Missed dose—If you miss a dose of this medicine, take it as soon as possible. However, if it is almost time for your next dose, skip the missed dose and go back to your regular dosing schedule. Do not double doses.

Storage—To store this medicine:
- Keep out of the reach of children.
- Store away from heat and direct light.
- Do not store in the bathroom, near the kitchen sink, or in other damp places. Heat or moisture may cause the medicine to break down.
- Do not keep outdated medicine or medicine no longer needed. Be sure that any discarded medicine is out of the reach of children.

Precautions While Using This Medicine

It is important that your doctor check your progress at regular visits to make sure that this medicine is working properly. This is especially important for elderly patients, who may be more sensitive to the effects of this medicine.

For patients *taking this medicine for high blood pressure:*

- *Do not take other medicines unless they have been discussed with your doctor.* This especially includes over-the-counter (nonprescription) medicines for appetite control, asthma, colds, cough, hay fever, or sinus problems, since they may tend to increase your blood pressure.

Dizziness, lightheadedness, or sudden fainting may occur after you take this medicine, especially when you get up from a lying or sitting position. These effects are more likely to occur when you take the first dose of this medicine. Taking the first dose at bedtime may prevent problems. However, *be especially careful if you need to get up during the night.* These effects may also occur with any doses you take after the first dose. Getting up slowly may help lessen this problem. *If you feel dizzy, lie down so that you do not faint.* Then sit for a few moments before standing to prevent the dizziness from returning.

The dizziness, lightheadedness, or sudden fainting is more likely to occur if you drink alcohol, stand for a long time, exercise, or if the weather is hot. *While you are taking this medicine, be careful to limit the amount of alcohol you drink. Also, use extra care during exercise or hot weather or if you must stand for a long time.*

Doxazosin may cause some people to become drowsy or less alert than they are normally. *Make sure you know how you react to this medicine before you drive, use machines, or do anything else that could be dangerous if you are dizzy, drowsy, or are not alert.* After you have taken several doses of this medicine, these effects should lessen.

Side Effects of This Medicine

Along with its needed effects, a medicine may cause some unwanted effects. Although not all of these side effects may occur, if they do occur they may need medical attention.

Check with your doctor as soon as possible if any of the following side effects occur:

More common

Dizziness or lightheadedness

Less common

Dizziness or lightheadedness when getting up from a lying or sitting position; fainting (sudden); fast and pounding heartbeat; irregular heartbeat; shortness of breath; swelling of feet or lower legs

Other side effects may occur that usually do not need medical attention. These side effects may go away during treatment as your body adjusts to the medicine. However, check with your doctor if any of the following side effects continue or are bothersome:

More common

Headache; unusual tiredness

Less common

Nausea; nervousness, restlessness, unusual irritability; runny nose; sleepiness or drowsiness

Other side effects not listed above may also occur in some patients. If you notice any other effects, check with your doctor.

ENCAINIDE   Systemic*†

A commonly used brand name is Enkaid.

*Not commercially available in the U.S.
†Not commercially available in Canada.

Description

Encainide (en-KAY-nide) belongs to the group of medicines known as antiarrhythmics. It is used to correct irregular heartbeats to a normal rhythm.

Encainide produces its helpful effects by slowing nerve impulses in the heart and making the heart tissue less sensitive.

There is a chance that encainide may cause new heart rhythm problems when it is used. Since it has been shown to cause severe problems in some patients, it is only used to treat serious heart rhythm problems. Discuss this possible effect with your doctor.

This medicine is available only from your doctor in the following dosage form:

Oral

- Capsules

Before Using This Medicine

In deciding to use a medicine, the risks of taking the medicine must be weighed against the good it will do. This is a decision you and your doctor will make. For encainide, the following should be considered:

Allergies—Tell your doctor if you have ever had any unusual or allergic reaction to encainide. Also tell your health care professional if you are allergic to any other substances, such as foods, preservatives, or dyes.

Pregnancy—Encainide has not been studied in pregnant women. However, this medicine has not been shown to cause birth defects or other problems in animal studies, but has been shown to reduce fertility in rats. Before taking encainide, make sure your doctor knows if you are pregnant or if you may become pregnant.

Breast-feeding—Encainide passes into the milk of some animals and may also pass into the milk of humans. However, this medicine has not been reported to cause problems in nursing babies.

Children—Studies on this medicine have been done only in adult patients. Therefore, be sure to discuss with your doctor the use of this medicine in children.

Older adults—Many medicines have not been tested in older people. Therefore, it may not be known whether they work exactly the same way they do in younger adults or if they cause different side effects or problems in older people. There is no specific information about the use of encainide in the elderly.

Other medical problems—The presence of other medical problems may affect the use of encainide. Make sure you tell your doctor if you have any other medical problems, especially:

- Diabetes mellitus—Encainide may raise blood sugar levels
- Kidney disease—Effects of encainide may be increased because of slower removal from the body
- Liver disease—Effects of encainide may be changed
- Recent heart attack—Risk of irregular heartbeats may be increased
- If you have a pacemaker—Encainide may interfere with the pacemaker and require more careful follow-up by the doctor

---

Proper Use of This Medicine

Take encainide exactly as directed by your doctor, even though you may feel well. Do not take more or less of it than your doctor ordered.

This medicine works best when there is a constant amount in the blood. *To help keep the amount constant, do not miss any doses. Also, it is best to take each dose at evenly spaced times day and night.* For example, if you are to take 3 doses a day, doses should be spaced about 8 hours apart. If you need help in planning the best times to take your medicine, check with your health care professional.

Dosing—The dose of encainide will be different for different patients. *Follow your doctor's orders or the directions on the label.* The following information includes only the average doses of encainide. *If your dose is different, do not change it* unless your doctor tells you to do so.

- For *oral* dosage form (capsules):
  —For irregular heartbeat:
    - Adults—25 to 50 milligrams (mg) every eight hours.
    - Children—Use and dose must be determined by your doctor.

Missed dose—If you miss a dose of encainide and remember within 4 hours, take it as soon as possible. However, if you do not remember until later, skip the missed dose and go back to your regular dosing schedule. Do not double doses.

Storage—To store this medicine:
- Keep out of the reach of children.
- Store away from heat and direct light.
- Do not store in the bathroom, near the kitchen sink, or in other damp places. Heat or moisture may cause the medicine to break down.
- Do not keep outdated medicine or medicine no longer needed. Be sure that any discarded medicine is out of the reach of children.

Precautions While Using This Medicine

It is important that your doctor check your progress at regular visits to make sure the medicine is working properly. This will allow changes to be made in the amount of medicine you are taking, if necessary.

Your doctor may want you to carry a medical identification card or bracelet stating that you are using this medicine.

Before having any kind of surgery (including dental surgery) or emergency treatment, tell the medical doctor or dentist in charge that you are taking this medicine.

Encainide may cause some people to become dizzy or lightheaded. Make sure you know how you react to this medicine before you drive, use machines, or do anything else that could be dangerous if you are dizzy.

Side Effects of This Medicine

Along with its needed effects, a medicine may cause some unwanted effects. Although not all of these side effects may occur, if they do occur they may need medical attention.

Check with your doctor as soon as possible if any of the following side effects occur:

More common

Chest pain; fast or irregular heartbeat

Rare

Shortness of breath; swelling of feet or lower legs; trembling or shaking

Other side effects may occur that usually do not need medical attention. These side effects may go away during treatment as your body adjusts to the medicine. However, check with your doctor if any of the following side effects continue or are bothersome:

Less common

Blurred or double vision; dizziness; headache; nausea; pain in arms or legs; skin rash; unusual tiredness or weakness

Other side effects not listed above may also occur in some patients. If you notice any other effects, check with your doctor.

ENOXAPARIN   Systemic

A commonly used brand name in the U.S. and Canada is Lovenox.

Description

Enoxaparin (e-nox-a-PA-rin) is used to prevent deep venous thrombosis, a condition in which harmful blood clots form in the blood vessels of the legs. This medicine is used for several days after hip or knee replacement surgery, while you are unable to walk. It is during this time that blood clots are most likely to form. Enoxaparin also may be used for other conditions as determined by your doctor.

Enoxaparin is available only with your doctor's prescription, in the following dosage form:

Parenteral
- Injection (U.S. and Canada)

Before Using This Medicine

In deciding to use a medicine, the risks of taking the medicine must be weighed against the good it will do. This is a decision you and your doctor will make. For enoxaparin, the following should be considered:

Allergies—Tell your doctor if you have ever had any unusual or allergic reaction to enoxaparin or to heparin. Also tell your health care professional if you are allergic to any other substances, such as foods, especially pork or pork products, preservatives, or dyes.

Pregnancy—Enoxaparin has not been studied in pregnant women. However, it has not been shown to cause birth defects or other problems in animal studies.

Breast-feeding—It is not known whether this medicine passes into breast milk. Although most medicines pass into breast milk in small amounts, many of them may be used safely while breast-feeding. Mothers who are using this medicine and who wish to breast-feed should discuss this with their doctor.

Children—Studies on this medicine have been done only in adult patients, and there is no specific information comparing use of enoxaparin in children with use in other age groups.

Older adults—This medicine has been tested and has not been shown to cause different side effects or problems in older people than it does in younger adults.

Other medicines—Although certain medicines should not be used together at all, in other cases two different medicines may be used together even if an interaction might occur. In these cases, your doctor may want to change the dose, or other precautions may be necessary. When you are using enoxaparin, it is especially important that your health care professional know if you are taking any of the following:

- Aspirin or
- Divalproex (e.g., Depakote) or
- Inflammation or pain medicine, except narcotics, or
- Plicamycin (e.g., Mithracin) or
- Sulfinpyrazone (e.g., Anturane) or
- Thrombolytic agents or
- Ticlopidine (e.g., Ticlid) or
- Valproic acid (e.g., Depakene)—Using any of these medicines together with enoxaparin may increase the risk of bleeding

Other medical problems—The presence of other medical problems may affect the use of enoxaparin. Make sure you tell your doctor if you have any other medical problems, especially:

- Blood disease or bleeding problems or
- Blood vessel problems or
- Heart infection or
- High blood pressure (hypertension) or

- Kidney disease or
- Liver disease or
- Stomach ulcer (active) or
- Threatened miscarriage—The risk of bleeding may be increased

Also, tell your doctor if you have received enoxaparin or heparin before and had a reaction to either of them called thrombocytopenia, or if new blood clots formed while you were receiving the medicine.

In addition, *tell your doctor if you have recently given birth, fallen or suffered a blow to the body or head, or had medical or dental surgery*. These events may increase the risk of serious bleeding when you are taking enoxaparin.

Proper Use of This Medicine

If you are using enoxaparin at home, your health care professional will teach you how to inject yourself with the medicine. *Be sure to follow the directions carefully. Check with your health care professional if you have any problems using the medicine.*

Put used syringes in a puncture-resistant, disposable container, or dispose of them as directed by your health care professional.

Dosing—The dose of enoxaparin will be different for different patients. *Follow your doctor's orders or the directions on the label.* The following information includes only the average doses of enoxaparin. *If your dose is different, do not change it* unless your doctor tells you to do so.

- For *injection* dosage form:
    - —For prevention of deep venous thrombosis:
        - Adults—30 milligrams (mg) every twelve hours for seven to ten days.

- Children—Use and dose must be determined by your doctor.

Missed dose—If you miss a dose of this medicine, use it as soon as possible. However, if it is almost time for your next dose, skip the missed dose and go back to your regular dosing schedule. Do not double doses.

Storage—To store this medicine:
- Keep out of the reach of children.
- Store away from heat and direct light.
- Keep the medicine from freezing. Do not refrigerate.
- Do not keep outdated medicine or medicine no longer needed. Be sure that any discarded medicine is out of the reach of children.

Precautions While Using This Medicine

Tell all your medical doctors and dentists that you are using this medicine.

Side Effects of This Medicine

Along with its needed effects, a medicine may cause some unwanted effects. Although not all of these side effects may occur, if they do occur they may need medical attention.

Stop using this medicine and check with your doctor immediately if any of the following side effects occur:

Less common

Blood in urine; bloody or black, tarry stools; bruising; chest discomfort; collection of blood under the skin; confusion; continuing bleeding or oozing from the nose and/or mouth, or surgical wound; convulsions; coughing up blood; fever; headache; irritability; lightheadedness; moderate to severe pain or numbness in the

arms, legs, hands, feet; nosebleed; shortness of breath;
swelling of hands and/or feet; unusual bleeding; unusual tiredness or weakness; vomiting of blood or material that looks like coffee grounds

Rare

Chest pain; dizziness or lightheadedness when getting up
from a lying or sitting position; fast or irregular heartbeat; skin rash or hives; sudden fainting; swelling of
the face, genitals, mouth, or tongue

Other side effects may occur that usually do not need
medical attention. These side effects may go away during
treatment as your body adjusts to the medicine. However,
check with your doctor if any of the following side effects
continue or are bothersome:

Less common

Increased menstrual bleeding; irritation, pain, or redness
at place of injection; nausea; vomiting

Other side effects not listed above may also occur in some
patients. If you notice any other effects, check with your
doctor.

ESTROGENS Systemic

Some commonly used brand names are:

In the U.S.—

Aquest[6]	Estrace[3]
Clinagen LA 40[3]	Estraderm[3]
Deladiol-40[3]	Estragyn 5[6]
Delestrogen[3]	Estragyn LA 5[3]
depGynogen[3]	Estra-L 40[3]
Depo-Estradiol[3]	Estratab[5]
Depogen[3]	Estro-A[6]
Dioval 40[3]	Estro-Cyp[3]
Dioval XX[3]	Estrofem[3]
Dura-Estrin[3]	Estroject-LA[3]
Duragen-20[3]	Estro-L.A.[3]
Duragen-40[3]	Estrone '5'[6]
E-Cypionate[3]	Estro-Span[3]
Estinyl[8]	Estrovis[9]

In the U.S. (cont'd)—

Gynogen L.A. 20[3]

Gynogen L.A. 40[3]

Kestrone-5[6]

Menaval-20[3]

Menest[5]

Ogen .625[7]

Ogen 1.25[7]

Ogen 2.5[7]

Ortho-Est[7]

Premarin[4]

Premarin Intravenous[4]

Stilphostrol[2]

TACE[1]

Valergen-10[3]

Valergen-20[3]

Valergen-40[3]

Wehgen[6]

In Canada—

C.E.S.[4]

Congest[4]

Delestrogen[3]

Estinyl[8]

Estrace[3]

Estraderm[3]

Femogex[3]

Honvol[2]

Neo-Estrone[5]

Ogen[7]

Premarin[4]

Premarin Intravenous[4]

Other commonly used names are:

DES[2]

Piperazine Estrone Sulfate[7]

Note: For quick reference, the following estrogens are numbered to match the corresponding brand names.

This information applies to the following medicines:

1. Chlorotrianisene (klor-oh-trye-AN-i-seen)†
2. Diethylstilbestrol (dye-eth-il-stil-BESS-trole)‡
3. Estradiol (ess-tra-DYE-ole)‡
4. Estrogens, Conjugated (ESS-troe-jenz, CON-ju-gate-ed)§
5. Estrogens, Esterified (ess-TAIR-i-fyed)
6. Estrone (ESS-trone)†‡
7. Estropipate (ess-troe-PI-pate)‡
8. Ethinyl Estradiol (ETH-in-il ess-tra-DYE-ole)
9. Quinestrol (quin-ESS-trole)†

---

†Not commercially available in Canada.

‡Generic name product may also be available in the U.S.

§Generic name product may also be available in Canada.

Description

Estrogens (ESS-troe-jenz) are female hormones. They are produced by the body and are necessary for the normal sexual development of the female and for the regulation of the menstrual cycle during the childbearing years.

The ovaries begin to produce less estrogen after menopause (the change of life). This medicine is prescribed to make up for the lower amount of estrogen. This should relieve signs of menopause, such as hot flashes and unusual sweating, chills, faintness, or dizziness.

Estrogens are prescribed for several reasons:
- to provide additional hormone when the body does not produce enough of its own, as during the menopause or following certain kinds of surgery.
- in the treatment of selected cases of breast cancer in men and women.
- in the treatment of men with certain kinds of cancer of the prostate.
- to help prevent weakening of bones (osteoporosis) in women past menopause.

Estrogens may also be used for other conditions as determined by your doctor.

There is *no* medical evidence to support the belief that the use of estrogens will keep the patient feeling young, keep the skin soft, or delay the appearance of wrinkles. Nor has it been proven that the use of estrogens during the menopause will relieve emotional and nervous symptoms, unless these symptoms are caused by other menopausal symptoms, such as hot flashes or hot flushes.

Estrogens are very useful medicines. However, in addition to their helpful effects in treating your medical problem, they sometimes have side effects that could be very serious. *A paper called "Information for the Patient" should be given to you with your prescription. Read this carefully.* Also, before you use an estrogen, you and your doctor should discuss the good that it will do as well as the risks of using it.

Estrogens are available only with your doctor's prescription, in the following dosage forms:

Oral

Chlorotrianisene
- Capsules (U.S.)

Diethylstilbestrol
- Tablets (U.S. and Canada)

Estradiol
- Tablets (U.S. and Canada)

Estrogens, Conjugated
- Tablets (U.S. and Canada)

Estrogens, Esterified
- Tablets (U.S. and Canada)

Estropipate
- Tablets (U.S. and Canada)

Ethinyl Estradiol
- Tablets (U.S. and Canada)

Quinestrol
- Tablets (U.S.)

Parenteral

Diethylstilbestrol
- Injection (U.S. and Canada)

Estradiol
- Injection (U.S. and Canada)

Estrogens, Conjugated
- Injection (U.S. and Canada)

Estrone
- Injection (U.S.)

Topical

Estradiol
- Transdermal system (stick-on patch) (U.S. and Canada)

Before Using This Medicine

In deciding to use a medicine, the risks of taking the medicine must be weighed against the good it will do. This is a decision you and your doctor will make. For estrogens, the following should be considered:

Allergies—Tell your doctor if you have ever had any unusual or allergic reaction to estrogens. Also tell your health care professional if you are allergic to any other substances, such as foods, preservatives, or dyes.

Pregnancy—Estrogens are not recommended for use during pregnancy, since some have been shown to cause serious birth defects in humans and animals. Some daughters of women who took diethylstilbestrol (DES) during pregnancy have developed reproductive (genital) tract problems and, rarely, cancer of the vagina or cervix (opening to the uterus) when they reached childbearing age. Some sons of women who took DES during pregnancy have developed urinary-genital tract problems.

Breast-feeding—Use of this medicine is not recommended in nursing mothers. Estrogens pass into the breast milk and their possible effect on the baby is not known.

Older adults—This medicine has been tested and has not been shown to cause different side effects or problems in older women than it does in younger women.

Other medicines—Although certain medicines should not be used together at all, in other cases two different medicines may be used together even if an interaction might occur. In these cases, your doctor may want to change the dose, or other precautions may be necessary. When you are taking estrogens, it is especially important that your health care professional know if you are taking any of the following:

- Acetaminophen (e.g., Tylenol) (with long-term, high-dose use) or
- Amiodarone (e.g., Cordarone) or
- Anabolic steroids (nandrolone [e.g., Anabolin], oxandrolone [e.g., Anavar], oxymetholone [e.g., Anadrol], stanozolol [e.g., Winstrol]) or
- Androgens (male hormones) or
- Anti-infectives by mouth or by injection (medicine for infection) or
- Antithyroid agents (medicine for overactive thyroid) or
- Carbamazepine (e.g., Tegretol) or
- Carmustine (e.g., BiCNU) or
- Chloroquine (e.g., Aralen) or
- Dantrolene (e.g., Dantrium) or
- Daunorubicin (e.g., Cerubidine) or

- Disulfiram (e.g., Antabuse) or
- Divalproex (e.g., Depakote) or
- Etretinate (e.g., Tegison) or
- Gold salts (medicine for arthritis) or
- Hydroxychloroquine (e.g., Plaquenil) or
- Mercaptopurine (e.g., Purinethol) or
- Methotrexate (e.g., Mexate) or
- Methyldopa (e.g., Aldomet) or
- Naltrexone (e.g., Trexan) (with long-term, high-dose use) or
- Oral contraceptives (birth control pills) containing estrogen or
- Phenothiazines (acetophenazine [e.g., Tindal], chlorpromazine [e.g., Thorazine], fluphenazine [e.g., Prolixin], mesoridazine [e.g., Serentil], perphenazine [e.g., Trilafon], prochlorperazine [e.g., Compazine], promazine [e.g., Sparine], promethazine [e.g., Phenergan], thioridazine [e.g., Mellaril], trifluoperazine [e.g., Stelazine], triflupromazine [e.g., Vesprin], trimeprazine [e.g., Temaril]) or
- Phenytoin (e.g., Dilantin) or
- Plicamycin (e.g., Mithracin) or
- Valproic acid (e.g., Depakene)—Estrogens and all of these medicines can cause liver damage. Your doctor may want you to have extra blood tests that tell about your liver, if you must take any of these medicines with estrogens
- Bromocriptine (e.g., Parlodel)—Estrogens may interfere with the effects of bromocriptine
- Cyclosporine (e.g., Sandimmune)—Estrogens can increase the chance of toxic effects to the kidney or liver from cyclosporine because estrogens can interfere with the body's ability to get the cyclosporine out of the bloodstream as it normally would

Other medical problems—The presence of other medical problems may affect the use of estrogens. Make sure you tell your doctor if you have any other medical problems, especially:

For all patients

- Blood clots (or history of during previous estrogen therapy)—Estrogens may worsen blood clots or cause new clots to form
- Breast cancer (active or suspected)—Estrogens may cause growth of the tumor in some cases

- Changes in vaginal bleeding of unknown causes—Some irregular vaginal bleeding is a sign that the lining of the uterus is growing too much or is a sign of cancer of the uterus lining; estrogens may make these conditions worse
- Endometriosis—Estrogens may worsen endometriosis by causing growth of endometriosis implants
- Fibroid tumors of the uterus—Estrogens may cause fibroid tumors to increase in size
- Gallbladder disease or gallstones (or history of)—Estrogens may possibly increase the risk of gallbladder disease or gallstones
- Jaundice (or history of during pregnancy)—Estrogens may worsen or cause jaundice in these patients
- Liver disease—Toxic drug effects may occur in patients with liver disease because the body is not able to get this medicine out of the bloodstream as it normally would
- Porphyria—Estrogens can make porphyria worse

For males treated for breast or prostate cancer

- Blood clots or
- Heart or circulation disease or
- Stroke—Males with these medical problems may be more likely to have clotting problems while taking estrogens; the doses of estrogens used to treat male breast or prostate cancer have been shown to increase the chances of heart attack, phlebitis (inflamed veins) caused by a blood clot, or blood clots in the lungs

---

Proper Use of This Medicine

For patients taking any of the estrogens by mouth:

- *Take this medicine only as directed by your doctor. Do not take more of it and do not take it for a longer time than your doctor ordered.* Try to take the medicine at the same time each day to reduce the possibility of side effects and to allow it to work better.
- Nausea may occur during the first few weeks after you start taking estrogens. This effect usually disappears with continued use. If the nausea is bothersome,

it can usually be prevented or reduced by taking each dose with food or immediately after food.

For patients using the transdermal (stick-on patch) form of estradiol:

- This medicine comes with patient directions. Read them carefully before using this medicine.
- Wash and dry your hands thoroughly before and after handling.
- Apply the patch to a clean, dry, non-oily skin area of your abdomen (stomach) or buttocks that has little or no hair and is free of cuts or irritation.
- *Do not apply to the breasts.* Also, do not apply to the waistline or anywhere else where tight clothes may rub the patch loose.
- Press the patch firmly in place with the palm of your hand for about 10 seconds. Make sure there is good contact, especially around the edges.
- If a patch becomes loose or falls off, you may reapply it or discard it and apply a new patch.
- Each dose is best applied to a different area of skin on your abdomen so that at least 1 week goes by before the same area is used again. This will help prevent skin irritation.

Dosing—The dose of these medicines will be different for different patients. *Follow your doctor's orders or the directions on the label.* The following information includes only the average doses of these medicines. *If your dose is different, do not change it* unless your doctor tells you to do so.

The number of capsules or tablets that you take or the amount of injection you use depends on the strength of the medicine. Also, *the number of doses you take or use each day, the time allowed between doses, and the length of time you take or use the medicine depend on the medical problem for which you are taking or using estrogen.*

For chlorotrianisene

- For *oral* dosage form (capsules):

    —For treating a genital skin condition (vulvar squamous hyperplasia), inflammation of the vagina (atrophic vaginitis), ovary disorders (female hypogonadism), or symptoms of menopause:

    - Adults—12 to 25 milligrams (mg) a day. Your doctor may want you to take this medicine every day or only on certain days each month.

    —For treating prostate cancer:

    - Adults—12 to 25 mg a day.

For conjugated estrogens

- For *oral* dosage form (tablets):

    —For treating a genital skin condition (vulvar squamous hyperplasia), inflammation of the vagina (atrophic vaginitis), or to prevent loss of bone (osteoporosis):

    - Adults—0.3 to 1.25 milligrams (mg) a day. Your doctor may want you to take the medicine each day or only on certain days of the month.

    —For treating ovary problems (female hypogonadism):

    - Adults—2.5 to 7.5 mg a day. This dose is divided up and taken in smaller doses. Your doctor may want you to take the medicine only on certain days of the month.

    —For treating symptoms of menopause:

    - Adults—0.625 to 1.25 mg a day. Your doctor may want you to take the medicine each day or only on certain days of the month.

    —For treating ovary problems (failure or removal of the ovary):

    - Adults—1.25 mg a day. Your doctor may want you to take the medicine each day or only on certain days of the month.

—For treating breast cancer in women after menopause and in men:

- Adults—10 mg three times a day for at least three months.

—For treating prostate cancer:

- Adults—1.25 to 2.5 mg three times a day.

• For *injection* dosage form:

—For controlling abnormal bleeding of the uterus:

- Adults—25 mg injected into a muscle or vein. This may be repeated in six to twelve hours if needed.

For diethylstilbestrol

• For *oral* dosage forms (tablets and enteric-coated tablets):

—For treating breast cancer in women after menopause and in men:

- Adults—15 milligrams (mg) a day.

—For treating prostate cancer:

- Adults—At first, 1 to 3 mg a day. Later, your doctor may decrease your dose to 1 mg a day.

For diethylstilbestrol diphosphate

• For *oral* dosage form (tablets):

—For treating prostate cancer:

- Adults—50 to 200 milligrams (mg) three times a day.

• For *injection* dosage form:

—For treating prostate cancer:

- Adults—At first, 500 mg mixed in solution with sodium chloride or dextrose injection and injected slowly into a vein. Your doctor may increase your dose to 1 gram a day for five or more straight days as needed. Then, your doctor may lower your dose to 250 to 500 mg one or two times a week.

For esterified estrogens

- For *oral* dosage form (tablets):

    —For treating a genital skin condition (vulvar squamous hyperplasia) or inflammation of the vagina (atrophic vaginitis):

    - Adults—0.3 to 1.25 milligrams (mg) a day. Your doctor may want you to take the medicine each day or only on certain days of the month.

    —For treating ovary problems (female hypogonadism):

    - Adults—2.5 to 7.5 mg a day. This dose may be divided up and taken in smaller doses. Your doctor may want you to take the medicine each day or only on certain days of the month.

    —For treating symptoms of menopause:

    - Adults—0.625 to 1.25 mg a day. Your doctor may want you to take the medicine each day or only on certain days of the month.

    —For treating ovary problems (failure or removal of the ovary):

    - Adults—1.25 mg a day. Your doctor may want you to take the medicine each day or only on certain days of the month.

    —For treating breast cancer in women after menopause and in men:

    - Adults—10 mg three times a day for at least three months.

    —For treating prostate cancer:

    - Adults—1.25 to 2.5 mg three times a day.

For estradiol

- For *oral* dosage form (tablets):

    —For treating a genital skin condition (vulvar squamous hyperplasia), inflammation of the vagina (atrophic vaginitis), ovary problems (female hypogonadism or failure or removal of the ovary), or symptoms of menopause:

• Adults—0.5 to 2 milligrams (mg) a day. Your doctor may want you to take the medicine each day or only on certain days of the month.

—For treating breast cancer in women after menopause and in men:

• Adults—10 mg three times a day for at least three months.

—For treating prostate cancer:

• Adults—1 to 2 mg three times a day.

—For preventing bone loss (osteoporosis):

• Adults—0.5 mg a day. Your doctor may want you to take the medicine each day or only on certain days of the month.

• For *transdermal* dosage form (patches):

—For treating a genital skin condition (vulvar squamous hyperplasia), inflammation of the vagina (atrophic vaginitis), symptoms of menopause, ovary problems (female hypogonadism or failure or removal of the ovary), or to prevent bone loss (osteoporosis):

• Adults—0.05 or 0.1 milligram (mg) (one patch) applied to the skin and worn for one-half of a week. Then, remove that patch and apply a new patch. A new patch should be applied two times a week.

For estradiol cypionate

• For *injectable* dosage form:

—For treating ovary problems (female hypogonadism):

• Adults—1.5 to 2 milligrams (mg) injected into a muscle once a month.

—For treating symptoms of menopause:

• Adults—1 to 5 mg injected into a muscle every three to four weeks.

For estradiol valerate

• For *injection* dosage form:

—For treating a genital skin condition (vulvar squamous hyperplasia), inflammation of the vagina (atrophic vaginitis), symptoms of menopause, or ovary problems (female hypogonadism or failure or removal of the ovary):

• Adults—10 to 20 milligrams (mg) injected into a muscle every four weeks as needed.

—For treating prostate cancer:

• Adults—30 mg injected into a muscle every one or two weeks.

For estrone

• For *injection* dosage form:

—For controlling abnormal bleeding of the uterus:

• Adults—2 to 5 milligrams (mg) a day, injected into a muscle for several days.

—For treating ovary problems (female hypogonadism, failure or removal of the ovary):

• Adults—0.1 to 2 mg a week. This is injected into a muscle as a single dose or divided into more than one dose. Your doctor may want you to receive the medicine each week or only during certain weeks of the month.

—For treating a genital skin condition (vulvar squamous hyperplasia), inflammation of the vagina (atrophic vaginitis), or symptoms of menopause:

• Adults—0.1 to 0.5 mg injected into a muscle two or three times a week. Your doctor may want you to receive the medicine each week or only during certain weeks of the month.

—For treating prostate cancer:

• Adults—2 to 4 mg injected into a muscle two or three times a week.

For estropipate

• For oral dosage form (tablets):

—For treating a genital skin condition (vulvar squamous hyperplasia), inflammation of the vagina (atrophic vaginitis), or symptoms of menopause:

- Adults—0.75 to 6 milligrams (mg) a day. Your doctor may want you to take the medicine each day or only on certain days of the month.

—For treating ovary problems (female hypogonadism, failure or removal of the ovary):

- Adults—1.5 to 9 mg a day. Your doctor may want you to take the medicine each day or only on certain days of the month.

For ethinyl estradiol

- For *oral* dosage form (tablets):

—For treating ovary problems (female hypogonadism):

- Adults—0.05 milligrams (mg) one to three times a day for three to six months. Your doctor may want you to take the medicine each day or only on certain days of the month.

—For treating symptoms of menopause:

- Adults—0.02 to 0.05 mg a day. Your doctor may want you to take the medicine each day or only on certain days of the month.

—For treating breast cancer in women after menopause:

- Adults—1 mg three times a day.

—For treating prostate cancer:

- Adults—0.15 to 3 mg a day.

For quinestrol

- For *oral* dosage form (tablets):

—For treating a genital skin condition (vulvar squamous hyperplasia), inflammation of the vagina (atrophic vaginitis), symptoms of menopause, or ovary problems (female hypogonadism, failure or removal of the ovary):

- Adults—At first, 100 micrograms (mcg) a day

for seven days. Then, no medicine is taken for seven days. After that, your doctor will lower your dose to 100 to 200 mcg taken once a week.

Missed dose—

- For patients taking any of the estrogens by mouth: If you miss a dose of this medicine, take it as soon as possible. However, if it is almost time for your next dose, skip the missed dose and go back to your regular dosing schedule. Do not double doses.

- For patients using the transdermal (stick-on patch) form of estradiol: If you forget to apply a new patch when you are supposed to, apply it as soon as possible. However, if it is almost time for the next patch, skip the missed one and go back to your regular schedule. Do not apply more than one patch at a time.

Storage—To store this medicine:

- Keep out of the reach of children.
- Store away from heat and direct light.
- Do not store in the bathroom medicine cabinet because the heat or moisture may cause the medicine to break down.
- Keep the injectable form of this medicine from freezing.
- Do not keep outdated medicine or medicine no longer needed. Be sure that any discarded medicine is out of the reach of children.

Precautions While Using This Medicine

It is very important that your doctor check your progress at regular visits to make sure this medicine does not cause unwanted effects. These visits will usually be every year, but some doctors require them more often.

It is not yet known whether the use of estrogens increases the risk of breast cancer in women. Therefore, it is very important that you regularly check your breasts for any unusual lumps or discharge. You should also have a mammogram (x-ray pictures of the breasts) done if your doctor recommends it. Because breast cancer has occurred in men taking estrogens, regular self-breast exams and exams by your doctor for any unusual lumps or discharge should be done.

In some patients using estrogens, tenderness, swelling, or bleeding of the gums may occur. Brushing and flossing your teeth carefully and regularly and massaging your gums may help prevent this. See your dentist regularly to have your teeth cleaned. Check with your medical doctor or dentist if you have any questions about how to take care of your teeth and gums, or if you notice any tenderness, swelling, or bleeding of your gums.

If you think that you may be pregnant, stop using the medicine immediately and check with your doctor. Continued use of some estrogens during pregnancy may cause birth defects in the child. DES may also increase the risk of vaginal cancer developing in daughters when they reach childbearing age.

Do not give this medicine to anyone else. Your doctor has prescribed it only for you after studying your health record and the results of your physical examination. Estrogens may be dangerous for other people because of differences in their health and body make-up.

Side Effects of This Medicine

Discuss these possible effects with your doctor:

- The prolonged use of estrogens has been reported to increase the risk of endometrial cancer (cancer of the lining of the uterus) in women after the menopause. This risk seems to increase as the dose and the length of use increase. When estrogens are used in low doses for less than 1 year, there is less risk. The risk is

also reduced if a progestin (another female hormone)
is added to, or replaces part of, your estrogen dose.
If the uterus has been removed by surgery (total hysterectomy), there is no risk of endometrial cancer.

• It is not yet known whether the use of estrogens increases the risk of breast cancer in women. Although
some large studies show an increased risk, most studies and information gathered to date do not support
this idea. Breast cancer has been reported in men
taking estrogens.

• In studies with oral contraceptives (birth control pills)
containing estrogens, cigarette smoking was shown to
cause an increased risk of serious side effects affecting the heart or blood circulation, such as dangerous
blood clots, heart attack, or stroke. The risk increased
as the amount of smoking and the age of the smoker
increased. Women aged 35 and over were at greatest
risk when they smoked while using oral contraceptives containing estrogens. It is not known if this risk
exists with the use of estrogens for symptoms of
menopause. However, smoking may make estrogens
less effective.

The following side effects may be caused by blood clots,
which could lead to stroke, heart attack, or death. These
side effects rarely occur, and when they do occur, they
occur in men treated for cancer using high doses of estrogens. *Get emergency help immediately* if any of the following side effects occur:

*Rare—For males being treated for breast or prostate
cancer only*

Headache (sudden or severe); loss of coordination (sudden); loss of vision or change of vision (sudden); pains
in chest, groin, or leg, especially in calf of leg; shortness of breath (sudden and unexplained); slurring of
speech (sudden); weakness or numbness in arm or leg

Also, check with your doctor as soon as possible if any
of the following side effects occur:

More common

Breast pain (in females and males); increased breast size (in females and males); swelling of feet and lower legs; weight gain (rapid)

Less common or rare

Changes in vaginal bleeding (spotting, breakthrough bleeding, prolonged or heavier bleeding, or complete stoppage of bleeding); lumps in, or discharge from, breast (in females and males); pains in stomach, side, or abdomen; uncontrolled jerky muscle movements; yellow eyes or skin

Other side effects may occur that usually do not need medical attention. These side effects may go away during treatment as your body adjusts to the medicine. However, check with your doctor if any of the following side effects continue or are bothersome:

More common

Bloating of stomach; cramps of lower stomach; loss of appetite; nausea; skin irritation or redness where skin patch was worn

Less common

Diarrhea (mild); dizziness (mild); headaches (mild); migraine headaches; problems in wearing contact lenses; unusual decrease in sexual desire (in males); unusual increase in sexual desire (in females); vomiting (usually with high doses)

Also, many women who are taking estrogens with a progestin (another female hormone) will start having monthly vaginal bleeding, similar to menstrual periods again. This effect will continue for as long as the medicine is taken. However, monthly bleeding will not occur in women who have had the uterus removed by surgery (total hysterectomy).

Other side effects not listed above may also occur in some patients. If you notice any other effects, check with your doctor.

Additional Information

Once a medicine has been approved for marketing for a certain use, experience may show that it is also useful for other medical problems. Although these uses are not included in product labeling, estrogen is used in certain patients with the following medical conditions:

- Osteoporosis caused by lack of estrogen before menopause
- Atherosclerotic disease (hardening of the arteries)
- Turner's syndrome (a genetic disorder)

Other than the above information, there is no additional information relating to proper use, precautions, or side effects for these uses.

FLECAINIDE   Systemic

A commonly used brand name in the U.S. and Canada is Tambocor.

Description

Flecainide (FLEK-a-nide) belongs to the group of medicines known as antiarrhythmics. It is used to correct irregular heartbeats to a normal rhythm.

Flecainide produces its helpful effects by slowing nerve impulses in the heart and making the heart tissue less sensitive.

There is a chance that flecainide may cause new or make worse existing heart rhythm problems when it is used. Since it has been shown to cause severe problems in some patients, it is only used to treat serious heart rhythm problems. Discuss this possible effect with your doctor.

This medicine is available only with your doctor's prescription, in the following dosage form:

Oral
- Tablets (U.S. and Canada)

Before Using This Medicine

In deciding to use a medicine, the risks of taking the medicine must be weighed against the good it will do. This is a decision you and your doctor will make. For flecainide, the following should be considered:

Allergies—Tell your doctor if you have ever had any unusual or allergic reaction to flecainide, lidocaine, tocainide, or anesthetics. Also tell your health care professional if you are allergic to any other substances, such as foods, preservatives, or dyes.

Pregnancy—Flecainide has not been studied in pregnant women. However, studies in one kind of rabbit given about 4 times the usual human dose have shown that flecainide causes birth defects. Before taking flecainide, make sure your doctor knows if you are pregnant or if you may become pregnant.

Breast-feeding—Flecainide passes into breast milk. However, this medicine has not been shown to cause problems in nursing babies.

Children—Studies on this medicine have been done only in adult patients, and there is no specific information comparing use of flecainide in children with use in other age groups.

Older adults—Elderly people are especially sensitive to the effects of flecainide. Flecainide may be more likely to cause irregular heartbeat in the elderly.

Other medicines—Although certain medicines should not be used together at all, in other cases two different medicines may be used together even if an interaction might occur. In these cases, your doctor may want to change the dose, or other precautions may be necessary. When you are taking flecainide it is especially important that your health care professional knows if you are taking any of the following:

- Other medicine for heart rhythm problems—Both wanted and unwanted effects on the heart may increase

Other medical problems—The presence of other medical problems may affect the use of flecainide. Make sure you tell your doctor if you have any other medical problems, especially:

- Congestive heart failure—Flecainide may make this condition worse
- Kidney disease or
- Liver disease—Effects of flecainide may be increased because of slower removal from the body
- Recent heart attack—Risk of irregular heartbeats may be increased
- If you have a pacemaker—Flecainide may interfere with the pacemaker and require more careful follow-up by the doctor

---

Proper Use of This Medicine

Take flecainide exactly as directed by your doctor, even though you may feel well. Do not take more medicine than ordered.

This medicine works best when there is a constant amount in the blood. *To help keep this amount constant, do not miss any doses. Also, it is best to take the doses 12 hours apart, in the morning and at night*, unless otherwise directed by your doctor. If you need help in planning the best times to take your medicine, check with your health care professional.

Dosing—The dose of flecainide will be different for different patients. *Follow your doctor's orders or the directions on the label.* The following information includes only the average doses of flecainide. *If your dose is different, do not change it* unless your doctor tells you to do so.

The number of tablets that you take depends on the strength of the medicine.

- For *oral* dosage form (tablets):
  —For correcting irregular heartbeat:
    - Adults—50 to 150 milligrams (mg) every twelve hours.
    - Children—Use and dose must be determined by your doctor.

Missed dose—If you miss a dose of flecainide and remember within 6 hours, take it as soon as possible. However, if you do not remember until later, skip the missed dose and go back to your regular dosing schedule. Do not double doses.

Storage—To store this medicine:

- Keep out of the reach of children.
- Store away from heat and direct light.
- Do not store in the bathroom, near the kitchen sink, or in other damp places. Heat or moisture may cause the medicine to break down.
- Do not keep outdated medicine or medicine no longer needed. Be sure that any discarded medicine is out of the reach of children.

Precautions While Using This Medicine

It is important that your doctor check your progress at regular visits to make sure the medicine is working properly. This will allow for changes to be made in the amount of medicine you are taking, if necessary.

Your doctor may want you to carry a medical identification card or bracelet stating that you are using this medicine.

Before having any kind of surgery (including dental surgery) or emergency treatment, tell the medical doctor or dentist in charge that you are taking this medicine.

Flecainide may cause some people to become dizzy, lightheaded, or less alert than they are normally. *Make sure you know how you react to this medicine before you drive, use machines, or do anything else that could be dangerous if you are dizzy or are not alert.*

If you have been using this medicine regularly for several weeks, do not suddenly stop using it. Check with your doctor for the best way to reduce gradually the amount you are taking before stopping completely.

Side Effects of This Medicine

Along with its needed effects, a medicine may cause some unwanted effects. Although not all of these side effects may occur, if they do occur they may need medical attention.

Check with your doctor as soon as possible if any of the following side effects occur:

Less common
> Chest pain; irregular heartbeat; shortness of breath; swelling of feet or lower legs; trembling or shaking

Rare
> Yellow eyes or skin

Other side effects may occur that usually do not need medical attention. These side effects may go away during treatment as your body adjusts to the medicine. However, check with your doctor if any of the following side effects continue or are bothersome:

More common
> Blurred vision or seeing spots; dizziness or lightheadedness

Less common
> Anxiety or mental depression; constipation; headache; nausea or vomiting; skin rash; stomach pain or loss of appetite; unusual tiredness or weakness

Other side effects not listed above may also occur in some

patients. If you notice any other effects, check with your doctor.

GEMFIBROZIL Systemic

A commonly used brand name in the U.S. and Canada is Lopid.

Description

Gemfibrozil (gem-FI-broe-zil) is used to lower cholesterol and triglyceride (fat-like substances) levels in the blood. This may help prevent medical problems caused by such substances clogging the blood vessels.

Gemfibrozil is available only with your doctor's prescription, in the following dosage forms:

Oral
- Capsules (Canada)
- Tablets (U.S. and Canada)

Before Using This Medicine

In addition to its helpful effects in treating your medical problem, this type of medicine may have some harmful effects.

Results of a large study using gemfibrozil seem to show that it may cause a higher rate of some cancers in humans. In addition, the action of gemfibrozil is similar to that of another medicine called clofibrate. Studies with clofibrate have suggested that it may increase the patient's risk of cancer, liver disease, pancreatitis (inflammation of the pancreas), gallstones and problems from gallbladder surgery, although it may also decrease the risk of heart attacks. Other studies have not found all of these effects.

Studies with gemfibrozil in rats found an increased risk of liver tumors when doses up to 10 times the human dose were given for a long time.

Be sure you have discussed this with your doctor before taking this medicine.

In deciding to use a medicine, the risks of taking the medicine must be weighed against the good it will do. This is a decision you and your doctor will make. For gemfibrozil, the following should be considered:

Allergies—Tell your doctor if you have ever had any unusual or allergic reaction to gemfibrozil. Also tell your health care professional if you are allergic to any other substances, such as foods, preservatives, or dyes.

Diet—Before prescribing medicine for your condition, your doctor will probably try to control your condition by prescribing a personal diet for you. Such a diet may be low in fats, sugars, and/or cholesterol. Many people are able to control their condition by carefully following their doctor's orders for proper diet and exercise. *Medicine is prescribed only when additional help is needed* and is effective only when a schedule of diet and exercise is properly followed.

Also, this medicine is less effective if you are greatly overweight. It may be very important for you to go on a reducing diet. However, check with your doctor before going on any diet.

Make certain your health care professional knows if you are on a low-sodium, low-sugar, or any other special diet. Most medicines contain more than their active ingredient.

Pregnancy—Gemfibrozil has not been studied in pregnant women. However, studies in animals have shown that high doses of gemfibrozil may increase the number of fetal deaths, decrease birth weight, or cause some skeletal defects. Before taking this medicine, make sure your doctor knows if you are pregnant or if you may become pregnant.

Breast-feeding—It is not known whether gemfibrozil passes into breast milk. However, studies in animals have shown that high doses of gemfibrozil may increase the risk of some kinds of tumors. Therefore, you should consider this when deciding whether to breast-feed your baby while taking this medicine.

Children—There is no specific information about the use of gemfibrozil in children. However, use is not recommended in children under 2 years of age since cholesterol is needed for normal development.

Older adults—Many medicines have not been studied specifically in older people. Therefore, it may not be known whether they work exactly the same way they do in younger adults or if they cause different side effects or problems in older people. There is no specific information comparing use of gemfibrozil in the elderly with use in other age groups.

Other medicines—Although certain medicines should not be used together at all, in other cases two different medicines may be used together even if an interaction might occur. In these cases, your doctor may want to change the dose, or other precautions may be necessary. When you are taking gemfibrozil it is especially important that your health care professional know if you are taking any of the following:

- Anticoagulants (blood thinners)—Use with gemfibrozil may increase the effect of the anticoagulant
- Lovastatin—Use with gemfibrozil may cause muscle or kidney problems or make them worse

Other medical problems—The presence of other medical problems may affect the use of gemfibrozil. Make sure you tell your doctor if you have any other medical problems, especially:

- Gallbladder disease or
- Gallstones—Gemfibrozil may make these conditions worse
- Kidney disease or

- Liver disease—Higher blood levels of gemfibrozil may result, which may increase the chance of side effects; a decrease in the dose of gemfibrozil may be needed

---

Proper Use of This Medicine

Use this medicine only as directed by your doctor. Do not use more or less of it, and do not use it more often or for a longer time than your doctor ordered.

This medicine is usually taken twice a day. If you are taking 2 doses a day, it is best to take the medicine 30 minutes before your breakfast and evening meal.

Follow carefully the special diet your doctor gave you. This is the most important part of controlling your condition and is necessary if the medicine is to work properly.

Dosing—The dose of gemfibrozil will be different for different patients. *Follow your doctor's orders or the directions on the label.* The following information includes only the average doses of gemfibrozil. *If your dose is different, do not change it* unless your doctor tells you to do so:

- For *oral* dosage forms (tablets):

  —Adults: 600 milligrams two times a day to be taken thirty minutes before the morning and evening meals.

Missed dose—If you miss a dose of this medicine, take it as soon as possible. However, if it is almost time for your next dose, skip the missed dose and go back to your regular dosing schedule. Do not double doses.

Storage—To store this medicine:

- Keep out of the reach of children.
- Store away from heat and direct light.
- Do not store in the bathroom, near the kitchen sink, or in other damp places. Heat or moisture may cause the medicine to break down.

• Do not keep outdated medicine or medicine no longer needed. Be sure that any discarded medicine is out of the reach of children.

Precautions While Using This Medicine

It is very important that your doctor check your progress at regular visits. This will allow your doctor to see if the medicine is working properly to lower your cholesterol and triglyceride levels and to decide if you should continue to take it.

Do not stop taking this medication without first checking with your doctor. When you stop taking this medicine, your blood cholesterol levels may increase again. Your doctor may want you to follow a special diet to help prevent this from happening.

Side Effects of This Medicine

Along with its needed effects, a medicine may cause some unwanted effects. Although not all of these side effects may occur, if they do occur they may need medical attention.

Check with your doctor immediately if any of the following side effects occur:

Rare

Cough or hoarseness; fever or chills; lower back or side pain; painful or difficult urination; stomach pain (severe) with nausea and vomiting

Check with your doctor as soon as possible if either of the following side effects occurs:

Rare

Muscle pain; unusual tiredness or weakness

Other side effects may occur that usually do not need medical attention. These side effects may go away during treatment as your body adjusts to the medicine. However, check with your doctor if any of the following side effects continue or are bothersome:

More common

Stomach pain, gas, or heartburn

Less common

Diarrhea; nausea or vomiting; skin rash

Other side effects not listed above may also occur in some patients. If you notice any other effects, check with your doctor.

GUANABENZ   Systemic†

A commonly used brand name in the U.S. is Wytensin.

†Not commercially available in Canada.

Description

Guanabenz (GWAHN-a-benz) belongs to the general class of medicines called antihypertensives. It is used to treat high blood pressure (hypertension).

High blood pressure adds to the workload of the heart and arteries. If it continues for a long time, the heart and arteries may not function properly. This can damage the blood vessels of the brain, heart, and kidneys, resulting in a stroke, heart failure, or kidney failure. High blood pressure may also increase the risk of heart attacks. These problems may be less likely to occur if blood pressure is controlled.

Guanabenz works by controlling nerve impulses along certain nerve pathways. As a result, it relaxes blood vessels so that blood passes through them more easily. This helps to lower blood pressure.

Guanabenz is available only with your doctor's prescription, in the following dosage form:

Oral
- Tablets (U.S.)

Before Using This Medicine

In deciding to use a medicine, the risks of taking the medicine must be weighed against the good it will do. This is a decision you and your doctor will make. For guanabenz, the following should be considered:

Allergies—Tell your doctor if you have ever had any unusual or allergic reaction to guanabenz. Also tell your health care professional if you are allergic to any other substance, such as foods, preservatives, or dyes.

Pregnancy—Guanabenz has not been studied in pregnant women. However, studies in rats have shown that guanabenz given in doses 9 to 10 times the maximum human dose caused a decrease in fertility. In addition, 3 to 6 times the maximum human dose caused birth defects (in the skeleton) in mice, and 6 to 9 times the maximum human dose caused death of the fetus in rats. Before taking this medicine, make sure your doctor knows if you are pregnant or if you may become pregnant.

Breast-feeding—It is not known whether guanabenz passes into the breast milk. However, this medicine has not been reported to cause problems in nursing babies.

Children—Studies on this medicine have been done only in adult patients, and there is no specific information comparing use of guanabenz in children with use in other age groups.

Older adults—Many medicines have not been studied specifically in older people. Therefore, it may not be known whether they work exactly the same way they do in younger adults or if they cause different side effects or problems in older people. There is no specific information comparing use of guanabenz in the elderly with use in other age groups. However, dizziness, faintness, or drowsiness may be more likely to occur in the elderly, who are usually more sensitive to the effects of guanabenz.

Other medicines—Although certain medicines should not be used together at all, in other cases two different medicines may be used together even if an interaction might occur. In these cases, your doctor may want to change the dose, or other precautions may be necessary. When you are taking guanabenz, it is especially important that your health care professional know if you are taking any of the following:

- Beta-blockers (acebutolol [e.g., Sectral], atenolol [e.g., Tenormin], betaxolol [Kerlone], carteolol [e.g., Cartrol], labetalol [e.g., Normodyne], metoprolol [e.g., Lopressor], nadolol [e.g., Corgard], oxprenolol [e.g., Trasicor], penbutolol [e.g., Levatol], pindolol [e.g., Visken], propranolol [e.g., Inderal], sotalol [e.g., Sotacor], timolol [e.g., Blocadren])—Effects on blood pressure may be increased. Also, the risk of unwanted effects when guanabenz treatment is stopped suddenly may be increased

Other medical problems—The presence of other medical problems may affect the use of guanabenz. Make sure you tell your doctor if you have any other medical problems, especially:

- Heart or blood vessel disease—Lowering blood pressure may make some conditions worse
- Kidney disease or
- Liver disease—Effects of guanabenz may be increased because of slower removal of guanabenz from the body

Proper Use of This Medicine

In addition to the use of the medicine your doctor has prescribed, treatment for your high blood pressure may include weight control and care in the types of foods you eat, especially foods high in sodium. Your doctor will tell you which of these are most important for you. You should check with your doctor before changing your diet.

Many patients who have high blood pressure will not notice any signs of the problem. In fact, many may feel normal. It is very important that you *take your medicine exactly as directed* and that you keep your appointments with your doctor even if you feel well.

Remember that this medicine will not cure your high blood pressure but it does help control it. Therefore, you must continue to take it as directed if you expect to lower your blood pressure and keep it down. *You may have to take high blood pressure medicine for the rest of your life.* If high blood pressure is not treated, it can cause serious problems such as heart failure, blood vessel disease, stroke, or kidney disease.

To help you remember to take your medicine, try to get into the habit of taking it at the same time each day.

Dosing—The dose of guanabenz will be different for different patients. *Follow your doctor's orders or the directions on the label.* The following information includes only the average doses of guanabenz. *If your dose is different, do not change it* unless your doctor tells you to do so.

The number of tablets that you take depends on the strength of the medicine.

- For *oral* dosage form (tablets):
    —For high blood pressure:
        - Adults—At first, 4 milligrams (mg) two times a day. Then, your doctor may gradually increase your dose.
        - Children—Use and dose must be determined by your doctor.

Missed dose—
- If you miss a dose of this medicine, take it as soon

as possible. However, if it is almost time for your next dose, skip the missed dose and go back to your regular dosing schedule. Do not double doses.

- If you miss two or more doses in a row, check with your doctor. If your body suddenly goes without this medicine, some unpleasant effects may occur. If you have any questions about this, check with your doctor.

Storage—To store this medicine:

- Keep out of the reach of children.
- Store away from heat and direct light.
- Do not store in the bathroom, near the kitchen sink, or in other damp places. Heat or moisture may cause the medicine to break down.
- Do not keep outdated medicine or medicine no longer needed. Be sure that any discarded medicine is out of the reach of children.

Precautions While Using This Medicine

It is important that your doctor check your progress at regular visits to make sure that this medicine is working properly.

Check with your doctor before you stop taking guanabenz. Your doctor may want you to reduce gradually the amount you are taking before stopping completely.

Before having any kind of surgery (including dental surgery) or emergency treatment, tell the medical doctor or dentist in charge that you are using this medicine.

Do not take other medicines unless they have been discussed with your doctor. This especially includes over-the-counter (nonprescription) medicines for appetite control, asthma, colds, cough, hay fever, or sinus problems, since they may tend to increase your blood pressure.

Guanabenz will add to the effects of alcohol and other CNS depressants (medicines that slow down the nervous system, possibly causing drowsiness). Some examples of CNS depressants are antihistamines or medicine for hay fever, other allergies, or colds; sedatives, tranquilizers, or sleeping medicine; prescription pain medicine or narcotics; barbiturates; medicine for seizures; muscle relaxants; or anesthetics, including some dental anesthetics. *Check with your doctor before taking any of the above while you are using this medicine.*

Guanabenz may cause some people to become dizzy, drowsy, or less alert than they are normally. *Make sure you know how you react to this medicine before you drive, use machines, or do anything else that could be dangerous if you are dizzy or are not alert.*

Guanabenz may cause dryness of the mouth, nose, and throat. For temporary relief of mouth dryness, use sugarless candy or gum, melt bits of ice in your mouth, or use a saliva substitute. However, if your mouth continues to feel dry for more than 2 weeks, check with your medical doctor or dentist. Continuing dryness of the mouth may increase the chance of dental disease, including tooth decay, gum disease, and fungus infections.

Side Effects of This Medicine

Along with its needed effects, a medicine may cause some unwanted effects. Although not all of these side effects may occur, if they do occur they may need medical attention.

Check with your doctor as soon as possible if any of the following side effects occur:

Signs and symptoms of overdose

Dizziness (severe); faintness; irritability; nervousness; pinpoint pupils; slow heartbeat; unusual tiredness or weakness

Other side effects may occur that usually do not need medical attention. These side effects may go away during treatment as your body adjusts to the medicine. However, check with your doctor if any of the following side effects continue or are bothersome:

More common
Dizziness; drowsiness; dryness of mouth; weakness

Less common or rare
Decreased sexual ability; headache; nausea

After you have been using this medicine for a while, unpleasant effects may occur if you stop taking it too suddenly. After you stop taking this medicine, check with your doctor if any of the following effects occur:

Anxiety or tenseness; chest pain; fast or irregular heartbeat; headache; increased salivation; increase in sweating; nausea or vomiting; nervousness or restlessness; shaking or trembling of hands or fingers; stomach cramps; trouble in sleeping

Other side effects not listed above may also occur in some patients. If you notice any other effects, check with your doctor.

GUANADREL   Systemic†

A commonly used brand name in the U.S. is Hylorel.

---

†Not commercially available in Canada.

Description

Guanadrel (GWAHN-a-drel) belongs to the general class of medicines called antihypertensives. It is used to treat high blood pressure (hypertension).

High blood pressure adds to the workload of the heart and arteries. If it continues for a long time, the heart and arteries may not function properly. This can damage the blood vessels of the brain, heart, and kidneys, resulting in a stroke, heart failure, or kidney failure. High blood pressure may also increase the risk of heart attacks. These problems may be less likely to occur if blood pressure is controlled.

Guanadrel works by controlling nerve impulses along certain nerve pathways. As a result, it relaxes the blood vessels so that blood passes through them more easily. This helps to lower blood pressure.

Guanadrel is available only with your doctor's prescription, in the following dosage form:

Oral
- Tablets (U.S.)

Before Using This Medicine

In deciding to use a medicine, the risks of taking the medicine must be weighed against the good it will do. This is a decision you and your doctor will make. For guanadrel, the following should be considered:

Allergies—Tell your doctor if you have ever had any unusual or allergic reaction to guanadrel. Also tell your health care professional if you are allergic to any other substance, such as foods, preservatives, or dyes.

Pregnancy—Guanadrel has not been studied in pregnant women. However, guanadrel has not been shown to cause birth defects or other problems in animal studies.

Breast-feeding—It is not known whether guanadrel passes into breast milk. However, it has not been reported to cause problems in nursing babies.

Children—Studies on this medicine have been done only in adult patients, and there is no specific information comparing use of guanadrel in children with use in other age groups.

Older adults—Dizziness or faintness may be more likely to occur in the elderly, who are usually more sensitive to the effects of guanadrel.

Other medicines—Although certain medicines should not be used together at all, in other cases two different medicines may be used together even if an interaction might occur. In these cases, your doctor may want to change the dose, or other precautions may be necessary. When you are taking guanadrel, it is especially important that your health care professional know if you are taking any of the following:

- Chlorprothixene (e.g., Taractan) or
- Loxapine (e.g., Loxitane) or
- Thiothixene (e.g., Navane) or
- Tricyclic antidepressants (amitriptyline [e.g., Elavil], amoxapine [e.g., Asendin], clomipramine [e.g., Anafranil], desipramine [e.g., Pertofrane], doxepin [e.g., Sinequan], imipramine [e.g., Tofranil], nortriptyline [e.g., Aventyl], protriptyline [e.g., Vivactil], trimipramine [e.g., Surmontil]) or
- Trimeprazine (e.g., Temaril)—May decrease the effects of guanadrel on blood pressure
- Monoamine oxidase (MAO) inhibitors (furazolidone [e.g., Furoxone], isocarboxazid [e.g., Marplan], phenelzine [e.g., Nardil], procarbazine [e.g., Matulane], selegiline [e.g., Eldepryl], tranylcypromine [e.g., Parnate])—Taking guanadrel while you are taking or within 2 weeks of taking MAO inhibitors may cause a severe increase in blood pressure

Other medical problems—The presence of other medical problems may affect the use of guanadrel. Make sure you tell your doctor if you have any other medical problems, especially:

- Asthma (history of) or
- Diarrhea or
- Pheochromocytoma or
- Stomach ulcer (history of)—May be worsened by guanadrel
- Fever—Effects of guanadrel may be increased
- Heart or blood vessel disease or

- Heart attack or stroke (recent)—Lowering blood pressure may make problems resulting from these conditions worse

---

Proper Use of This Medicine

In addition to the use of the medicine your doctor has prescribed, treatment for your high blood pressure may include weight control and care in the types of foods you eat, especially foods high in sodium. Your doctor will tell you which of these are most important for you. You should check with your doctor before changing your diet.

Many patients who have high blood pressure will not notice any signs of the problem. In fact, many may feel normal. It is very important that you *take your medicine exactly as directed* and that you keep your appointments with your doctor even if you feel well.

Remember that guanadrel will not cure your high blood pressure, but it does help control it. Therefore, you must continue to take it as directed if you expect to lower your blood pressure and keep it down. *You may have to take high blood pressure medicine for the rest of your life.* If high blood pressure is not treated, it can cause serious problems such as heart failure, blood vessel disease, stroke, or kidney disease.

To help you remember to take your medicine, try to get into the habit of taking it at the same time each day.

Dosing—The dose of guanadrel will be different for different patients. *Follow your doctor's orders or the directions on the label.* The following information includes only the average doses of guanadrel. *If your dose is different, do not change it* unless your doctor tells you to do so.

The number of tablets that you take depends on the strength of the medicine.

- For *oral* dosage form (tablets):
  - —For high blood pressure:
    - Adults—At first, 5 milligrams (mg) two times a day. Then, your doctor may increase your dose to 20 to 75 mg a day, divided into two to four doses.
    - Children—Use and dose must be determined by your doctor.

Missed dose—If you miss a dose of guanadrel, take it as soon as possible. However, if it is almost time for your next dose, skip the missed dose and go back to your regular dosing schedule. Do not double doses.

Storage—To store this medicine:
- Keep out of the reach of children.
- Store away from heat and direct light.
- Do not store in the bathroom, near the kitchen sink, or in other damp places. Heat or moisture may cause the medicine to break down.
- Do not keep outdated medicine or medicine no longer needed. Be sure that any discarded medicine is out of the reach of children.

Precautions While Using This Medicine

It is important that your doctor check your progress at regular visits to make sure that this medicine is working properly.

Dizziness, lightheadedness, or fainting may occur, especially when you get up from a lying or sitting position. This may be more likely to occur in the morning. *Getting up slowly may help.* If you feel dizzy, sit or lie down. When you get up from lying down, sit on the edge of the bed with your feet dangling for 1 or 2 minutes. Then stand up slowly. If the problem continues or gets worse, check with your doctor.

The dizziness, lightheadedness, or fainting is also more likely to occur if you drink alcohol, stand for long periods of time, exercise, or if the weather is hot. *While you are taking guanadrel, be careful to limit the amount of alcohol you drink. Also, use extra care during exercise or hot weather or if you must stand for long periods of time.*

Do not take other medicines unless they have been discussed with your doctor. This especially includes over-the-counter (nonprescription) medicines for appetite control, asthma, colds, cough, hay fever, or sinus problems, since they may tend to increase your blood pressure.

Before having any kind of surgery (including dental surgery) or emergency treatment, tell the medical doctor or dentist in charge that you are taking guanadrel.

Tell your doctor if you get a fever since that may change the amount of medicine you have to take.

Side Effects of This Medicine

Along with its needed effects, a medicine may cause some unwanted effects. Although not all of these side effects may occur, if they do occur they may need medical attention.

Check with your doctor immediately if either of the following side effects occurs since they may be symptoms of an overdose:

Rare

Blurred vision; dizziness or faintness (severe)

Check with your doctor as soon as possible if any of the following side effects occur:

More common

Swelling of feet or lower legs

Less common or rare

Chest pain; shortness of breath

Other side effects may occur that usually do not need medical attention. These side effects may go away during treatment as your body adjusts to the medicine. However, check with your doctor if any of the following side effects continue or are bothersome:

More common

Difficulty in ejaculating; dizziness, lightheadedness, or fainting, especially when getting up from a lying or sitting position; drowsiness or tiredness

Less common or rare

Diarrhea or increase in bowel movements; dryness of mouth; headache; muscle pain or tremors; nighttime urination

Other side effects not listed above may also occur in some patients. If you notice any other effects, check with your doctor.

GUANETHIDINE Systemic

Some commonly used brand names are:

In the U.S.—

Ismelin

Generic name product may also be available.

In Canada—

Apo-Guanethidine

Ismelin

Description

Guanethidine (gwahn-ETH-i-deen) belongs to the general class of medicines called antihypertensives. It is used to treat high blood pressure (hypertension).

High blood pressure adds to the workload of the heart and arteries. If it continues for a long time, the heart and arteries may not function properly. This can damage the blood vessels of the brain, heart, and kidneys, resulting in a stroke, heart failure, or kidney failure. High blood pressure may also increase the risk of heart attacks. These problems may be less likely to occur if blood pressure is controlled.

Guanethidine works by controlling nerve impulses along certain nerve pathways. As a result, it relaxes the blood vessels so that blood passes through them more easily. This helps to lower blood pressure.

Guanethidine is available only with your doctor's prescription, in the following dosage form:

Oral
- Tablets (U.S. and Canada)

Before Using This Medicine

In deciding to use a medicine, the risks of taking the medicine must be weighed against the good it will do. This is a decision you and your doctor will make. For guanethidine, the following should be considered:

Allergies—Tell your doctor if you have ever had any unusual or allergic reaction to guanethidine. Also tell your health care professional if you are allergic to any other substance, such as foods, preservatives, or dyes.

Pregnancy—Studies on effects in pregnancy have not been done in either humans or animals.

Breast-feeding—Small amounts of guanethidine pass into breast milk. However, this medicine has not been reported to cause problems in nursing babies.

Children—Although there is no specific information comparing use of guanethidine in children with use in other age groups, this medicine is not expected to cause different side effects or problems in children than it does in adults.

Older adults—Many medicines have not been studied specifically in older people. Therefore, it may not be known whether they work exactly the same way they do in younger adults. Although there is no specific information comparing use of guanethidine in the elderly with use in other age groups, dizziness, lightheadedness, or fainting may be more likely to occur in the elderly, who are more sensitive to the effects of guanethidine.

Other medicines—Although certain medicines should not be used together at all, in other cases two different medicines may be used together even if an interaction might occur. In these cases, your doctor may want to change the dose, or other precautions may be necessary. When you are taking guanethidine, it is especially important that your health care professional knows if you are taking any of the following:

- Antidiabetics, oral (diabetes medicine you take by mouth)— Effects may be increased by guanethidine
- Loxapine (e.g., Loxitane) or
- Thioxanthenes (chlorprothixene [e.g., Taractan], thiothixene [e.g., Navane]) or
- Tricyclic antidepressants (amitriptyline [e.g., Elavil], amoxapine [e.g., Asendin], clomipramine [e.g., Anafranil], desipramine [e.g., Pertofrane], doxepin [e.g., Sinequan], imipramine [e.g., Tofranil], nortriptyline [e.g., Aventyl], protriptyline [e.g., Vivactil], trimipramine [e.g., Surmontil]) or
- Trimeprazine (e.g., Temaril)—May decrease the effects of guanethidine on blood pressure
- Minoxidil (e.g., Loniten)—Effects on blood pressure may be greatly increased
- Monoamine oxidase (MAO) inhibitors (furazolidone [e.g., Furoxone], isocarboxazid [e.g., Marplan], phenelzine [e.g., Nardil], procarbazine [e.g., Matulane], selegiline [e.g., Eldepryl], tranylcypromine [e.g., Parnate])—Taking guanethidine while you are taking or within 2 weeks of taking MAO inhibitors may cause a severe increase in blood pressure

Other medical problems—The presence of other medical problems may affect the use of guanethidine. Make sure

you tell your doctor if you have any other medical problems, especially:

- Asthma (history of) or
- Diarrhea or
- Pheochromocytoma or
- Stomach ulcer (history of)—May be worsened by guanethidine
- Diabetes mellitus (sugar diabetes)—Effects of medicine used to treat this may be increased by guanethidine
- Fever—Effects of guanethidine may be increased
- Heart or blood vessel disease or
- Heart attack or stroke (recent)—Lowering blood pressure may make problems resulting from these conditions worse
- Kidney disease—May be worsened. Also, effects of guanethidine may be increased because of slower removal of this medicine from the body
- Liver disease—Effects of guanethidine may be increased because of slower removal from the body

---

Proper Use of This Medicine

In addition to the use of the medicine your doctor has prescribed, treatment for your high blood pressure may include weight control and care in the types of foods you eat, especially foods high in sodium. Your doctor will tell you which of these are most important for you. You should check with your doctor before changing your diet.

Many patients who have high blood pressure will not notice any signs of the problem. In fact, many may feel normal. It is very important that you *take your medicine exactly as directed* and that you keep your appointments with your doctor even if you feel well.

Remember that guanethidine will not cure your high blood pressure but it does help control it. Therefore, you must continue to take it as directed if you expect to lower your blood pressure and keep it down. *You may have to take high blood pressure medicine for the rest of your life.* If high blood pressure is not treated, it can cause serious problems such as heart failure, blood vessel disease, stroke, or kidney disease.

To help you remember to take your medicine, try to get into the habit of taking it at the same time each day.

Dosing—The dose of guanethidine will be different for different patients. *Follow your doctor's orders or the directions on the label.* The following information includes only the average doses of guanethidine. *If your dose is different, do not change it* unless your doctor tells you to do so.

The number of tablets that you take depends on the strength of the medicine.

* For *oral* dosage form (tablets):
    —For high blood pressure:
    * Adults—At first, 10 or 12.5 milligrams (mg) once a day. Then, your doctor may increase your dose to 25 to 50 mg once a day.
    * Children—The dose is based on body weight. The usual dose is 200 micrograms (mcg) per kilogram (kg) (90.9 mcg per pound) of body weight a day. Then, your doctor may increase your dose as needed.

Missed dose—If you miss a dose of guanethidine, take it as soon as possible. However, if it is almost time for your next dose, skip the missed dose and go back to your regular dosing schedule. Do not double doses.

Storage—To store this medicine:
* Keep out of the reach of children.
* Store away from heat and direct light.
* Do not store in the bathroom, near the kitchen sink, or in other damp places. Heat or moisture may cause the medicine to break down.
* Do not keep outdated medicine or medicine no longer

needed. Be sure that any discarded medicine is out of the reach of children.

Precautions While Using This Medicine

It is important that your doctor check your progress at regular visits to make sure that this medicine is working properly.

Dizziness, lightheadedness, or fainting may occur, especially when you get up from a lying or sitting position. This is more likely to occur in the morning. *Getting up slowly may help.* When you get up from lying down, sit on the edge of the bed with your feet dangling for 1 or 2 minutes. Then stand up slowly. If the problem continues or gets worse, check with your doctor.

The dizziness, lightheadedness, or fainting is also more likely to occur if you drink alcohol, stand for long periods of time, exercise, or if the weather is hot. *While you are taking this medicine, be careful in the amount of alcohol you drink. Also, use extra care during exercise or hot weather or if you must stand for long periods of time.*

Do not take other medicines unless they have been discussed with your doctor. This especially includes over-the-counter (nonprescription) medicines for appetite control, asthma, colds, cough, hay fever, or sinus problems, since they may tend to increase your blood pressure.

Before having any kind of surgery (including dental surgery) or emergency treatment, tell the medical doctor or dentist in charge that you are taking this medicine.

Tell your doctor if you get a fever since that may change the amount of medicine you have to take.

Side Effects of This Medicine

Along with its needed effects, a medicine may cause some unwanted effects. Although not all of these side effects

may occur, if they do occur they may need medical attention.

Check with your doctor as soon as possible if any of the following side effects occur:

More common

Swelling of feet or lower legs

Less common or rare

Chest pain; shortness of breath

Other side effects may occur that usually do not need medical attention. These side effects may go away during treatment as your body adjusts to the medicine. However, check with your doctor if any of the following side effects continue or are bothersome:

More common

Diarrhea or increase in bowel movements; dizziness, lightheadedness, or fainting, especially when getting up from a lying or sitting position; sexual problems in males; slow heartbeat; stuffy nose; unusual tiredness or weakness

Less common or rare

Blurred vision; drooping eyelids; dryness of mouth; headache; loss of hair on scalp; muscle pain or tremors; nausea or vomiting; nighttime urination; skin rash

Other side effects not listed above may also occur in some patients. If you notice any other effects, check with your doctor.

GUANETHIDINE AND HYDROCHLOROTHIAZIDE Systemic

Some commonly used brand names are:

In the U.S.—
Esimil

In Canada—
Ismelin-Esidrix

Amiloride and Hydrochlorothiazide

5/50 mg

Tablets
MSD: *Moduretic*

Amiodarone*

200 mg

Tablets
Wyeth-Ayerst: *Cordarone*

Atenolol and Chlorthalidone

50/25 mg   100/25 mg

Tablets
Mutual

50/25 mg   100/25 mg

Tablets
Schein/Danbury
(continued)

Atenolol and Chlorthalidone *(continued)*

50/25 mg   100/25 mg

Tablets
ZENECA: *Tenoretic*

Bisoprolol and Hydrochlorothiazide*

2.5/6.25 mg   5/6.25 mg   10/6.25 mg

Tablets
Lederle: *Ziac*

Captopril and Hydrochlorothiazide*

25/15 mg   25/25 mg

50/15 mg   50/25 mg

Tablets
Squibb: *Capozide*

Clonidine and Chlorthalidone

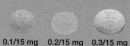

0.1/15 mg   0.2/15 mg   0.3/15 mg

Tablets
Boehringer Ingelheim:
Combipres

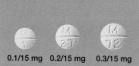

0.1/15 mg   0.2/15 mg   0.3/15 mg

Tablets
Mylan

Dipyridamole

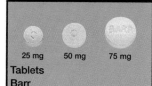

25 mg   50 mg   75 mg

Tablets
Barr

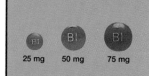

25 mg   50 mg   75 mg

Tablets
Boehringer Ingelheim:
Persantine

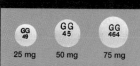

Dipyridamole *(continued)*

25 mg   50 mg   75 mg

Tablets
Geneva

25 mg   50 mg   75 mg

Tablets
Purepac

Enalapril and Hydrochlorothiazide*

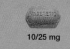

10/25 mg

Tablets
Merck: *Vaseretic*

Gemfibrozil

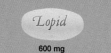

600 mg

Tablets
PD: *Lopid*

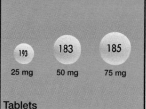

(continued)

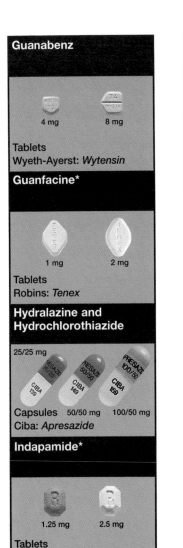

Guanabenz

4 mg 8 mg

Tablets
Wyeth-Ayerst: *Wytensin*

Guanfacine*

1 mg 2 mg

Tablets
Robins: *Tenex*

Hydralazine and Hydrochlorothiazide

25/25 mg

Capsules 50/50 mg 100/50 mg
Ciba: *Apresazide*

Indapamide*

1.25 mg 2.5 mg

Tablets
Rhône-Poulenc Rorer: *Lozol*

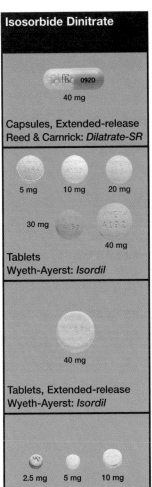

Isosorbide Dinitrate

40 mg

Capsules, Extended-release
Reed & Carnrick: *Dilatrate-SR*

5 mg 10 mg 20 mg

30 mg 40 mg

Tablets
Wyeth-Ayerst: *Isordil*

40 mg

Tablets, Extended-release
Wyeth-Ayerst: *Isordil*

2.5 mg 5 mg 10 mg

Tablets, Sublingual
Wyeth-Ayerst: *Isordil*

(continued)

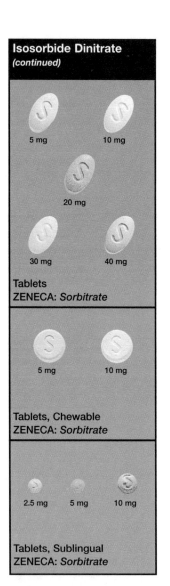

Isosorbide Dinitrate
(continued)

5 mg | 10 mg

20 mg

30 mg | 40 mg

Tablets
ZENECA: *Sorbitrate*

5 mg | 10 mg

Tablets, Chewable
ZENECA: *Sorbitrate*

2.5 mg | 5 mg | 10 mg

Tablets, Sublingual
ZENECA: *Sorbitrate*

Isosorbide Mononitrate

20 mg

Tablets
Wyeth-Ayerst: *ISMO*

Lisinopril and Hydrochlorothiazide

20/12.5 mg | 20/25 mg

Tablets
Merck: *Prinzide*

20/12.5 mg | 20/25 mg

Tablets
Stuart: *Zestoretic*

Methyldopa and Hydrochlorothiazide

250/15 mg | 250/25 mg

Tablets
Geneva

(continued)

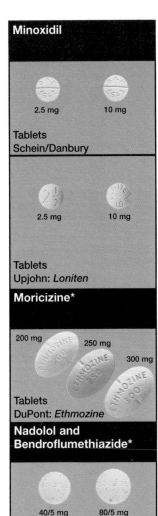

Methyldopa and Hydrochlorothiazide
(continued)

500/30 mg   500/50 mg
Tablets
Geneva

250/15 mg   250/25 mg

500/30 mg   500/50 mg

Tablets
Merck: *Aldoril*

Metoprolol and Hydrochlorothiazide*

50/25 mg   100/25 mg   100/50 mg
Tablets
Geigy: *Lopressor HCT*

Minoxidil

2.5 mg   10 mg

Tablets
Schein/Danbury

2.5 mg   10 mg

Tablets
Upjohn: *Loniten*

Moricizine*

200 mg   250 mg   300 mg

Tablets
DuPont: *Ethmozine*

Nadolol and Bendroflumethiazide*

40/5 mg   80/5 mg

Tablets
Bristol: *Corzide*

Niacin

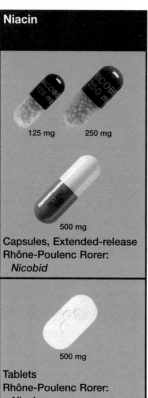

125 mg   250 mg

500 mg

Capsules, Extended-release
Rhône-Poulenc Rorer:
Nicobid

500 mg

Tablets
Rhône-Poulenc Rorer:
Nicolar

250 mg
500 mg
750 mg

Tablets, Extended-release
Upsher-Smith: *Slo-Niacin*

Nitroglycerin

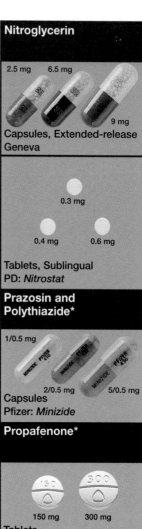

2.5 mg   6.5 mg

9 mg

Capsules, Extended-release
Geneva

0.3 mg

0.4 mg   0.6 mg

Tablets, Sublingual
PD: *Nitrostat*

Prazosin and Polythiazide*

1/0.5 mg

2/0.5 mg   5/0.5 mg

Capsules
Pfizer: *Minizide*

Propafenone*

150 mg   300 mg

Tablets
Knoll: *Rythmol*

Propranolol and Hydrochlorothiazide

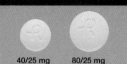

40/25 mg   80/25 mg

Tablets
Purepac

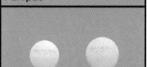

40/25 mg   80/25 mg

Tablets
Rugby

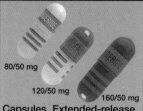

80/50 mg

120/50 mg   160/50 mg

Capsules, Extended-release
Wyeth-Ayerst: *Inderide LA*

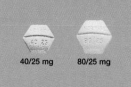

40/25 mg   80/25 mg

Tablets
Wyeth-Ayerst: *Inderide*

Reserpine and Chlorthalidone

0.125/25 mg

Tablets
Rhône-Poulenc Rorer:
Demi-Regroton

0.25/50 mg

Tablets
Rhône-Poulenc Rorer:
Regroton

Reserpine, Hydralazine, and Hydrochlorothiazide

0.1/25/15 mg

Tablets
Ciba: *Ser-Ap-Es*

Spironolactone and Hydrochlorothiazide

25/25 mg

Tablets
Geneva

(continued)

Spironolactone and Hydrochlorothiazide
(continued)

25/25 mg

Tablets
Schein/Danbury

25/25 mg   50/50 mg

Tablets
Searle: *Aldactazide*

Tocainide*

400 mg   600 mg

Tablets
Merck: *Tonocard*

Triamterene and Hydrochlorothiazide

75/50 mg

Tablets
Barr

Triamterene and Hydrochlorothiazide
(continued)

75/50 mg

Tablets
Geneva

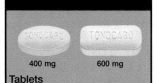

37.5/25 mg   75/50 mg

Tablets
Lederle: *Maxzide*

75/50 mg

Tablets
Schein/Danbury

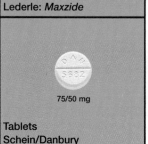

37.5/25 mg

Capsules
SmithKline Beecham:
Dyazide

(continued)

Description

Guanethidine (gwahn-ETH-i-deen) and hydrochlorothiazide (hye-droe-klor-oh-THYE-a-zide) combination is used to treat high blood pressure (hypertension).

High blood pressure adds to the workload of the heart and arteries. If it continues for a long time, the heart and arteries may not function properly. This can damage the blood vessels of the brain, heart, and kidneys, resulting in a stroke, heart failure, or kidney failure. High blood pressure may also increase the risk of heart attacks. These problems may be less likely to occur if blood pressure is controlled.

Guanethidine works by controlling nerve impulses along certain nerve pathways. As a result, it relaxes the blood vessels so that blood passes through them more easily. The hydrochlorothiazide in this combination is a thiazide diuretic (water pill) that helps reduce the amount of water in the body by increasing the flow of urine.

Guanethidine and hydrochlorothiazide combination is available only with your doctor's prescription, in the following dosage form:

Oral
   • Tablets (U.S. and Canada)

Before Using This Medicine

In deciding to use a medicine, the risks of taking the medicine must be weighed against the good it will do. This is a decision you and your doctor will make. For guanethidine and hydrochlorothiazide, the following should be considered:

Allergies—Tell your doctor if you have ever had any unusual or allergic reaction to guanethidine, sulfonamides (sulfa drugs), hydrochlorothiazide, bumetanide, furosemide, acetazolamide, dichlorphenamide, methazolamide, or to other thiazide diuretics (water pills). Also tell your health care professional if you are allergic to any other substance, such as foods, preservatives, or dyes.

Pregnancy—When hydrochlorothiazide is used during pregnancy, it may cause side effects including jaundice, blood problems, and low potassium in the newborn infant. However, this medicine has not been shown to cause birth defects.

Breast-feeding—Guanethidine and hydrochlorothiazide pass into breast milk. However, this medicine has not been reported to cause problems in nursing babies.

Children—Although there is no specific information about the use of this medicine in children, it is not expected to cause different side effects or problems in children than it does in adults. However, extra caution may be necessary in infants with jaundice, because thiazide diuretics can make the condition worse.

Older adults—Dizziness, lightheadedness, fainting, or signs and symptoms of too much potassium loss may be more likely to occur in the elderly, who are more sensitive to the effects of guanethidine and hydrochlorothiazide.

Other medicines—Although certain medicines should not be used together at all, in other cases two different medicines may be used together even if an interaction might occur. In these cases, your doctor may want to change the dose, or other precautions may be necessary. When you are taking guanethidine and hydrochlorothiazide, it is especially important that your health care professional know if you are taking any of the following:

- Antidiabetics, oral (diabetes medicine you take by mouth)—
  Effects may be increased by guanethidine

- Cholestyramine or
- Colestipol—Use with thiazide diuretics may prevent the di-

uretic from working properly; take the diuretic at least 1 hour before or 4 hours after cholestyramine or colestipol

- Digitalis glycosides (heart medicine)—Hydrochlorothiazide may cause low potassium in the blood, which can lead to symptoms of digitalis toxicity
- Lithium (e.g., Lithane)—Risk of lithium overdose, even at usual doses, may be increased
- Loxapine (e.g., Loxitane) or
- Thioxanthenes (chlorprothixene [e.g., Taractan], thiothixene [e.g., Navane]) or
- Tricyclic antidepressants (amitriptyline [e.g., Elavil], amoxapine [e.g., Asendin], clomipramine [e.g., Anafranil], desipramine [e.g., Pertofrane], doxepin [e.g., Sinequan], imipramine [e.g., Tofranil], nortriptyline [e.g., Aventyl], protriptyline [e.g., Vivactil], trimipramine [e.g., Surmontil]) or
- Trimeprazine (e.g., Temaril)—May decrease the effects of guanethidine on blood pressure
- Monoamine oxidase (MAO) inhibitors (furazolidone [e.g., Furoxone], isocarboxazid [e.g., Marplan], phenelzine [e.g., Nardil], procarbazine [e.g., Matulane], selegiline [e.g., Eldepryl], tranylcypromine [e.g., Parnate])—Taking guanethidine while you are taking or within 2 weeks of taking MAO inhibitors may cause a severe increase in blood pressure

Other medical problems—The presence of other medical problems may affect the use of guanethidine and hydrochlorothiazide. Make sure you tell your doctor if you have any other medical problems, especially:

- Asthma (history of) or
- Diarrhea or
- Pheochromocytoma or
- Stomach ulcer (history of)—May be worsened by guanethidine
- Diabetes mellitus (sugar diabetes)—Effects of medicine used to treat this may be increased by guanethidine. Hydrochlorothiazide may change the amount of diabetes medicine needed
- Fever—Effects of guanethidine may be increased

- Gout (history of)—Hydrochlorothiazide may increase the amount of uric acid in the blood, which can lead to gout
- Heart or blood vessel disease or
- Heart attack or stroke (recent)—Lowering blood pressure may make problems resulting from these conditions worse
- Kidney disease—May be worsened. Also, effects may be increased because of slower removal of guanethidine from the body
- Liver disease—Effects may be increased because of slower removal of guanethidine from the body
- Lupus erythematosus (history of)—Hydrochlorothiazide may worsen the condition
- Pancreatitis (inflammation of the pancreas)

Proper Use of This Medicine

This medicine may cause you to have an unusual feeling of tiredness when you begin to take it. You may also notice an increase in the amount of urine or in your frequency of urination. After taking the medicine for a while, these effects should lessen. In general, in order to keep the increase in urine from affecting your sleep:

- If you are to take a single dose a day, take it in the morning after breakfast.
- If you are to take more than one dose a day, take the last dose no later than 6 p.m., unless otherwise directed by your doctor.

However, it is best to plan your dose or doses according to a schedule that will least affect your personal activities and sleep. Ask your health care professional to help you plan the best time to take this medicine.

In addition to the use of the medicine your doctor has prescribed, treatment for your high blood pressure may include weight control and care in the types of foods you eat, especially foods high in sodium. Your doctor will tell you which of these are most important for you. You should check with your doctor before changing your diet.

Many patients who have high blood pressure will not notice any signs of the problem. In fact, many may feel normal. It is very important that you *take your medicine exactly as directed* and that you keep your appointments with your doctor even if you feel well.

Remember that this medicine will not cure your high blood pressure, but it does help control it. Therefore, you must continue to take it as directed if you expect to lower your blood pressure and keep it down. *You may have to take high blood pressure medicine for the rest of your life.* If high blood pressure is not treated, it can cause serious problems such as heart failure, blood vessel disease, stroke, or kidney disease.

To help you remember to take your medicine, try to get into the habit of taking it at the same time each day.

Dosing—The dose of guanethidine and hydrochlorothiazide combination will be different for different patients. *Follow your doctor's orders or the directions on the label.* The following information includes only the average dose of guanethidine and hydrochlorothiazide combination. *If your dose is different, do not change it* unless your doctor tells you to do so.

- For *oral* dosage form (tablets):
  —For high blood pressure:
    - Adults—2 tablets a day.
    - Children—Dose must be determined by your doctor.

Missed dose—If you miss a dose of this medicine, take it as soon as possible. However, if it is almost time for your next dose, skip the missed dose and go back to your regular dosing schedule. Do not double doses.

Storage—To store this medicine:
- Keep out of the reach of children.
- Store away from heat and direct light.
- Do not store in the bathroom, near the kitchen sink,

or in other damp places. Heat or moisture may cause the medicine to break down.

- Do not keep outdated medicine or medicine no longer needed. Be sure that any discarded medicine is out of the reach of children.

Precautions While Using This Medicine

It is important that your doctor check your progress at regular visits to make sure that this medicine is working properly.

Do not take other medicines unless they have been discussed with your doctor. This especially includes over-the-counter (nonprescription) medicines for appetite control, asthma, colds, cough, hay fever, or sinus problems, since they may tend to increase your blood pressure.

This medicine may cause a loss of potassium from your body.

- To help prevent this, your doctor may want you to:
  —eat or drink foods that have a high potassium content (for example, orange or other citrus fruit juices), or

  —take a potassium supplement, or

  —take another medicine to help prevent the loss of the potassium in the first place.

- It is very important to follow these directions. Also, it is important not to change your diet on your own. This is more important if you are already on a special diet (as for diabetes), or if you are taking a potassium supplement or a medicine to reduce potassium loss. Extra potassium may not be necessary and, in some cases, too much potassium could be harmful.

Check with your doctor if you become sick and have severe or continuing vomiting or diarrhea. These problems may cause you to lose additional water and potassium.

Dizziness, lightheadedness, or fainting may occur, especially when you get up from a lying or sitting position. This is more likely to occur in the morning. *Getting up slowly* may help. When you get up from lying down, sit on the edge of the bed with your feet dangling for 1 or 2 minutes. Then stand up slowly. If the problem continues or gets worse, check with your doctor.

The dizziness, lightheadedness, or fainting is also more likely to occur if you drink alcohol, stand for long periods of time or exercise, or if the weather is hot. *While you are taking this medicine, be careful in the amount of alcohol you drink. Also, use extra care during exercise or hot weather or if you must stand for long periods of time.*

For *diabetic patients*:

- This medicine may raise blood sugar levels. While you are using this medicine, be especially careful in testing for sugar in your blood or urine. If you have any questions about this, check with your doctor.

Some people who take this medicine may become more sensitive to sunlight than they are normally. Exposure to sunlight, even for brief periods of time, may cause severe sunburn; skin rash, redness, itching, or discoloration; or vision changes. When you begin taking this medicine:

- Stay out of direct sunlight, especially between the hours of 10:00 a.m. and 3:00 p.m., if possible.
- Wear protective clothing, including a hat and sunglasses.
- Apply a sun block product that has a skin protection factor (SPF) of at least 15. Some patients may require a product with a higher SPF number, especially if they have a fair complexion. If you have any questions about this, check with your health care professional.
- Do not use a sunlamp or tanning bed or booth.

If you have a severe reaction from the sun, check with your doctor.

Tell your doctor if you get a fever since that may change the amount of medicine you have to take.

Before having any kind of surgery (including dental surgery) or emergency treatment, tell the medical doctor or dentist in charge that you are taking this medicine.

Side Effects of This Medicine

Along with its needed effects, a medicine may cause some unwanted effects. Although not all of these side effects may occur, if they do occur they may need medical attention.

Check with your doctor as soon as possible if any of the following side effects occur, especially since some of them may mean that your body is losing too much potassium:

Signs and symptoms of too much potassium loss

> Dryness of mouth; increased thirst; irregular heartbeats; mood or mental changes; muscle cramps or pain; nausea or vomiting; unusual tiredness or weakness; weak pulse

Signs and symptoms of too much sodium loss

> Confusion; convulsions; decreased mental activity; irritability; muscle cramps; unusual tiredness or weakness

Less common

> Chest pain

Rare

> Black, tarry stools; blood in urine or stools; cough or hoarseness; fever or chills; joint pain; lower back or side pain; painful or difficult urination; pinpoint red spots on skin; skin rash or hives; sore throat and fever; stomach pain (severe) with nausea and vomiting; unusual bleeding or bruising; yellow eyes or skin

Other side effects may occur that usually do not need medical attention. These side effects may go away during treatment as your body adjusts to the medicine. However,

check with your doctor if any of the following side effects
continue or are bothersome:

More common

> Diarrhea or increase in bowel movements; dizziness, light-
> headedness, or fainting, especially when getting up
> from a lying or sitting position; sexual problems in
> males; slow heartbeat; stuffy nose

Less common or rare

> Blurred vision; drooping eyelids; headache; increased sen-
> sitivity of skin to sunlight; loss of appetite; loss of hair;
> nighttime urination

Other side effects not listed above may also occur in some
patients. If you notice any other effects, check with your
doctor.

GUANFACINE   Systemic†

A commonly used brand name in the U.S. is Tenex.

†Not commercially available in Canada.

Description

Guanfacine (GWAHN-fa-seen) belongs to the general class
of medicines called antihypertensives. It is used to treat
high blood pressure (hypertension).

High blood pressure adds to the workload of the heart and
arteries. If it continues for a long time, the heart and arteries may not function properly. This can damage the blood
vessels of the brain, heart, and kidneys, resulting in a
stroke, heart failure, or kidney failure. High blood pressure
may also increase the risk of heart attacks. These problems
may be less likely to occur if blood pressure is controlled.

Guanfacine works by controlling nerve impulses along certain nerve pathways. As a result, it relaxes blood vessels

so that blood passes through them more easily. This helps
to lower blood pressure.

Guanfacine is available only with your doctor's prescription, in the following dosage form:

Oral
 • Tablets (U.S.)

Before Using This Medicine

In deciding to use a medicine, the risks of taking the
medicine must be weighed against the good it will do.
This is a decision you and your doctor will make. For
guanfacine, the following should be considered:

Allergies—Tell your doctor if you have ever had any unusual or allergic reaction to guanfacine. Also tell your
health care professional if you are allergic to any other
substance, such as foods, preservatives, or dyes.

Pregnancy—Guanfacine has not been studied in pregnant
women. However, guanfacine has not been shown to cause
birth defects or other problems in rats or rabbits given
many times the human dose. In rats and rabbits given
extremely high doses (up to 200 times the human dose),
there was an increase in deaths of the animal fetus.

Breast-feeding—It is not known whether guanfacine
passes into breast milk. However, this medicine has not
been reported to cause problems in nursing babies.

Children—Studies on this medicine have been done only
in adult patients, and there is no specific information comparing use of guanfacine in children with use in other
age groups.

Older adults—Dizziness, drowsiness, or faintness may be
more likely to occur in the elderly, who are more sensitive
to the effects of guanfacine.

Other medicines—Although certain medicines should not be used together at all, in other cases two different medicines may be used together even if an interaction might occur. In these cases, your doctor may want to change the dose, or other precautions may be necessary. Tell your health care professional if you are taking any other prescription or nonprescription (over-the-counter [OTC]) medicine.

Other medical problems—The presence of other medical problems may affect the use of guanfacine. Make sure you tell your doctor if you have any other medical problems, especially:

- Heart disease or
- Heart attack or stroke (recent)—Lowering blood pressure may make problems resulting from these conditions worse
- Liver disease—Effects may be increased because of slower removal of guanfacine from the body
- Mental depression—Guanfacine may cause mental depression

Proper Use of This Medicine

In addition to the use of the medicine your doctor has prescribed, treatment for your high blood pressure may include weight control and care in the types of foods you eat, especially foods high in sodium. Your doctor will tell you which of these are most important for you. You should check with your doctor before changing your diet.

Many patients who have high blood pressure will not notice any signs of the problem. In fact, many may feel normal. It is very important that you *take your medicine exactly as directed* and that you keep your appointments with your doctor even if you feel well.

Remember that this medicine will not cure your high blood pressure, but it does help control it. Therefore, you must continue to use it as directed if you expect to lower your blood pressure and keep it down. *You may have to take high blood pressure medicine for the rest of your life.* If high blood pressure is not treated, it can cause serious problems such as heart failure, blood vessel disease, stroke, or kidney disease.

Take your daily dose of guanfacine at bedtime. (If you are taking more than one dose a day, take your last dose at bedtime.) Taking it this way will help lessen daytime drowsiness.

Dosing—The dose of guanfacine will be different for different patients. *Follow your doctor's orders or the directions on the label.* The following information includes only the average doses of guanfacine. *If your dose is different, do not change it* unless your doctor tells you to do so.

The number of tablets that you take depends on the strength of the medicine.

*   For *oral* dosage form (tablets):
    —For high blood pressure:
        *   Adults—At first, 1 milligram (mg) once a day at bedtime. Then, your doctor may gradually increase your dose up to 3 mg a day, if needed.
        *   Children—Dose must be determined by your doctor.

Missed dose—If you miss a dose of this medicine, take it as soon as possible. However, if it is almost time for your next dose, skip the missed dose and go back to your regular dosing schedule. Do not double doses. *If you miss taking guanfacine for two or more days in a row, check with your doctor.* If your body suddenly goes without this medicine, some unwanted effects may occur. If you have any questions about this, check with your doctor.

Storage—To store this medicine:

*   Keep out of the reach of children.
*   Store away from heat and direct light.
*   Do not store in the bathroom, near the kitchen sink,

or in other damp places. Heat or moisture may cause the medicine to break down.

- Do not keep outdated medicine or medicine no longer needed. Be sure any discarded medicine is out of the reach of children.

Precautions While Using This Medicine

It is important that your doctor check your progress at regular visits to make sure this medicine is working properly.

Check with your doctor before you stop taking guanfacine. Your doctor may want you to reduce gradually the amount you are taking before stopping completely.

Make sure that you have enough guanfacine on hand to last through weekends, holidays, and vacations. You should not miss any doses. You may want to ask your doctor for another written prescription for guanfacine to carry in your wallet or purse. You can then have it filled if you run out when you are away from home.

Before having any kind of surgery (including dental surgery) or emergency treatment, tell the medical doctor or dentist in charge that you are using this medicine.

Do not take other medicines unless they have been discussed with your doctor. This especially includes over-the-counter (nonprescription) medicines for appetite control, asthma, colds, cough, hay fever, or sinus problems, since they may tend to increase your blood pressure.

Guanfacine will add to the effects of alcohol and other CNS depressants (medicines that slow down the nervous system, possibly causing drowsiness). Some examples of CNS depressants are antihistamines or medicine for hay fever, other allergies, or colds; sedatives, tranquilizers, or sleeping medicine; prescription pain medicine or narcotics; barbiturates; medicine for seizures; muscle relaxants; or anesthetics, including some dental anesthetics. *Check with your doctor before taking any of the above while you are using this medicine.*

Guanfacine may cause some people to become dizzy, drowsy, or less alert than they are normally. *Make sure you know how you react to this medicine before you drive, use machines, or do anything else that could be dangerous if you are dizzy or are not alert.*

Guanfacine may cause dryness of the mouth, nose, and throat. For temporary relief of mouth dryness, use sugarless candy or gum, melt bits of ice in your mouth, or use a saliva substitute. However, if dry mouth continues for more than 2 weeks, check with your physician or dentist. Continuing dryness of the mouth may increase the chance of dental disease, including tooth decay, gum disease, and fungus infections.

Side Effects of This Medicine

Along with its needed effects, a medicine may cause some unwanted effects. Although not all of these side effects may occur, if they do occur they may need medical attention.

Check with your doctor as soon as possible if any of the following side effects occur:

Less common
    Confusion; mental depression

Signs and symptoms of overdose
    Difficulty in breathing; dizziness (extreme) or faintness; slow heartbeat; unusual tiredness or weakness (severe)

Other side effects may occur that usually do not need medical attention. These side effects may go away during treatment as your body adjusts to the medicine. However, check with your doctor if any of the following side effects continue or are bothersome:

More common

Constipation; dizziness; drowsiness; dryness of mouth

Less common

Decreased sexual ability; dry, itching, or burning eyes; headache; nausea or vomiting; trouble in sleeping; unusual tiredness or weakness

After you have been using this medicine for a while, unwanted effects may occur if you stop taking it too suddenly. After you stop taking this medicine, check with your doctor if any of the following side effects occur:

Anxiety or tenseness; chest pain; fast or irregular heartbeat; headache; increased salivation; nausea or vomiting; nervousness or restlessness; shaking or trembling of hands and fingers; stomach cramps; sweating; trouble in sleeping

Other side effects not listed above may also occur in some patients. If you notice any other effects, check with your doctor.

HEPARIN   Systemic

Some commonly used brand names are:

In the U.S.—

Calciparine	Liquaemin

Generic name product may also be available.

In Canada—

Calcilean	Hepalean
Calciparine	Heparin Leo

Generic name product may also be available.

Description

Heparin (HEP-a-rin) is an anticoagulant. It is used to decrease the clotting ability of the blood and help prevent harmful clots from forming in the blood vessels. This medicine is sometimes called a blood thinner, although it does not actually thin the blood. Heparin will not dissolve blood clots that have already formed, but it may prevent the clots from becoming larger and causing more serious problems.

Heparin is often used as a treatment for certain blood vessel, heart, and lung conditions. Heparin is also used to prevent blood clotting during open-heart surgery, bypass surgery, and dialysis. It is also used in low doses to prevent the formation of blood clots in certain patients, especially those who must have certain types of surgery or who must remain in bed for a long time.

Heparin is available only with your doctor's prescription, in the following dosage form:

Parenteral
- Injection (U.S. and Canada)

Before Using This Medicine

In deciding to use a medicine, the risks of taking the medicine must be weighed against the good it will do. This is a decision you and your doctor will make. For heparin, the following should be considered:

Allergies—Tell your doctor if you have ever had any unusual or allergic reaction to heparin, to beef, or to pork. Also tell your health care professional if you are allergic to any other substances, such as foods, preservatives, or dyes.

Pregnancy—Heparin has not been shown to cause birth defects or bleeding problems in the baby. However, use during the last 3 months of pregnancy or during the month following the baby's delivery may cause bleeding problems in the mother.

Breast-feeding—Heparin does not pass into the breast milk. However, heparin can rarely cause bone problems in the nursing mother. This effect has been reported to occur when heparin is used for 2 weeks or more. Be sure to discuss this with your doctor.

Children—Heparin has been tested in children and, in effective doses, has not been shown to cause different side effects or problems than it does in adults.

Older adults—Bleeding problems may be more likely to occur in elderly patients, especially women, who are usually more sensitive than younger adults to the effects of heparin.

Other medicines—Although certain medicines should not be used together at all, in other cases two different medicines may be used together even if an interaction might occur. In these cases, your doctor may want to change the dose, or other precautions may be necessary. When you are taking heparin, it is especially important that your health care professional know if you are taking any of the following:

- Aspirin or
- Carbenicillin by injection (e.g., Geopen) or
- Cefamandole (e.g., Mandol) or
- Cefoperazone (e.g., Cefobid) or
- Cefotetan (e.g., Cefotan) or
- Dipyridamole (e.g., Persantine) or
- Divalproex (e.g., Depakote) or
- Medicine for inflammation or pain, except narcotics, or
- Medicine for overactive thyroid or
- Pentoxifylline (e.g., Trental) or
- Plicamycin (e.g., Mithracin) or
- Probenecid (e.g., Benemid) or
- Sulfinpyrazone (e.g., Anturane) or
- Ticarcillin (e.g., Ticar) or
- Valproic acid (e.g., Depakene)—Using any of these medicines together with heparin may increase the risk of bleeding

Also, tell your doctor if you are now receiving any kind of medicine by intramuscular (IM) injection.

Other medical problems—The presence of other medical problems may affect the use of heparin. Make sure you tell your doctor if you have any other medical problems, especially:

- Allergies or asthma (history of)—The risk of an allergic reaction to heparin may be increased
- Blood disease or bleeding problems or
- Colitis or stomach ulcer (or history of) or
- Diabetes mellitus (sugar diabetes) (severe) or
- High blood pressure (hypertension) or
- Kidney disease or
- Liver disease or
- Tuberculosis (active)—The risk of bleeding may be increased

Also, tell your doctor if you have received heparin before and had a reaction to it called thrombocytopenia, or if new blood clots formed while you were receiving the medicine.

In addition, it is important that you tell your doctor if you have recently had any of the following conditions or medical procedures:

- Childbirth or
- Falls or blows to the body or head or
- Heavy or unusual menstrual bleeding or
- Insertion of intrauterine device (IUD) or
- Medical or dental surgery or
- Spinal anesthesia or
- X-ray (radiation) treatment—The risk of serious bleeding may be increased

---

Proper Use of This Medicine

If you are using these injections at home, make sure your doctor has explained exactly how this medicine is to be given.

To obtain the best results without causing serious bleeding, *use this medicine exactly as directed by your doctor. Be certain that you are using the right amount of heparin, and that you use it according to schedule.* Be especially careful that you do not use more of it, do not use it more often, and do not use it for a longer time than your doctor ordered.

Your doctor should check your progress at regular visits. A blood test must be taken regularly to see how fast your blood is clotting so that your doctor can decide on the proper amount of heparin you should be receiving each day.

Dosing—The dose of heparin will be different for different patients and must be determined by your doctor. The dose you receive will be based on the type of heparin you receive, the condition for which you are receiving heparin, and your body weight.

Missed dose—If you miss a dose of this medicine, use it as soon as possible. However, if it is almost time for your next dose, do not use the missed dose at all and do not double the next one. *Doubling the dose may cause bleeding.* Instead, go back to your regular dosing schedule. It is best to keep a record of each dose as you use it to avoid mistakes. Be sure to give your doctor a record of any doses you miss. If you have any questions about this, check with your doctor.

Storage—To store this medicine:

- Keep out of the reach of children.
- Store away from heat and direct light.
- Keep the medicine from freezing.
- Do not keep outdated medicine or medicine no longer needed. Be sure that any discarded medicine is out of the reach of children.

Precautions While Using This Medicine

Do not take aspirin while using this medicine. Many non-prescription (over-the-counter [OTC]) medicines and some prescription medicines contain aspirin. Check the labels of all medicines you take. Also, do not take ibuprofen unless it has been ordered by your doctor. In addition, there are many other medicines that may change the way heparin works or increase the chance of bleeding if they are used together with heparin. It is best to check with your health care professional before taking any other medicine while you are using heparin.

Tell all medical doctors and dentists you visit that you are using this medicine.

It is recommended that you carry identification stating that you are using heparin. If you have any questions about what kind of identification to carry, check with your health care professional.

While you are using this medicine, it is very important that you avoid sports and other activities that may cause you to be injured. Report to your doctor any falls, blows to the body or head, or other injuries, since serious bleeding inside the body may occur without your knowing about it.

Take special care in brushing your teeth and in shaving. Use a soft toothbrush and floss gently. Also, it is best to use an electric shaver rather than a blade.

Side Effects of This Medicine

Since many things can affect the way your body reacts to this medicine, you should always watch for signs of unusual bleeding. Unusual bleeding may mean that your body is getting more heparin than it needs.

Along with its needed effects, a medicine may cause some unwanted effects. Although not all of these side effects may occur, if they do occur they may need medical attention.

Check with your doctor immediately if any of the following signs and symptoms of bleeding inside the body occur:

  Abdominal or stomach pain or swelling; back pain or backaches; blood in urine; bloody or black, tarry stools; constipation; coughing up blood; dizziness; headaches (severe or continuing); joint pain, stiffness, or swelling; vomiting of blood or material that looks like coffee grounds

Also, *check with your doctor immediately* if any of the following side effects occur, since they may mean that you are having a serious allergic reaction to the medicine:

Changes in the skin color of the face; fast or irregular breathing; puffiness or swelling of the eyelids or around the eyes; shortness of breath, troubled breathing, tightness in chest, and/or wheezing; skin rash, hives, and/or itching

Also, check with your doctor as soon as possible if any of the following occur:

Bleeding from gums when brushing teeth; heavy bleeding or oozing from cuts or wounds; unexplained bruising or purplish areas on skin; unexplained nosebleeds; unusually heavy or unexpected menstrual bleeding

Other side effects that may need medical attention may occur while you are using this medicine. Check with your doctor as soon as possible if any of the following side effects occur:

Less common or rare

Back or rib pain (with long-term use only); change in skin color, especially near the place of injection or in the fingers, toes, arms, or legs; chest pain; chills and/or fever; collection of blood under skin (blood blister) at place of injection; decrease in height (with long-term use only); frequent or persistent erection; irritation, pain, redness, or ulcers at place of injection; itching and burning feeling, especially on the bottom of the feet; nausea and/or vomiting; numbness or tingling in hands or feet; pain, coldness, or blue color of skin of arms or legs; peeling of skin; runny nose; tearing of eyes; unusual hair loss (with long-term use only)

Other side effects not listed above may also occur in some patients. If you notice any other effects, check with your doctor.

HMG-CoA REDUCTASE INHIBITORS   Systemic

Some commonly used brand names are:

In the U.S.—
    Lescol[1]   Pravachol[3]
    Mevacor[2]   Zocor[4]

In Canada—
    Mevacor[2]   Zocor[4]
    Pravachol[3]

Other commonly used names are:

    Epistatin[4]   Mevinolin[2]
    Eptastatin[3]   Synvinolin[4]

Note: For quick reference, the following HMG-CoA reductase inhibitors are numbered to match the corresponding brand names.

This information applies to the following medicines:

1. Fluvastatin (FLOO-va-sta-tin)†
2. Lovastatin (LOE-va-sta-tin)
3. Pravastatin (PRA-va-stat-in)
4. Simvastatin (SIM-va-stat-in)

---

†Not commercially available in Canada.

Description

Fluvastatin, lovastatin, pravastatin, and simvastatin are used to lower levels of cholesterol and other fats in the blood. This may help prevent medical problems caused by cholesterol clogging the blood vessels.

These medicines belong to the group of medicines called 3-hydroxy-3-methylglutaryl coenzyme A (HMG-CoA) reductase inhibitors. They work by blocking an enzyme that is needed by the body to make cholesterol. Thus, less cholesterol is made.

HMG-CoA reductase inhibitors are available only with your doctor's prescription, in the following dosage forms:

Oral

Fluvastatin
- Capsules (U.S.)

Lovastatin
- Tablets (U.S. and Canada)

Pravastatin
- Tablets (U.S. and Canada)

Simvastatin
- Tablets (U.S and Canada)

Before Using This Medicine

In deciding to use a medicine, the risks of taking the medicine must be weighed against the good it will do. This is a decision you and your doctor will make. For HMG-CoA reductase inhibitors, the following should be considered:

Allergies—Tell your doctor if you have ever had any unusual or allergic reaction to HMG-CoA reductase inhibitors. Also tell your health care professional if you are allergic to any other substances, such as foods, preservatives, or dyes.

Diet—Before prescribing medicines to lower your cholesterol, your doctor will probably try to control your condition by prescribing a personal diet for you. Such a diet will be lower in total fat, particularly saturated fat, and dietary cholesterol. Many people are able to control their condition by carefully following their doctor's orders for proper diet and exercise. *Medicine is prescribed only when additional help is needed* and is effective only when a schedule of diet and exercise is properly followed.

Also, this medicine is less effective if you are greatly overweight. It may be very important for you to go on a reducing diet. However, check with your doctor before going on any diet.

Pregnancy—HMG-CoA reductase inhibitors should not be used during pregnancy or by women who plan to become pregnant in the near future. These medicines block formation of cholesterol, which is necessary for the fetus to develop properly. HMG-CoA reductase inhibitors may cause birth defects or other problems in the baby if taken during pregnancy. An effective form of birth control should be used during treatment with these medicines. *Check with your doctor immediately if you think you have become pregnant while taking this medicine.* Be sure you have discussed this with your doctor.

Breast-feeding—These medicines are not recommended for use during breast-feeding because they may cause unwanted effects in nursing babies.

Children—Studies on this medicine have been done only in adult patients, and there is no specific information comparing use of HMG-CoA reductase inhibitors in children with use in other age groups. However, lovastatin and simvastatin have been used in a limited number of children under 18 years of age. Early information seems to show that these medicines may be effective in children, but their long-term safety has not been studied.

Older adults—This medicine has been tested in a limited number of patients 65 years of age or older and has not been shown to cause different side effects or problems in older people than it does in younger adults.

Other medicines—Although certain medicines should not be used together at all, in other cases two different medicines may be used together even if an interaction might occur. In these cases, your doctor may want to change the dose, or other precautions may be necessary. When you are taking HMG-CoA reductase inhibitors, it is especially important that your health care professional know if you are taking any of the following:

- Cyclosporine (e.g., Sandimmune) or
- Gemfibrozil (e.g., Lopid) or
- Niacin—Use of these medicines with an HMG-CoA reductase inhibitor may increase the risk of developing muscle problems and kidney failure

Other medical problems—The presence of other medical problems may affect the use of HMG-CoA reductase inhibitors. Make sure you tell your doctor if you have any other medical problems, especially:

- Alcohol abuse (or history of) or
- Liver disease—Use of this medicine may make liver problems worse
- Convulsions (seizures), not well-controlled, or
- Organ transplant with therapy to prevent transplant rejection or
- If you have recently had major surgery—Patients with these conditions may be at risk of developing problems that may lead to kidney failure

---

Proper Use of This Medicine

Use this medicine only as directed by your doctor. Do not use more or less of it, and do not use it more often or for a longer time than your doctor ordered.

Remember that this medicine will not cure your condition, but it does help control it. Therefore, you must continue to take it as directed if you expect to keep your cholesterol levels down.

Follow carefully the special diet your doctor gave you. This is the most important part of controlling your condition, and is necessary if the medicine is to work properly.

For patients taking *lovastatin:*

- This medicine works better when it is taken with food. If you are taking this medicine once a day, take it with the evening meal. If you are taking more than one dose a day, take each dose with a meal or snack.

Dosing—The dose of these medicines will be different for different patients. *Follow your doctor's orders or the directions on the label.* The following information includes only the average doses of these medicines. *If your dose is* *different, do not change it* unless your doctor tells you to do so.

The number of capsules or tablets that you take depends on the strength of the medicine.

For fluvastatin

- For *oral* dosage form (capsules):

  —For high cholesterol:

    - Adults—20 to 40 milligrams (mg) once a day in the evening.

    - Children—Use and dose must be determined by your doctor.

For lovastatin

- For *oral* dosage form (tablets):

  —For high cholesterol:

    - Adults—20 to 80 milligrams (mg) a day taken as a single dose or divided into smaller doses. Take with meals.

    - Children—Use and dose must be determined by your doctor.

For pravastatin

- For *oral* dosage form (tablets):

  —For high cholesterol:

    - Adults—10 to 40 mg once a day at bedtime.

    - Children—Use and dose must be determined by your doctor.

For simvastatin

- For *oral* dosage form (tablets):

  —For high cholesterol:

    - Adults—5 to 40 mg once a day in the evening.

    - Children—Use and dose must be determined by your doctor.

Missed dose—If you miss a dose of this medicine, take it as soon as possible. However, if it is almost time for

your next dose, skip the missed dose and go back to your regular dosing schedule. Do not double doses.

Storage—To store this medicine:
- Keep out of the reach of children.
- Store away from heat and direct light.
- Do not store in the bathroom, near the kitchen sink, or in other damp places. Heat or moisture may cause the medicine to break down.
- Keep the medicine from freezing. Do not refrigerate.
- Do not keep outdated medicine or medicine no longer needed. Be sure that any discarded medicine is out of the reach of children.

Precautions While Using This Medicine

It is very important that your doctor check your progress at regular visits. This will allow your doctor to see if the medicine is working properly to lower your cholesterol levels and that it does not cause unwanted effects.

Check with your doctor immediately if you think that you may be pregnant. HMG-CoA reductase inhibitors may cause birth defects or other problems in the baby if taken during pregnancy.

Do not stop taking this medicine without first checking with your doctor. When you stop taking this medicine, your blood cholesterol levels may increase again. Your doctor may want you to follow a special diet to help prevent this from happening.

Before having any kind of surgery (including dental surgery) or emergency treatment, tell the medical doctor or dentist in charge that you are taking this medicine.

Side Effects of This Medicine

Along with its needed effects, a medicine may cause some unwanted effects. Although not all of these side effects

may occur, if they do occur they may need medical attention.

Check with your doctor as soon as possible if any of the following side effects occur:

Less common or rare

Fever; muscle aches or cramps; severe stomach pain; unusual tiredness or weakness

Other side effects may occur that usually do not need medical attention. These side effects may go away during treatment as your body adjusts to the medicine. However, check with your doctor if any of the following side effects continue or are bothersome:

More common

Constipation; diarrhea; dizziness; gas; headache; heartburn; nausea; skin rash; stomach pain

Rare

Decreased sexual ability; trouble in sleeping

Other side effects not listed above may also occur in some patients. If you notice any other effects, check with your doctor.

HYDRALAZINE   Systemic

Some commonly used brand names are:
In the U.S.—
Apresoline
Generic name product may also be available.
In Canada—
Apresoline
Novo-Hylazin

Description

Hydralazine (hye-DRAL-a-zeen) belongs to the general class of medicines called antihypertensives. It is used to treat high blood pressure (hypertension).

High blood pressure adds to the workload of the heart and arteries. If it continues for a long time, the heart and arteries may not function properly. This can damage the blood vessels of the brain, heart, and kidneys, resulting in a stroke, heart failure, or kidney failure. High blood pressure may also increase the risk of heart attacks. These problems may be less likely to occur if blood pressure is controlled.

Hydralazine works by relaxing blood vessels and increasing the supply of blood and oxygen to the heart while reducing its work load.

Hydralazine may also be used for other conditions as determined by your doctor.

Hydralazine is available only with your doctor's prescription, in the following dosage forms:

Oral
- Tablets (U.S. and Canada)

Parenteral
- Injection (U.S.)

Before Using This Medicine

In deciding to use a medicine, the risks of taking the medicine must be weighed against the good it will do. This is a decision you and your doctor will make. For hydralazine, the following should be considered:

Allergies—Tell your doctor if you have ever had any unusual or allergic reaction to hydralazine. Also tell your health care professional if you are allergic to any other substance, such as foods, preservatives, or dyes.

Pregnancy—Hydralazine has not been studied in pregnant women. However, blood problems have been reported in infants of mothers who took hydralazine during pregnancy. In addition, studies in mice have shown that hydralazine causes birth defects (cleft palate, defects in head and face bones). These birth defects may also occur in rabbits, but do not occur in rats. Before taking this medicine, make sure your doctor knows if you are pregnant or if you may become pregnant.

Breast-feeding—It is not known whether hydralazine passes into breast milk.

Children—Although there is no specific information comparing use of hydralazine in children with use in other age groups, this medicine is not expected to cause different side effects or problems in children than it does in adults.

Older adults—Many medicines have not been studied specifically in older people. Therefore, it may not be known whether they work exactly the same way they do in younger adults. Although there is no specific information comparing use of hydralazine in the elderly with use in other age groups, this medicine is not expected to cause different side effects or problems in older people than it does in younger adults. However, dizziness or lightheadedness may be more likely to occur in the elderly, who are more sensitive to the effects of hydralazine.

Other medicines—Although certain medicines should not be used together at all, in other cases two different medicines may be used together even if an interaction might occur. In these cases, your doctor may want to change the dose, or other precautions may be necessary. When you are taking hydralazine, it is especially important that your health care professional know if you are taking the following:

• Diazoxide (e.g., Proglycem)—Effect on blood pressure may be increased

Other medical problems—The presence of other medical problems may affect the use of hydralazine. Make sure you tell your doctor if you have any other medical problems, especially:

• Heart or blood vessel disease or

- Stroke—Lowering blood pressure may make problems resulting from these conditions worse
- Kidney disease—Effects may be increased because of slower removal of hydralazine from the body

---

Proper Use of This Medicine

For patients taking this medicine *for high blood pressure:*

- In addition to the use of the medicine your doctor has prescribed, treatment for your high blood pressure may include weight control and care in the types of foods you eat, especially foods high in sodium. Your doctor will tell you which of these are most important for you. You should check with your doctor before changing your diet.

- Many patients who have high blood pressure will not notice any signs of the problem. In fact, many may feel normal. It is very important that you *take your medicine exactly as directed* and that you keep your appointments with your doctor even if you feel well.

- Remember that hydralazine will not cure your high blood pressure but it does help control it. Therefore, you must continue to take it as directed if you expect to lower your blood pressure and keep it down. *You may have to take high blood pressure medicine for the rest of your life.* If high blood pressure is not treated, it can cause serious problems such as heart failure, blood vessel disease, stroke, or kidney disease.

To help you remember to take your medicine, try to get into the habit of taking it at the same time each day.

Dosing—The dose of hydralazine will be different for different patients. *Follow your doctor's orders or the directions on the label.* The following information includes only the average doses of hydralazine. *If your dose is different, do not change it* unless your doctor tells you to do so.

The number of tablets that you take depends on the strength of the medicine.

- For *oral* dosage form (tablets):

    —For high blood pressure:

    - Adults—10 to 50 milligrams (mg) four times a day.

    - Children—Dose is based on body weight or size. The usual dose is 0.75 to 7.5 mg per kilogram (kg) (0.34 to 3.4 mg per pound) of body weight a day. This is divided into two to four doses.

- For *injection* dosage form:

    —For high blood pressure:

    - Adults—10 to 40 mg injected into a muscle or a vein. Your doctor may repeat the dose as needed.

    - Children—Dose is based on body weight or size. The usual dose is 1.7 to 3.5 mg per kg (0.77 to 1.6 mg per pound) of body weight a day. This is divided into four to six doses and injected into a muscle or a vein.

Missed dose—If you miss a dose of this medicine, take it as soon as possible. However, if it is almost time for your next dose, skip the missed dose and go back to your regular dosing schedule. Do not double doses.

Storage—To store this medicine:

- Keep out of the reach of children.

- Store away from heat and direct light.

- Do not store in the bathroom, near the kitchen sink, or in other damp places. Heat or moisture may cause the medicine to break down.

- Do not keep outdated medicine or medicine no longer needed. Be sure that any discarded medicine is out of the reach of children.

Precautions While Using This Medicine

It is important that your doctor check your progress at regular visits to make sure that this medicine is working properly.

For patients taking this medicine *for high blood pressure:*

- *Do not take other medicines unless they have been discussed with your doctor.* This especially includes over-the-counter (nonprescription) medicines for appetite control, asthma, colds, cough, hay fever, or sinus problems, since they may tend to increase your blood pressure.

Hydralazine may cause some people to have headaches or to feel dizzy. *Make sure you know how you react to this medicine before you drive, use machines, or do anything else that could be dangerous if you are dizzy or are not alert.*

Side Effects of This Medicine

Along with its needed effects, a medicine may cause some unwanted effects. Although not all of these side effects may occur, if they do occur they may need medical attention.

In general, side effects with hydralazine are rare at lower doses. However, check with your doctor as soon as possible if any of the following occur:

Less common

Blisters on skin; chest pain; general feeling of discomfort or illness or weakness; joint pain; numbness, tingling, pain, or weakness in hands or feet; skin rash or itching; sore throat and fever; swelling of feet or lower legs; swelling of the lymph glands

Other side effects may occur that usually do not need medical attention. These side effects may go away during treatment as your body adjusts to the medicine. However,

check with your doctor if any of the following side effects continue or are bothersome:

More common

   Diarrhea; fast or irregular heartbeat; headache; loss of appetite; nausea or vomiting; pounding heartbeat

Less common

   Constipation; dizziness or lightheadedness; redness or flushing of face; shortness of breath; stuffy nose; watering or irritated eyes

Other side effects not listed above may also occur in some patients. If you notice any other effects, check with your doctor.

Additional Information

Once a medicine has been approved for marketing for a certain use, experience may show that it is also useful for other medical problems. Although this use is not specifically included in product labeling, hydralazine is used in certain patients with the following medical condition:

• Congestive heart failure

Other than the above information, there is no additional information relating to proper use, precautions, or side effects for this use.

HYDRALAZINE AND HYDRO-CHLOROTHIAZIDE   Systemic†

Some commonly used brand names are:

In the U.S.—

Apresazide	Aprozide
Apresoline-Esidrix	Hydra-zide

Generic name product may also be available.

---

†Not commercially available in Canada.

Description

Hydralazine (hye-DRAL-a-zeen) and hydrochlorothiazide (hye-droe-klor-oh-THYE-a-zide) combination is used to treat high blood pressure (hypertension).

High blood pressure adds to the workload of the heart and arteries. If it continues for a long time, the heart and arteries may not function properly. This can damage the blood vessels of the brain, heart, and kidneys, resulting in a stroke, heart failure, or kidney failure. High blood pressure may also increase the risk of heart attacks. These problems may be less likely to occur if blood pressure is controlled.

Hydralazine works by relaxing blood vessels and increasing the supply of blood and oxygen to the heart while reducing its workload. The hydrochlorothiazide in this combination helps reduce the amount of water in the body by acting on the kidneys to increase the flow of urine.

This medicine is available only with your doctor's prescription, in the following dosage forms:

Oral
- Capsules (U.S.)
- Tablets (U.S.)

Before Using This Medicine

In deciding to use a medicine, the risks of taking the medicine must be weighed against the good it will do. This is a decision you and your doctor will make. For hydralazine and hydrochlorothiazide, the following should be considered:

Allergies—Tell your doctor if you have ever had any unusual or allergic reaction to hydralazine, sulfonamides (sulfa drugs), indapamide, or any of the thiazide diuretics (water pills). Also tell your health care professional if you are allergic to any other substance, such as foods, preservatives, or dyes.

Pregnancy—When hydrochlorothiazide is used during pregnancy, it may cause side effects including jaundice, blood problems, and low potassium in the newborn infant.

Studies with hydralazine have not been done in humans. However, blood problems have been reported in infants of mothers who took hydralazine during pregnancy. In addition, studies in mice have shown that hydralazine causes birth defects (cleft palate, defects in head and face bones); these birth defects may also occur in rabbits, but do not occur in rats.

Breast-feeding—Hydrochlorothiazide passes into breast milk. However, neither hydralazine nor hydrochlorothiazide has been reported to cause problems in nursing babies.

Children—Although there is no specific information comparing use of this medicine in children with use in other age groups, this medicine is not expected to cause different side effects or problems in children than it does in adults. However, extra caution may be necessary in infants with jaundice, because thiazide diuretics can make this condition worse.

Older adults—Many medicines have not been studied specifically in older people. Therefore, it may not be known whether they work exactly the same way they do in younger adults. Although there is no specific information comparing use of hydralazine and hydrochlorothiazide combination in the elderly with use in other age groups, this medicine is not expected to cause different side effects or problems in older people than it does in younger adults. However, dizziness or lightheadedness or symptoms of too much potassium loss may be more likely to occur in the elderly, who are usually more sensitive to the effects of this medicine. Also, this medicine may reduce tolerance to cold temperatures in elderly patients.

Other medicines—Although certain medicines should not be used together at all, in other cases two different medicines may be used together even if an interaction might occur. In these cases, your doctor may want to change the dose, or other precautions may be necessary. When you are taking hydralazine and hydrochlorothiazide, it is especially important that your health care professional know if you are taking any of the following:

- Cholestyramine or
- Colestipol—Use with thiazide diuretics may prevent the diuretic from working properly; take the diuretic at least 1 hour before or 4 hours after cholestyramine or colestipol
- Diazoxide (e.g., Proglycem)—Effect on blood pressure may be increased
- Digitalis glycosides (heart medicine)—Hydrochlorothiazide may cause low potassium in the blood, which can lead to symptoms of digitalis toxicity
- Lithium (e.g., Lithane)—Risk of lithium overdose, even at usual doses, may be increased

Other medical problems—The presence of other medical problems may affect the use of hydralazine and hydrochlorothiazide. Make sure you tell your doctor if you have any other medical problems, especially:

- Diabetes mellitus (sugar diabetes)—Hydrochlorothiazide may change the amount of diabetes medicine needed
- Gout (history of)—Hydrochlorothiazide may increase the amount of uric acid in the blood, which can lead to gout
- Heart or blood vessel disease or
- Stroke (recent)—Lowering blood pressure may make problems resulting from these conditions worse
- Kidney disease—Hydrochlorothiazide may worsen this condition. Also, the blood-pressure-lowering effects may be increased because of slower removal of hydralazine from the body
- Liver disease—If hydrochlorothiazide causes loss of too

much water from the body, liver disease can become much worse

- Lupus erythematosus (history of)—Hydrochlorothiazide may worsen the condition
- Pancreatitis (inflammation of the pancreas)

Proper Use of This Medicine

This medicine may cause you to have an unusual feeling of tiredness when you begin to take it. You may also notice an increase in the amount of urine or in your frequency of urination. After taking the medicine for a while, these effects should lessen. To keep the increase in urine from affecting your sleep:

- If you are to take a single dose a day, take it in the morning after breakfast.
- If you are to take more than one dose a day, take the last dose no later than 6 p.m., unless otherwise directed by your doctor.

However, it is best to plan your dose or doses according to a schedule that will least affect your personal activities and sleep. Ask your health care professional to help you plan the best time to take this medicine.

In addition to the use of the medicine your doctor has prescribed, treatment for your high blood pressure may include weight control and care in the types of foods you eat, especially foods high in sodium. Your doctor will tell you which of these are most important for you. You should check with your doctor before changing your diet.

Many patients who have high blood pressure will not notice any signs of the problem. In fact, many may feel normal. It is very important that you *take your medicine exactly as directed* and that you keep your appointments with your doctor even if you feel well.

Remember that this medicine will not cure your high blood pressure but it does help control it. Therefore, you must continue to take it as directed if you expect to lower your blood pressure and keep it down. *You may have to take high blood pressure medicine for the rest of your life.* If high blood pressure is not treated, it can cause serious problems such as heart failure, blood vessel disease, stroke, or kidney disease.

To help you remember to take your medicine, try to get into the habit of taking it at the same time each day.

Dosing—The dose of hydralazine and hydrochlorothiazide combination will be different for different patients. *Follow your doctor's orders or the directions on the label.* The following information includes only the average dose of hydralazine and hydrochlorothiazide combination. *If your dose is different, do not change it* unless your doctor tells you to do so.

The number of capsules or tablets that you take depends on the strength of the medicine.

- For *oral* dosage forms (capsules or tablets):
  - —For high blood pressure:
    - Adults—1 capsule or tablet two times a day.
    - Children—Dose must be determined by your doctor.

Missed dose—If you miss a dose of this medicine, take it as soon as possible. However, if it is almost time for your next dose, skip the missed dose and go back to your regular dosing schedule. Do not double doses.

Storage—To store this medicine:

- Keep out of the reach of children.
- Store away from heat and direct light.
- Do not store in the bathroom, near the kitchen sink, or in other damp places. Heat or moisture may cause the medicine to break down.
- Do not keep outdated medicine or medicine no longer needed. Be sure that any discarded medicine is out of the reach of children.

Precautions While Using This Medicine

It is important that your doctor check your progress at regular visits to make sure that this medicine is working properly.

Do not take other medicines unless they have been discussed with your doctor. This especially includes over-the-counter (nonprescription) medicines for appetite control, asthma, colds, cough, hay fever, or sinus problems, since they may tend to increase your blood pressure.

This medicine may cause some people to have headaches or to feel dizzy. *Make sure you know how you react to this medicine before you drive, use machines, or do anything else that could be dangerous if you are dizzy or are not alert.*

Dizziness, lightheadedness, or fainting may occur, especially when you get up from a lying or sitting position. This is more likely to occur in the morning. *Getting up slowly may help.* When you get up from lying down, sit on the edge of the bed with your feet dangling for 1 or 2 minutes. Then stand up slowly. If the problem continues or gets worse, check with your doctor.

The dizziness, lightheadedness, or fainting is also more likely to occur if you drink alcohol, stand for a long time, exercise, or if the weather is hot. *While you are taking this medicine, be careful in the amount of alcohol you drink. Also, use extra care during exercise or hot weather or if you must stand for a long time.*

This medicine may cause a loss of potassium from your body.
- To help prevent this, your doctor may want you to:
    —eat or drink foods that have a high potassium content (for example, orange or other citrus fruit juices), or
    —take a potassium supplement, or

—take another medicine to help prevent the loss of the potassium in the first place.

- It is very important to follow these directions. Also, it is important not to change your diet on your own. This is more important if you are already on a special diet (as for diabetes), or if you are taking a potassium supplement or a medicine to reduce potassium loss. Extra potassium may not be necessary and, in some cases, too much potassium could be harmful.

Check with your doctor if you become sick and have severe or continuing nausea, vomiting, or diarrhea. These problems may cause you to lose additional water and potassium.

For *diabetic patients*:

- Thiazide diuretics may raise blood sugar levels. While you are using this medicine, be especially careful in testing for sugar in your blood or urine. If you have any questions about this, check with your doctor.

Some people who take this medicine may become more sensitive to sunlight than they are normally. Exposure to sunlight, even for brief periods of time, may cause severe sunburn; skin rash, redness, itching, or discoloration; or vision changes. When you begin taking this medicine:

- Stay out of direct sunlight, especially between the hours of 10:00 a.m. and 3:00 p.m., if possible.
- Wear protective clothing, including a hat and sunglasses.
- Apply a sun block product that has a skin protection factor (SPF) of at least 15. Some patients may require a product with a higher SPF number, especially if they have a fair complexion. If you have any questions about this, check with your health care professional.
- Do not use a sunlamp or tanning bed or booth.

If you have a severe reaction from the sun, check with your doctor.

Side Effects of This Medicine

Along with its needed effects, a medicine may cause some unwanted effects. Although not all of these side effects may occur, if they do occur they may need medical attention.

Check with your doctor as soon as possible if any of the following side effects occur:

Signs and symptoms of too much potassium loss

Dryness of mouth; increased thirst; irregular heartbeat; mood or mental changes; muscle cramps or pain; weak pulse

Signs and symptoms of too much sodium loss

Confusion; convulsions; decreased mental activity; irritability; muscle cramps; unusual tiredness or weakness

Less common

Blisters on skin; chest pain; general feeling of discomfort or illness or weakness; joint pain; numbness, tingling, pain, or weakness in hands or feet; skin rash or itching; sore throat and fever; swelling of the lymph glands

Rare

Lower back or side pain; severe stomach pain with nausea and vomiting; unusual bleeding or bruising; yellow eyes or skin

Other side effects may occur that usually do not need medical attention. These side effects may go away during treatment as your body adjusts to the medicine. However, check with your doctor if any of the following side effects continue or are bothersome:

More common

Diarrhea; fast or irregular heartbeat; headache; loss of appetite; nausea or vomiting

Less common

Constipation; decreased sexual ability; dizziness or light-headedness, especially when getting up from a lying or sitting position; increased sensitivity of skin to sunlight; redness or flushing of face; shortness of breath with exercise or work; stuffy nose; watering or irritated eyes

Other side effects not listed above may also occur in some patients. If you notice any other effects, check with your doctor.

INDAPAMIDE Systemic

Some commonly used brand names are:
In the U.S.—
Lozol
In Canada—
Lozide

Description

Indapamide (in-DAP-a-mide) belongs to the group of medicines known as diuretics. It is commonly used to treat high blood pressure (hypertension).

High blood pressure adds to the workload of the heart and arteries. If it continues for a long time, the heart and arteries may not function properly. This can damage the blood vessels of the brain, heart, and kidneys, resulting in a stroke, heart failure, or kidney failure. High blood pressure may also increase the risk of heart attacks. These problems may be less likely to occur if blood pressure is controlled.

Indapamide is also used to help reduce the amount of water in the body by increasing the flow of urine.

Indapamide is available only with your doctor's prescription, in the following dosage form:

Oral
- Tablets (U.S. and Canada)

Before Using This Medicine

In deciding to use a medicine, the risks of taking the medicine must be weighed against the good it will do. This is a decision you and your doctor will make. For indapamide, the following should be considered:

Allergies—Tell your doctor if you have ever had any unusual or allergic reaction to indapamide or other sulfonamide-type medicines. Also tell your health care professional if you are allergic to any other substances, such as foods, preservatives, or dyes.

Pregnancy—Indapamide has not been studied in pregnant women. However, indapamide has not been shown to cause birth defects or other problems in animal studies.

In general, diuretics are not useful for normal swelling of feet and hands that occurs during pregnancy. Diuretics should not be taken during pregnancy unless recommended by your doctor.

Breast-feeding—It is not known whether indapamide passes into breast milk. However, this medicine has not been reported to cause problems in nursing babies.

Children—Studies on this medicine have been done only in adult patients, and there is no specific information comparing use of indapamide in children with use in other age groups.

Older adults—Dizziness or lightheadedness and signs and symptoms of too much potassium loss are more likely to occur in the elderly, who are usually more sensitive than younger adults to the effects of indapamide.

Other medicines—Although certain medicines should not be used together at all, in other cases two different medicines may be used together even if an interaction might occur. In these cases, your doctor may want to change the dose, or other precautions may be necessary. When you are taking indapamide, it is especially important that your health care professional know if you are taking any of the following:

- Digitalis glycosides (heart medicine)—Use with indapamide may increase the chance of side effects of digitalis glycosides
- Lithium (e.g., Lithane)—Use with indapamide may cause high blood levels of lithium, which may increase the chance of side effects

Other medical problems—The presence of other medical problems may affect the use of indapamide. Make sure you tell your doctor if you have any other medical problems, especially:

- Diabetes mellitus (sugar diabetes) or
- Gout (history of)—Indapamide may make these conditions worse
- Kidney disease—May prevent indapamide from working properly
- Liver disease—Higher blood levels of indapamide may occur, which may increase the chance of side effects

---

Proper Use of This Medicine

Indapamide may cause you to have an unusual feeling of tiredness when you begin to take it. You may also notice an increase in the amount of urine or in your frequency of urination. After taking the medicine for a while, these effects should lessen. In general, to keep the increase in urine from affecting your sleep:

- If you are to take a single dose a day, take it in the morning after breakfast.
- If you are to take more than one dose a day, take the last dose no later than 6 p.m., unless otherwise directed by your doctor.

However, it is best to plan your dose or doses according to a schedule that will least affect your personal activities and sleep. Ask your health care professional to help you plan the best time to take this medicine.

To help you remember to take indapamide, try to get into the habit of taking it at the same time each day.

For patients taking indapamide for *high blood pressure:*

- In addition to the use of the medicine your doctor has prescribed, treatment for your high blood pressure may include weight control and care in the types of foods you eat, especially foods high in sodium. Your doctor will tell you which of these are most important for you. You should check with your doctor before changing your diet.

- Many patients who have high blood pressure will not notice any signs of the problem. In fact, many may feel normal. It is very important that you *take your medicine exactly as directed* and that you keep your appointments with your doctor even if you feel well.

- Remember that this medicine will not cure your high blood pressure, but it does help control it. Therefore, you must continue to take it as directed if you expect to lower your blood pressure and keep it down. *You may have to take high blood pressure medicine for the rest of your life.* If high blood pressure is not treated, it can cause serious problems such as heart failure, blood vessel disease, stroke, or kidney disease.

Dosing—The dose of indapamide will be different for different patients. *Follow your doctor's orders or the directions on the label.* The following information includes only the average doses of indapamide. *If your dose is different, do not change it* unless your doctor tells you to do so:

- For *oral* dosage forms (tablets):

    —Adults: 2.5 to 5 milligrams once a day.

Missed dose—If you miss a dose of this medicine, take it as soon as possible. However, if it is almost time for

your next dose, skip the missed dose and go back to your regular dosing schedule. Do not double doses.

Storage—To store this medicine:

- Keep out of the reach of children.
- Store away from heat and direct light.
- Do not store in the bathroom, near the kitchen sink, or in other damp places. Heat or moisture may cause the medicine to break down.
- Do not keep outdated medicine or medicine no longer needed. Be sure that any discarded medicine is out of the reach of children.

Precautions While Using This Medicine

It is important that your doctor check your progress at regular visits to make sure that indapamide is working properly.

This medicine may cause a loss of potassium from your body:

- To help prevent this, your doctor may want you to:

   —eat or drink foods that have a high potassium content (for example, orange or other citrus fruit juices), or

   —take a potassium supplement, or

   —take another medication to help prevent the loss of the potassium in the first place.

- It is very important to follow these directions. Also, it is important not to change your diet on your own. This is more important if you are already on a special diet (as for diabetes), or if you are taking a potassium supplement or a medicine to reduce potassium loss. Extra potassium may not be necessary and, in some cases, too much potassium could be harmful.

Check with your doctor if you become sick and have severe or continuing vomiting or diarrhea. These problems may cause you to lose additional water and potassium.

For patients taking this medicine for *high blood pressure:*

• *Do not take other medicines unless they have been discussed with your doctor.* This especially includes over-the-counter (nonprescription) medicines for appetite control, asthma, colds, hay fever, or sinus problems, since they may tend to increase your blood pressure.

Side Effects of This Medicine

Along with its needed effects, a medicine may cause some unwanted effects. Although not all of these side effects may occur, if they do occur they may need medical attention.

Check with your doctor as soon as possible if any of the following side effects occur:

Dryness of mouth; increased thirst; irregular heartbeat; mood or mental changes; muscle cramps or pain; nausea or vomiting; unusual tiredness or weakness; weak pulse

Rare

Skin rash, itching, or hives

Other side effects may occur that usually do not need medical attention. These side effects may go away during treatment as your body adjusts to the medicine. However, check with your doctor if any of the following side effects continue or are bothersome:

Less common or rare

Diarrhea; dizziness or lightheadedness, especially when getting up from a lying or sitting position; headache; loss of appetite; trouble in sleeping; stomach upset

Other side effects not listed above may also occur in some patients. If you notice any other effects, check with your doctor.

ISOXSUPRINE Systemic

A commonly used brand name in the U.S. and Canada is Vasodilan.

Generic name product may also be available in the U.S.

Description

Isoxsuprine (eye-SOX-syoo-preen) belongs to the group of medicines called vasodilators. Vasodilators increase the size of blood vessels. Isoxsuprine is used to treat problems resulting from poor blood circulation.

It may also be used for other conditions as determined by your doctor.

Isoxsuprine is available only with your doctor's prescription, in the following dosage forms:

Oral
- Tablets (U.S. and Canada)

Parenteral
- Injection (Canada)

Before Using This Medicine

In deciding to use a medicine, the risks of taking the medicine must be weighed against the good it will do. This is a decision you and your doctor will make. For isoxsuprine, the following should be considered:

Allergies—Tell your doctor if you have ever had any unusual or allergic reaction to isoxsuprine. Also tell your health care professional if you are allergic to any other substances, such as foods, preservatives, or dyes.

Pregnancy—Isoxsuprine has not been shown to cause birth defects in humans. However, isoxsuprine given shortly before delivery may cause fast heartbeat and other problems (low blood sugar, bowel problems, low blood pressure) in the newborn.

Breast-feeding—Isoxsuprine has not been reported to cause problems in nursing babies.

Older adults—Many medicines have not been studied specifically in older people. Therefore, it may not be known whether they work exactly the same way they do in younger adults or if they cause different side effects or problems in older people. There is no specific information comparing use of isoxsuprine in the elderly with use in other age groups. However, isoxsuprine may reduce tolerance to cold temperatures in elderly patients.

Other medicines—Although certain medicines should not be used together at all, in other cases two different medicines may be used together even if an interaction might occur. In these cases, your doctor may want to change the dose, or other precautions may be necessary. Tell your health care professional if you are taking any other prescription or nonprescription (over-the-counter [OTC]) medicine, or if you smoke.

Other medical problems—The presence of other medical problems may affect the use of isoxsuprine. Make sure you tell your doctor if you have any other medical problems, especially:
- Angina (chest pain) or
- Bleeding problems or
- Glaucoma or
- Hardening of the arteries or
- Heart attack (recent) or
- Stroke (recent)—The chance of side effects may be increased

---

Proper Use of This Medicine

If this medicine upsets your stomach, it may be taken with meals, milk, or antacids.

Dosing—The dose of isoxsuprine will be different for different patients. *Follow your doctor's orders or the directions on the label.* The following information includes only the average doses of isoxsuprine. *If your dose is different, do not change it* unless your doctor tells you to do so.

The number of tablets that you take depends on the strength of the medicine.

- For *oral* dosage form (tablets):
  —For poor blood circulation:
    - Adults—10 to 20 milligrams (mg) three or four times a day.

Missed dose—If you miss a dose of this medicine, take it as soon as possible. However, if it is almost time for your next dose, skip the missed dose and go back to your regular dosing schedule. Do not double doses.

Storage—To store this medicine:

- Keep out of the reach of children.
- Store away from heat and direct light.
- Do not store in the bathroom, near the kitchen sink, or in other damp places. Heat or moisture may cause the medicine to break down.
- Do not keep outdated medicine or medicine no longer needed. Be sure that any discarded medicine is out of the reach of children.

Precautions While Using This Medicine

It may take some time for this medicine to work. If you feel that the medicine is not working, do not stop taking it on your own. Instead, check with your doctor.

The helpful effects of this medicine may be decreased if you smoke. If you have any questions about this, check with your doctor.

Dizziness may occur, especially when you get up from a lying or sitting position or climb stairs. Getting up slowly may help. If this problem continues or gets worse, check with your doctor.

Side Effects of This Medicine

Along with its needed effects, a medicine may cause some unwanted effects. Although not all of these side effects may occur, if they do occur they may need medical attention.

Check with your doctor as soon as possible if any of the following side effects occur:

> *Rare*
>> Chest pain; dizziness or faintness (more common for injection); fast heartbeat (more common for injection); shortness of breath; skin rash

Other side effects may occur that usually do not need medical attention. These side effects may go away during treatment as your body adjusts to the medicine. However, check with your doctor if the following side effects continue or are bothersome:

> *Less common*
>> Nausea or vomiting (more common for injection)

Other side effects not listed above may also occur in some patients. If you notice any other effects, check with your doctor.

Additional Information

Although this use is not included in U.S. product labeling, isoxsuprine is used in certain women to stop premature labor.

In addition to the above information, the following infor-

mation applies when this medicine is used to stop premature labor:

- Before you begin treatment with this medicine, tell your doctor if you have any of the following medical problems:

  Asthma
  Diabetes mellitus (sugar diabetes)
  Heart disease
  High blood pressure
  Overactive thyroid

- *Check with your doctor immediately:*

  —if your contractions begin again or your water breaks.

  —if you notice chest pain or shortness of breath while taking isoxsuprine.

LIDOCAINE—For Self-injection
Systemic†

A commonly used brand name in the U.S. is LidoPen.

This information does *not* apply to any other dosage forms or brand names of lidocaine.

†Not commercially available in Canada.

Description

Lidocaine (LYE-doe-kane) belongs to the group of medicines called antiarrhythmics. It is used to change an abnormal rhythm in the heart back to normal. Lidocaine produces its helpful effects by slowing abnormal nerve impulses in the heart and reducing irritability of heart tissues.

Lidocaine is usually given by a health care professional when a rapid effect is needed. However, this dosage form has been prescribed by your doctor as part of the early management of a heart attack when certain abnormal heart rhythms occur. It is designed to be used by the patient under instructions from a doctor.

This form of lidocaine is available only with your doctor's prescription and *is to be administered only under direct orders from your doctor*. It is available in the following dosage form:

Parenteral
- Injection (U.S.)

Before Using This Medicine

In deciding to use a medicine, the risks of taking the medicine must be weighed against the good it will do. This is a decision you and your doctor will make. For lidocaine, the following should be considered:

Allergies—Tell your doctor if you have ever had any unusual or allergic reaction to lidocaine, flecainide, tocainide, or anesthetics.

Pregnancy—Lidocaine has not been studied in pregnant women. However, this medicine may reduce the blood supply to the unborn baby.

Breast-feeding—It is not known whether lidocaine passes into breast milk. However, this medicine has not been reported to cause problems in nursing babies.

Children—Although there is no specific information comparing use of lidocaine in children with use in other age groups, this medicine is not expected to cause different side effects or problems in children than it does in adults.

Older adults—Elderly people are especially sensitive to the effects of lidocaine. This may increase the chance of side effects during treatment.

Other medicines—Although certain medicines should not be used together at all, in other cases two different medicines may be used together even if an interaction might occur. In these cases, your doctor may want to change the dose, or other precautions may be necessary. When you are receiving lidocaine it is especially important that your health care professional know if you are taking any of the following:

- Ethotoin (e.g., Peganone) or
- Mephenytoin (e.g., Mesantoin) or
- Phenytoin (e.g., Dilantin)—Risk of slow heartbeat may be increased. Other effects of lidocaine may be decreased because these medicines may cause it to be removed from the body more quickly

Other medical problems—The presence of other medical problems may affect the use of lidocaine. Make sure you tell your doctor if you have any other medical problems, especially:

- Congestive heart failure or
- Kidney disease or
- Liver disease—Effects may be increased because of slower removal of lidocaine from the body

---

Proper Use of This Medicine

This medicine should be kept within easy reach, along with your doctor's telephone number. Check the expiration date on the lidocaine regularly. Replace the medicine before it expires.

Be familiar with possible symptoms of a heart attack and how to recognize them. If they occur, *telephone your doctor immediately*. The special device your doctor gave you will transmit your electrocardiogram (ECG or EKG) over the telephone. Your doctor will look at your ECG and tell you whether you need to use this medicine.

Lidocaine comes with patient directions. Read them carefully before you actually need to use this medicine. Then, when an emergency arises, you will know how to inject the lidocaine.

To use the lidocaine self-injector:

- Remove the gray safety cap.
- Place the black end of the self-injector on the thickest part of your thigh and press hard until the injector functions. You should feel a needle prick.
- Hold the device firmly in place for 10 seconds, then remove it. Massage the injection area for 10 seconds.

Dosing—The dose of lidocaine will be different for different patients. *Follow your doctor's orders or the directions on the label.* The following information includes only the average doses of lidocaine. *If your dose is different, do not change it* unless your doctor tells you to do so.

- For *injection* dosage form:
  —For arrhythmia (abnormal heart rhythm):
    - Adults—4.3 milligrams (mg) per kilogram (kg) (1.95 mg per pound) of body weight injected into the muscle. The dose may be repeated after sixty to ninety minutes if needed.
    - Children—Dose must be determined by your doctor. Use is not recommended in children weighing less than 50 kg (23 pounds).

Storage—To store this medicine:

- Keep out of the reach of children.
- Store away from heat and direct light.
- Keep the medicine from freezing.

Precautions While Using This Medicine

Do not administer this injection unless instructed to do so by your doctor. Your doctor is trained to read the electrocardiogram and decide whether an abnormal heart rhythm is occurring.

Unless it is absolutely necessary, *do not attempt to drive after using this medicine.* Follow your doctor's instructions about what to do next, including going to the doctor's office or hospital emergency room, if necessary.

Side Effects of This Medicine

Along with its needed effects, a medicine may cause some unwanted effects. Although not all of these side effects may occur, if they do occur they may need medical attention.

Check with your doctor immediately if any of the following side effects occur:

Rare

Convulsions (seizures); difficulty in breathing; itching; skin rash; swelling of skin

Check with your doctor as soon as possible if any of the following side effects occur:

Signs and symptoms of overdose

Blurred or double vision; dizziness (severe) or fainting; nausea or vomiting; ringing in ears; slow heartbeat; tremors or twitching

Other side effects may occur that usually do not need medical attention. However, check with your doctor if the following side effects continue or are bothersome:

Less common or rare

Anxiety or nervousness; dizziness; drowsiness; feelings of coldness, heat, or numbness; pain at place of injection

Other side effects not listed above may also occur in some patients. If you notice any other effects, check with your doctor.

MECAMYLAMINE Systemic†

A commonly used brand name in the U.S. is Inversine.

†Not commercially available in Canada.

Description

Mecamylamine (mek-a-MILL-a-meen) belongs to the general class of medicines called antihypertensives. It is used to treat high blood pressure (hypertension).

High blood pressure adds to the workload of the heart and arteries. If it continues for a long time, the heart and arteries may not function properly. This can damage the blood vessels of the brain, heart, and kidneys, resulting in a stroke, heart failure, or kidney failure. High blood pressure may also increase the risk of heart attacks. These problems may be less likely to occur if blood pressure is controlled.

Mecamylamine works by controlling impulses along certain nerve pathways. As a result, it relaxes blood vessels so that blood passes through them more easily. This helps to lower blood pressure.

Mecamylamine is available only with your doctor's prescription, in the following dosage form:

Oral
- Tablets (U.S.)

Before Using This Medicine

In deciding to use a medicine, the risks of taking the medicine must be weighed against the good it will do. This is a decision you and your doctor will make. For mecamylamine, the following should be considered:

Allergies—Tell your doctor if you have ever had any unusual or allergic reaction to mecamylamine. Also tell your

health care professional if you are allergic to any other substances, such as foods, preservatives, or dyes.

Pregnancy—Studies on effects in pregnancy have not been done in either humans or animals. However, in general, use of this medicine during pregnancy is not recommended because pregnant women may be more sensitive to its effects. In addition, mecamylamine may cause bowel problems in the unborn baby.

Breast-feeding—It is not known whether mecamylamine passes into breast milk. However, this medicine has not been reported to cause problems in nursing babies.

Children—Studies on this medicine have been done only in adult patients, and there is no specific information comparing use of mecamylamine in children with use in other age groups.

Older adults—Dizziness or lightheadedness may be more likely to occur in the elderly, who are more sensitive to the effects of mecamylamine.

Other medicines—Although certain medicines should not be used together at all, in many cases two different medicines may be used together even if an interaction might occur. In these cases, changes in dose or other precautions may be necessary. When taking mecamylamine it is especially important that your health care professional know if you are taking any of the following:

- Antibiotics or
- Sulfonamides (sulfa medicine)—Patients with chronic pyelonephritis being treated with these medications should not be treated with mecamylamine
- Antimyasthenics (ambenonium [e.g., Mytelase], neostigmine [e.g., Prostigmin], pyridostigmine [e.g., Mestinon])—Effects of these medicines may be decreased by mecamylamine
- Urinary alkalizers (medicine that makes the urine less acid, such as acetazolamide [e.g., Diamox], calcium- and/or magnesium-containing antacids, dichlorphenamide [e.g.,

Daranide], methazolamide [e.g., Neptazane], potassium or sodium citrate and/or citric acid, sodium bicarbonate [baking soda])—Effects of mecamylamine may be increased because these medicines cause it to be removed more slowly from the body

Other medical problems—The presence of other medical problems may affect the use of mecamylamine. Make sure you tell your doctor if you have any other medical problems, especially:

- Bladder or prostate problems—Mecamylamine may interfere with urination
- Bowel problems—Patients with bowel problems who take mecamylamine may be at inceased risk for serious bowel side effects of mecamylamine
- Diarrhea or
- Fever or infection or
- Nausea or vomiting—Effects of mecamylamine on blood pressure may be increased
- Glaucoma—Mecamylamine may make this condition worse
- Heart or blood vessel disease or
- Heart attack or stroke (recent)—Lowering of blood pressure by mecamylamine may make problems resulting from these conditions worse
- Kidney disease—Effects of mecamylamine may be increased because of slower removal of mecamylamine from the body

---

Proper Use of This Medicine

In addition to the use of the medicine your doctor has prescribed, treatment for your high blood pressure may include weight control and care in the types of foods you eat, especially foods high in sodium. Your doctor will tell you which of these are most important for you. You should check with your doctor before changing your diet.

Many patients who have high blood pressure will not notice any signs of the problem. In fact, many may feel normal. *It is very important that you take your medicine exactly as directed and that you keep your appointments with your doctor* even if you feel well.

Remember that this medicine will not cure your high blood pressure but it does help control it. Therefore, you must continue to take it as directed if you expect to lower your blood pressure and keep it down. *You may have to take high blood pressure medicine for the rest of your life.* If high blood pressure is not treated, it can cause serious problems such as heart failure, blood vessel disease, stroke, or kidney disease.

To help you remember to take your medicine, try to get into the habit of taking it at the same time each day.

Dosing—The dose of mecamylamine will be different for different patients. *Follow your doctor's orders or the directions on the label.* The following information includes only the average doses of mecamylamine. *If your dose is different, do not change it* unless your doctor tells you to do so:

* For *oral* dosage forms (tablets):
  —Adults: 2.5 milligrams two times a day to 25 milligrams three times a day.

Missed dose—If you miss a dose of this medicine, take it as soon as possible. Then go back to your regular dosing schedule. *If you miss two or more doses in a row, check with your doctor right away.* If your body goes without this medicine for too long, your blood pressure may go up to a dangerously high level.

Storage—To store this medicine:

* Keep out of the reach of children.
* Store away from heat and direct light.
* Do not store in the bathroom, near the kitchen sink, or in other damp places. Heat or moisture may cause the medicine to break down.
* Do not keep outdated medicine or medicine no longer

needed. Be sure that any discarded medicine is out of the reach of children.

Precautions While Using This Medicine

It is important that your doctor check your progress at regular visits to make sure that this medicine is working properly.

Check with your doctor before you stop taking this medicine. Your doctor may want you to reduce gradually the amount you are taking before stopping completely.

Make sure that you have enough medicine on hand to last through weekends, holidays, or vacations. You should not miss taking any doses. You may want to ask your doctor for another written prescription for mecamylamine to carry in your wallet or purse. You can then have it filled if you run out of medicine when you are away from home.

Do not take other medicines unless they have been discussed with your doctor. This especially includes over-the-counter (nonprescription) medicines for appetite control, asthma, colds, cough, hay fever, or sinus problems, since they may tend to increase your blood pressure.

Dizziness, lightheadedness, or fainting may occur, especially when you get up from a lying or sitting position. This is more likely to occur in the morning. *Getting up slowly may help.* When you get up from lying down, sit on the edge of the bed with your feet dangling for one or two minutes. Then stand up slowly. If you feel dizzy, sit or lie down. If the problem continues or gets worse, check with your doctor.

The dizziness, lightheadedness, or fainting is also more likely to occur if you drink alcohol, stand for a long time, exercise, or if the weather is hot. *While you are taking this medicine, be careful to limit the amount of alcohol you drink. Also, use extra care during exercise or hot weather or if you must stand for a long time.*

Sodium bicarbonate (commonly known as baking soda) may cause you to get a greater than normal effect from this medicine. To prevent problems, check with your health care professional before using an antacid or medicine for heartburn since some of these contain sodium bicarbonate.

Tell your doctor if you get a fever or infection since that may change the amount of medicine you have to take.

Mecamylamine may cause dryness of the mouth, nose, and throat. For temporary relief of mouth dryness, use sugarless candy or gum, melt bits of ice in your mouth, or use a saliva substitute. However, if your mouth continues to feel dry for more than 2 weeks, check with your medical doctor or dentist. Continuing dryness of the mouth may increase the chance of dental disease, including tooth decay, gum disease, and fungus infections.

Before having any kind of surgery (including dental surgery) or emergency treatment, tell the medical doctor or dentist in charge that you are taking this medicine.

Side Effects of This Medicine

Along with its needed effects, a medicine may cause some unwanted effects. Although not all of these side effects may occur, if they do occur they may need medical attention.

Check with your doctor as soon as possible if any of the following side effects occur:

More common

Dizziness or lightheadedness, especially when getting up from a lying or sitting position

Less common

Difficult urination

Rare

Bloating and frequent loose stools; confusion or excitement; constipation (severe); convulsions (seizures); mental depression; shortness of breath; trembling; uncontrolled movements of face, hands, arms, or legs

Other side effects may occur that usually do not need medical attention. These side effects may go away during treatment as your body adjusts to the medicine. However, check with your doctor if any of the following side effects continue or are bothersome:

More common

Constipation; drowsiness; unusual tiredness

Less common or rare

Blurred vision; decreased sexual ability or interest in sex; dryness of mouth; enlarged pupils; loss of appetite; nausea and vomiting; weakness

Other side effects not listed above may also occur in some patients. If you notice any other effects, check with your doctor.

METHYLDOPA   Systemic

Some commonly used brand names are:

In the U.S.—

Aldomet

Generic name product may also be available.

In Canada—

Aldomet   Dopamet

Apo-Methyldopa   Novomedopa

Generic name product may also be available.

Description

Methyldopa (meth-ill-DOE-pa) belongs to the general class of medicines called antihypertensives. It is used to treat high blood pressure (hypertension).

High blood pressure adds to the workload of the heart and arteries. If it continues for a long time, the heart and arteries may not function properly. This can damage the blood vessels of the brain, heart, and kidneys, resulting in a stroke, heart failure, or kidney failure. High blood pressure may also increase the risk of heart attacks. These problems may be less likely to occur if blood pressure is controlled.

Methyldopa works by controlling impulses along certain nerve pathways. As a result, it relaxes blood vessels so that blood passes through them more easily. This helps to lower blood pressure.

Methyldopa is available only with your doctor's prescription, in the following dosage forms:

Oral
- Oral suspension (U.S.)
- Tablets (U.S. and Canada)

Parenteral
- Injection (U.S. and Canada)

Before Using This Medicine

In deciding to use a medicine, the risks of taking the medicine must be weighed against the good it will do. This is a decision you and your doctor will make. For methyldopa, the following should be considered:

Allergies—Tell your doctor if you have ever had any unusual or allergic reaction to methyldopa. Also tell your health care professional if you are allergic to any other substances, such as foods, sulfites or other preservatives, or dyes. Some methyldopa products may contain sulfites. Your health care professional can help you avoid products that may cause a problem.

Pregnancy—Methyldopa has not been studied in pregnant women in the first and second trimesters (the first 6

months of pregnancy). However, studies in pregnant
women during the third trimester (the last 3 months of
pregnancy) have not shown that methyldopa causes birth
defects or other problems.

Breast-feeding—Although methyldopa passes into breast
milk, it has not been reported to cause problems in nursing babies.

Children—Although there is no specific information comparing use of methyldopa in children with use in other age
groups, this medicine is not expected to cause different
side effects or problems in children than it does in adults.

Older adults—Dizziness or lightheadedness and drowsiness may be more likely to occur in the elderly, who are
more sensitive to the effects of methyldopa.

Other medicines—Although certain medicines should not
be used together at all, in other cases two different medicines may be used together even if an interaction might
occur. In these cases, your doctor may want to change the
dose, or other precautions may be necessary. When you
are taking methyldopa, it is especially important that your
health care professional know if you are taking any of
the following:

- Monoamine oxidase (MAO) inhibitors (furazolidone [e.g.,
  Furoxone], isocarboxazid [e.g., Marplan], phenelzine [e.g.,
  Nardil], procarbazine [e.g., Matulane], selegiline [e.g., El-
  depryl], tranylcypromine [e.g., Parnate])—Taking methyldopa while you are taking or within 2 weeks of taking
  MAO inhibitors may cause nervousness in patients receiving MAO inhibitors; headache, severe high blood pressure,
  and hallucinations have been reported

Other medical problems—The presence of other medical
problems may affect the use of methyldopa. Make sure
you tell your doctor if you have any other medical problems, especially:

- Angina (chest pain)—Methyldopa may worsen the condition

- Kidney disease or
- Liver disease—Effects of methyldopa may be increased because of slower removal from the body
- Mental depression (history of)—Methyldopa can cause mental depression
- Parkinson's disease—Methyldopa may worsen condition
- Pheochromocytoma—Methyldopa may interfere with tests for the condition; in addition, there have been reports of increased blood pressure
- If you have taken methyldopa in the past and developed liver problems

Proper Use of This Medicine

In addition to the use of the medicine your doctor has prescribed, treatment for your high blood pressure may include weight control and care in the types of foods you eat, especially foods high in sodium. Your doctor will tell you which of these are most important for you. You should check with your doctor before changing your diet.

Many patients who have high blood pressure will not notice any signs of the problem. In fact, many may feel normal. It is very important that you *take your medicine exactly as directed* and that you keep your appointments with your doctor even if you feel well.

Remember that methyldopa will not cure your high blood pressure but it does help control it. Therefore, you must continue to take it as directed if you expect to lower your blood pressure and keep it down. *You may have to take high blood pressure medicine for the rest of your life.* If high blood pressure is not treated, it can cause serious problems such as heart failure, blood vessel disease, stroke, or kidney disease.

To help you remember to take your medicine, try to get into the habit of taking it at the same time each day.

Dosing—The dose of methyldopa will be different for different patients. *Follow your doctor's orders or the directions on the label.* The following information includes only the average doses of methyldopa. *If your dose is different, do not change it* unless your doctor tells you to do so.

The number of tablets or teaspoonfuls of suspension that you take depends on the strength of the medicine.

- For *oral* dosage form (suspension or tablets):
  —For high blood pressure:
  - Adults—250 milligrams (mg) to 2 grams a day. This is divided into two to four doses.
  - Children—Dose is based on body weight or size and must be determined by your doctor. The usual dose is 10 mg per kilogram (kg) (4.5 mg per pound) of body weight a day. This is divided into two to four doses. Your doctor may increase the dose as needed.
- For *injection* dosage form:
  —For high blood pressure:
  - Adults—250 to 500 mg mixed in 100 milliliters (mL) of solution (5% dextrose) and slowly injected into a vein every six hours as needed.
  - Children—Dose is based on body weight and must be determined by your doctor. The usual dose is 5 to 10 mg per kg (2.3 to 4.5 mg per pound) of body weight. This is mixed in a solution (5% dextrose) and slowly injected into a vein every six hours as needed.

Missed dose—If you miss a dose of this medicine, take it as soon as possible. However, if it is almost time for your next dose, skip the missed dose and go back to your regular dosing schedule. Do not double doses.

Storage—To store this medicine:
- Keep out of the reach of children.
- Store away from heat and direct light.
- Do not store in the bathroom, near the kitchen sink,

or in other damp places. Heat or moisture may cause the medicine to break down.

- Keep the oral liquid form of this medicine from freezing.
- Do not keep outdated medicine or medicine no longer needed. Be sure that any discarded medicine is out of the reach of children.

Precautions While Using This Medicine

It is important that your doctor check your progress at regular visits to make sure that this medicine is working properly.

Do not take other medicines unless they have been discussed with your doctor. This especially includes over-the-counter (nonprescription) medicines for appetite control, asthma, colds, cough, hay fever, or sinus problems, since they may tend to increase your blood pressure.

If you have a fever and there seems to be no reason for it, check with your doctor. This is especially important during the first few weeks you take methyldopa, since fever may be a sign of a serious reaction to this medicine.

Before having any kind of surgery (including dental surgery) or emergency treatment, make sure the medical doctor or dentist in charge knows that you are taking this medicine.

Methyldopa may cause some people to become drowsy or less alert than they are normally. This is more likely to happen when you begin to take it or when you increase the amount of medicine you are taking. *Make sure you know how you react to this medicine before you drive, use machines, or do anything else that could be dangerous if you are not alert.*

Dizziness, lightheadedness, or fainting may occur, especially when you get up from a lying or sitting position.

Getting up slowly may help, but if the problem continues or gets worse, check with your doctor.

Methyldopa may cause dryness of the mouth. For temporary relief, use sugarless candy or gum, melt bits of ice in your mouth, or use a saliva substitute. However, if your mouth continues to feel dry for more than 2 weeks, check with your medical doctor or dentist. Continuing dryness of the mouth may increase the chance of dental disease, including tooth decay, gum disease, and fungus infections.

Tell the doctor in charge that you are taking this medicine before you have any medical tests. The results of some tests may be affected by this medicine.

Side Effects of This Medicine

Along with its needed effects, a medicine may cause some unwanted effects. Although not all of these side effects may occur, if they do occur they may need medical attention.

Check with your doctor immediately if the following side effect occurs:

Less common

Fever, shortly after starting to take this medicine

Check with your doctor as soon as possible if any of the following side effects occur:

More common

Swelling of feet or lower legs

Less common

Mental depression or anxiety; nightmares or unusually vivid dreams

Rare

Dark or amber urine; diarrhea or stomach cramps (severe or continuing); fever, chills, troubled breathing, and fast heartbeat; general feeling of discomfort or illness or weakness; joint pain; pale stools; skin rash or itching;

   stomach pain (severe) with nausea and vomiting; tiredness or weakness after having taken this medicine for
   several weeks (continuing); yellow eyes or skin

Other side effects may occur that usually do not need
medical attention. These side effects may go away during
treatment as your body adjusts to the medicine. However,
check with your doctor if any of the following side effects
continue or are bothersome:

 More common
   Drowsiness; dryness of mouth; headache

 Less common
   Decreased sexual ability or interest in sex; diarrhea; dizziness or lightheadedness when getting up from a lying
   or sitting position; nausea or vomiting; numbness, tingling, pain, or weakness in hands or feet; slow heartbeat; stuffy nose; swelling of breasts or unusual milk
   production

Other side effects not listed above may also occur in some
patients. If you notice any other effects, check with your
doctor.

METHYLDOPA AND THIAZIDE
DIURETICS   Systemic

Some commonly used brand names are:

In the U.S.—
 Aldoclor[1]   Aldoril[2]

In Canada—
 Aldoril[2]   PMS Dopazide[2]
 Novodoparil[2]   Supres[1]

Note: For quick reference, the following medicines are numbered to
   match the corresponding brand names.

This information applies to the following medicines:

 1. Methyldopa (meth-ill-DOE-pa) and Chlorothiazide (klor-oh-THYE-
   a-zide)‡
 2. Methyldopa and Hydrochlorothiazide (hye-droe-klor-oh-THYE-a-
   zide)‡

‡Generic name product may also be available in the U.S.

Description

Combinations of methyldopa and a thiazide diuretic (chlorothiazide or hydrochlorothiazide) are used to treat high blood pressure (hypertension).

High blood pressure adds to the workload of the heart and arteries. If it continues for a long time, the heart and arteries may not function properly. This can damage the blood vessels of the brain, heart, and kidneys, resulting in a stroke, heart failure, or kidney failure. High blood pressure may also increase the risk of heart attacks. These problems may be less likely to occur if blood pressure is controlled.

Methyldopa works by controlling nerve impulses along certain nerve pathways. As a result, it relaxes blood vessels so that blood passes through them more easily. Thiazide diuretics help reduce the amount of water in the body by increasing the flow of urine. These actions help to lower blood pressure.

This medicine is available only with your doctor's prescription, in the following dosage forms:

Oral

Methyldopa and Chlorothiazide
  • Tablets (U.S. and Canada)
Methyldopa and Hydrochlorothiazide
  • Tablets (U.S. and Canada)

Before Using This Medicine

In deciding to use a medicine, the risks of taking the medicine must be weighed against the good it will do. This is a decision you and your doctor will make. For methyldopa and thiazide diuretics, the following should be considered:

Allergies—Tell your doctor if you have ever had any unusual or allergic reaction to methyldopa, sulfonamides (sulfa drugs), bumetanide, furosemide, indapamide, aceta-zolamide, dichlorphenamide, methazolamide, or thiazide diuretics (water pills). Also tell your health care professional if you are allergic to any other substances, such as foods, sulfites or other preservatives, or dyes.

Pregnancy—Studies in humans have not shown that methyldopa causes birth defects or other problems. However, when thiazide diuretics are used during pregnancy, they may cause side effects including jaundice, blood problems, and low potassium in the newborn infant. Thiazide diuretics have not been shown to cause birth defects.

Breast-feeding—This medicine passes into breast milk. Thiazide diuretics may decrease the flow of breast milk. Therefore, you should avoid use of thiazide diuretics during the first month of breast-feeding.

Children—Although there is no specific information comparing use of this medicine in children with use in other age groups, it is not expected to cause different side effects or problems in children than it does in adults.

Older adults—Dizziness or lightheadedness, drowsiness, or signs of too much potassium loss may be more likely to occur in the elderly, who are more sensitive to the effects of methyldopa and thiazide diuretics.

Other medicines—Although certain medicines should not be used together at all, in other cases two different medicines may be used together even if an interaction might occur. In these cases, your doctor may want to change the dose, or other precautions may be necessary. When you are taking methyldopa and thiazide diuretics, it is especially important that your health care professional know if you are taking any of the following:

- Digitalis glycosides (heart medicine)—Thiazide diuretics may cause low potassium in the blood, which can lead to symptoms of digitalis toxicity
- Lithium (e.g., Lithane)—Risk of lithium overdose, even at usual doses, may be increased

- Monoamine oxidase (MAO) inhibitors (furazolidone [e.g., Furoxone], isocarboxazid [e.g., Marplan], phenelzine [e.g., Nardil], procarbazine [e.g., Matulane], selegiline [e.g., Eldepryl], tranylcypromine [e.g., Parnate])—Taking methyldopa while you are taking or within 2 weeks of taking MAO inhibitors may cause nervousness; headache, severe high blood pressure, and hallucinations have been reported

Other medical problems—The presence of other medical problems may affect the use of methyldopa and thiazide diuretics. Make sure you tell your doctor if you have any other medical problems, especially:

- Angina (chest pain)—Methyldopa may worsen the condition
- Diabetes mellitus (sugar diabetes)—Thiazide diuretics may change the amount of diabetes medicine needed
- Gout (history of)—Thiazide diuretics may increase the amount of uric acid in the blood, which can lead to gout
- High cholesterol—Thiazide diuretics may raise cholesterol levels
- Kidney disease—Effects of methyldopa and thiazide diuretics may be increased because of slower removal from the body. If severe, thiazide diuretics may not work
- Liver disease—Effects of methyldopa may be increased because of slower removal from the body. If thiazide diuretics cause loss of too much water from the body, liver disease can become much worse
- Lupus erythematosus (history of)—Thiazide diuretics may worsen the condition
- Mental depression (history of)—Methyldopa can cause mental depression
- Pancreatitis (inflammation of the pancreas)
- Parkinson's disease—Methyldopa may worsen the condition
- Pheochromocytoma—Methyldopa may interfere with tests for the condition; in addition, there have been reports of increased blood pressure
- If you have taken methyldopa in the past and developed liver problems

Proper Use of This Medicine

In addition to the use of the medicine your doctor has prescribed, appropriate treatment for your high blood pressure may include weight control and care in the types of foods you eat, especially foods high in sodium. Your doctor will tell you which factors are most important for you. You should check with your doctor before changing your diet.

Many patients who have high blood pressure will not notice any signs of the problem. In fact, many may feel normal. It is very important *that you take your medicine exactly as directed* and that you keep your appointments with your doctor even if you feel well.

Remember that this medicine will not cure your high blood pressure, but it does help control it. Therefore, you must continue to take it as directed if you expect to lower your blood pressure and keep it down. *You may have to take high blood pressure medicine for the rest of your life.* If high blood pressure is not treated, it can cause serious problems such as heart failure, blood vessel disease, stroke, or kidney disease.

This medicine may cause you to have an unusual feeling of tiredness when you begin to take it. You may also notice an increase in the amount of urine or in your frequency of urination. After taking the medicine for a while, these effects should lessen. In general, to keep the increase in urine from affecting your sleep:

- If you are to take a single dose a day, take it in the morning after breakfast.
- If you are to take more than one dose a day, take the last dose no later than 6 p.m., unless otherwise directed by your doctor.

However, it is best to plan your dose or doses according to a schedule that will least affect your personal activities and sleep. Ask your health care professional to help you plan the best time to take this medicine.

To help you remember to take your medicine, try to get into the habit of taking it at the same time each day.

Dosing—The dose of methyldopa and thiazide diuretic combinations will be different for different patients. *Follow your doctor's orders or the directions on the label.* The following information includes only the average doses of methyldopa and thiazide diuretic combinations. *If your dose is different, do not change it* unless your doctor tells you to do so:

For methyldopa and chlorothiazide

• For *oral* dosage form (tablets):

—Adults: Two to four tablets a day, taken as a single dose or in divided doses.

—Children: Dose must be determined by your doctor.

For methyldopa and hydrochlorothiazide

• For *oral* dosage form (tablets):

—Adults: Two to four tablets a day, taken as a single dose or in divided doses.

—Children: Dose must be determined by your doctor.

Missed dose—If you miss a dose of this medicine, take it as soon as possible. However, if it is almost time for your next dose, skip the missed dose and go back to your regular dosing schedule. Do not double doses.

Storage—To store this medicine:

• Keep out of the reach of children.

• Store away from heat and direct light.

• Do not store in the bathroom, near the kitchen sink, or in other damp places. Heat or moisture may cause the medicine to break down.

• Do not keep outdated medicine or medicine no longer

needed. Be sure that any discarded medicine is out of the reach of children.

Precautions While Using This Medicine

It is important that your doctor check your progress at regular visits to make sure that this medicine is working properly.

Do not take other medicines unless they have been discussed with your doctor. This especially includes over-the-counter (nonprescription) medicines for appetite control, asthma, colds, cough, hay fever, or sinus problems, since they may tend to increase your blood pressure.

This medicine may cause a loss of potassium from your body:

- To help prevent this, your doctor may want you to:
  —eat or drink foods that have a high potassium content (for example, orange or other citrus fruit juices), or
  —take a potassium supplement, or
  —take another medicine to help prevent the loss of the potassium in the first place.
- It is very important to follow these directions. Also, it is important not to change your diet on your own. This is more important if you are already on a special diet (as for diabetes), or if you are taking a potassium supplement or a medicine to reduce potassium loss. Extra potassium may not be necessary and, in some cases, too much potassium could be harmful.

Check with your doctor if you become sick and have severe or continuing vomiting or diarrhea. These problems may cause you to lose additional water and potassium.

Before having any kind of surgery (including dental surgery) or emergency treatment, tell the medical doctor or dentist in charge that you are taking this medicine.

If you have a fever and there seems to be no reason for it, check with your doctor. This is especially important during the first few weeks you take this medicine since fever may be a sign of a serious reaction to methyldopa.

This medicine may cause some people to become drowsy or less alert than they are normally. This is more likely to happen when you begin to take it or when you increase the amount of medicine you are taking. *Make sure you know how you react to this medicine before you drive, use machines, or do anything else that could be dangerous if you are not alert.*

Dizziness, lightheadedness, or fainting may occur, especially when you get up from a lying or sitting position. Getting up slowly may help, but if the problem continues or gets worse, check with your doctor.

The dizziness, lightheadedness, or fainting is also more likely to occur if you drink alcohol, stand for long periods of time, exercise, or if the weather is hot. Drinking alcoholic beverages may also make the drowsiness worse. *While you are taking this medicine, be careful in the amount of alcohol you drink.* Also, use extra care during exercise or hot weather or if you must stand for long periods of time.

For *diabetic patients*:

- This medicine may raise blood sugar levels. While you are using this medicine, be especially careful in testing for sugar in your urine. If you have any questions about this, check with your doctor.

This medicine may cause dryness of the mouth. For temporary relief, use sugarless candy or gum, melt bits of ice in your mouth, or use a saliva substitute. However, if your mouth continues to feel dry for more than 2 weeks, check with your medical doctor or dentist. Continuing dryness of the mouth may increase the chance of dental disease, including tooth decay, gum disease, and fungus infections.

Thiazide diuretics may cause your skin to be more sensitive to sunlight than it is normally. Exposure to sunlight, even for brief periods of time, may cause a skin rash, itching, redness or other discoloration of the skin, or a severe sunburn. When you begin taking this medicine:

- Stay out of direct sunlight, especially between the hours of 10:00 a.m. and 3:00 p.m., if possible.
- Wear protective clothing, including a hat. Also, wear sunglasses.
- Apply a sun block product that has a skin protection factor (SPF) of at least 15. Some patients may require a product with a higher SPF number, especially if they have a fair complexion. If you have any questions about this, check with your health care professional.
- Apply a sun block lipstick that has an SPF of at least 15 to protect your lips.
- Do not use a sunlamp or tanning bed or booth.

If you have a severe reaction from the sun, check with your doctor.

Before you have any medical tests, tell the doctor in charge that you are taking this medicine. The results of some tests may be affected by this medicine.

Side Effects of This Medicine

Along with its needed effects, a medicine may cause some unwanted effects. Although not all of these side effects may occur, if they do occur they may need medical attention.

Check with your doctor immediately if the following side effect occurs:

Rare

Unexplained fever shortly after starting to take this medicine

Check with your doctor as soon as possible if any of the following side effects occur, especially since some of them may mean that your body is losing too much potassium:

Signs and symptoms of too much potassium loss

Dry mouth; increased thirst; irregular heartbeats; muscle cramps or pain; nausea or vomiting; unusual tiredness or weakness; weak pulse

Less common

Mental depression or anxiety; nightmares or unusually vivid dreams

Rare

Cough or hoarseness; dark or amber urine; diarrhea or stomach cramps (severe or continuing); fever, chills, troubled breathing, and fast heartbeat; general feeling of discomfort or illness or weakness; joint pain; lower back or side pain; painful or difficult urination; pale stools; skin rash, hives, or itching; stomach pain (severe) with nausea and vomiting; tiredness or weakness after having taken this medicine for several weeks (continuing); yellow eyes or skin

Other side effects may occur that usually do not need medical attention. These side effects may go away during treatment as your body adjusts to the medicine. However, check with your doctor if any of the following side effects continue or are bothersome:

More common

Dizziness or lightheadedness when getting up from a lying or sitting position; drowsiness; dryness of mouth; headache

Less common

Decreased sexual ability or interest in sex; diarrhea; increased sensitivity of skin to sunlight (skin rash, itching, redness or other discoloration of skin or severe sunburn after exposure to sunlight); loss of appetite; numbness, tingling, pain, or weakness in hands or feet; slow heartbeat; stuffy nose; swelling of breasts or unusual milk production

Other side effects not listed above may also occur in some

patients. If you notice any other effects, check with your doctor.

METYROSINE Systemic†

A commonly used brand name in the U.S. is Demser.

†Not commercially available in Canada.

Description

Metyrosine (me-TYE-roe-seen) belongs to the general class of medicines called antihypertensives. It is used to treat high blood pressure (hypertension) caused by a disease called pheochromocytoma (a noncancerous tumor of the adrenal gland).

Metyrosine reduces the amount of certain chemicals in the body. When these chemicals are present in large amounts, they cause high blood pressure.

Metyrosine is available only with your doctor's prescription, in the following dosage form:

Oral
- Capsules (U.S.)

Before Using This Medicine

In deciding to use a medicine, the risks of taking the medicine must be weighed against the good it will do. This is a decision you and your doctor will make. For metyrosine, the following should be considered:

Allergies—Tell your doctor if you have ever had any unusual or allergic reaction to metyrosine. Also tell your health care professional if you are allergic to any other substances, such as foods, sulfites or other preservatives, or dyes.

Pregnancy—Studies on effects in pregnancy have not been done in either humans or animals.

Breast-feeding—It is not known whether metyrosine passes into breast milk. However, this medicine has not been reported to cause problems in nursing babies.

Children—Studies on this medicine have been done only in adult patients, and there is no specific information comparing use of metyrosine in children with use in other age groups.

Older adults—Many medicines have not been studied specifically in older people. Therefore, it may not be known whether they work exactly the same way they do in younger adults or if they cause different side effects or problems in older people. There is no specific information comparing use of metyrosine in the elderly with use in other age groups.

Other medicines—Although certain medicines should not be used together at all, in other cases two different medicines may be used together even if an interaction might occur. In these cases, your doctor may want to change the dose, or other precautions may be necessary. Tell your health care professional if you are taking any other prescription or nonprescription (over-the-counter [OTC]) medicine.

Other medical problems—The presence of other medical problems may affect the use of metyrosine. Make sure you tell your doctor if you have any other medical problems, especially:

- Kidney disease or
- Liver disease—Effects of metyrosine may be increased because of slower removal from the body
- Mental depression (or history of) or
- Parkinson's disease—Metyrosine may make these conditions worse

Proper Use of This Medicine

Take this medicine only as directed by your doctor. Do not take more or less of it than your doctor ordered.

To help you remember to take your medicine, try to get into the habit of taking it at the same times each day.

Dosing—The dose of metyrosine will be different for different patients. *Follow your doctor's orders or the directions on the label.* The following information includes only the average doses of metyrosine. *If your dose is different, do not change it* unless your doctor tells you to do so:

- For *oral* dosage forms (capsules):
  —Adults and children 12 years of age and older: 1000 milligrams to 3000 milligrams (1 to 3 grams) a day, divided into four doses.

Missed dose—If you miss a dose of this medicine, take it as soon as possible. However, if it is almost time for your next dose, skip the missed dose and go back to your regular dosing schedule. Do not double doses.

Storage—To store this medicine:

- Keep out of the reach of children.
- Store away from heat and direct light.
- Do not store in the bathroom, near the kitchen sink, or in other damp places. Heat or moisture may cause the medicine to break down.
- Do not keep outdated medicine or medicine no longer needed. Be sure that any discarded medicine is out of the reach of children.

Precautions While Using This Medicine

It is important that your doctor check your progress at regular visits to make sure that this medicine is working properly and to check for unwanted effects.

While taking this medicine, it is important that you drink plenty of fluids and urinate often. This will help prevent kidney problems and keep your kidneys working well. If you have any questions about how much you should drink, check with your doctor.

This medicine will add to the effects of alcohol and other CNS depressants (medicines that slow down the nervous system, possibly causing drowsiness). Some examples of CNS depressants are antihistamines or medicine for hay fever, other allergies, or colds; sedatives, tranquilizers, or sleeping medicine; prescription pain medicine or narcotics; barbiturates; medicine for seizures; tricyclic antidepressants (medicine for depression); muscle relaxants; or anesthetics, including some dental anesthetics. *Check with your doctor before taking any of the above while you are taking this medicine.*

Before having any kind of surgery (including dental surgery), tell the medical doctor or dentist in charge that you are taking this medicine.

This medicine may cause most people to become drowsy or less alert than they are normally. *Make sure you know how you react to this medicine before you drive, use machines, or do anything else that could be dangerous if you are not alert.*

Side Effects of This Medicine

Along with its needed effects, a medicine may cause some unwanted effects. Although not all of these side effects may occur, if they do occur they may need medical attention.

Check with your doctor as soon as possible if any of the following side effects occur:

More common

    Diarrhea; drooling; trembling and shaking of hands and fingers; trouble in speaking

Less common

> Anxiety; confusion; hallucinations (seeing, hearing, or feeling things that are not there); mental depression

Rare

> Black, tarry stools; blood in urine or stools; unusual bleeding or bruising; muscle spasms, especially of neck and back; painful urination; pinpoint red spots on skin; restlessness; shortness of breath; shuffling walk; skin rash and itching; swelling of feet or lower legs; tic-like (jerky) movements of head, face, mouth, and neck; unusual tiredness or weakness

Other side effects may occur that usually do not need medical attention. These side effects may go away during treatment as your body adjusts to the medicine. However, check with your doctor if any of the following side effects continue or are bothersome:

More common

> Drowsiness

Less common

> Decreased sexual ability in men; dryness of mouth; nausea, vomiting, or stomach pain; stuffy nose; swelling of breasts or unusual milk production

After you stop taking this medicine, it may still produce some side effects that need attention. During this period of time check with your doctor if you notice the following side effect:

> Diarrhea

Also, after you stop taking this medicine, you may have feelings of increased energy or you may have trouble sleeping. However, these effects should last only for two or three days.

Other side effects not listed above may also occur in some patients. If you notice any other effects, check with your doctor.

MEXILETINE   Systemic

A commonly used brand name in the U.S. and Canada is Mexitil.

Description

Mexiletine (MEX-i-le-teen) belongs to the group of medicines known as antiarrhythmics. It is used to correct irregular heartbeats to a normal rhythm.

Mexiletine produces its helpful effects by slowing nerve impulses in the heart and making the heart tissue less sensitive.

Mexiletine is available only with your doctor's prescription, in the following dosage form:

Oral

- Capsules (U.S. and Canada)

Before Using This Medicine

In deciding to use a medicine, the risks of taking the medicine must be weighed against the good it will do. This is a decision you and your doctor will make. For mexiletine, the following should be considered:

Allergies—Tell your doctor if you have ever had any unusual or allergic reaction to mexiletine, lidocaine, or tocainide. Also tell your health care professional if you are allergic to any other substance, such as foods, preservatives, or dyes.

Pregnancy—Mexiletine has not been studied in pregnant women. However, studies in animals have shown that mexiletine causes a decrease in successful pregnancies but no birth defects. Before taking this medicine, make sure your doctor knows if you are pregnant or if you may become pregnant.

Breast-feeding—Mexiletine passes into breast milk. Because this medicine may cause serious side effects, breast-feeding is generally not recommended while you are receiving it. Be sure you have discussed this with your doctor before taking mexiletine.

Children—Studies on this medicine have been done only in adult patients, and there is no specific information comparing use of mexiletine in children with use in other age groups.

Older adults—Many medicines have not been studied specifically in older people. Therefore, it may not be known whether they work exactly the same way they do in younger adults or if they cause different side effects or problems in older people. There is no specific information comparing use of mexiletine in the elderly with use in other age groups.

Other medicines—Although certain medicines should not be used together at all, in other cases two different medicines may be used together even if an interaction might occur. In these cases, your doctor may want to change the dose, or other precautions may be necessary. Tell your health care professional if you are taking any other prescription or nonprescription (over-the-counter [OTC]) medicine.

Smoking—Smoking may decrease the effects of mexiletine.

Other medical problems—The presence of other medical problems may affect the use of mexiletine. Make sure you tell your doctor if you have any other medical problems, especially:

- Congestive heart failure or
- Low blood pressure—Mexiletine may make these conditions worse
- Heart attack (severe) or
- Liver disease—Effects may last longer because of slower removal of mexiletine from the body
- Seizures (history of)—Mexiletine can cause seizures

Proper Use of This Medicine

Take mexiletine exactly as directed by your doctor, even though you may feel well. Do not take more medicine than ordered.

To lessen the possibility of stomach upset, mexiletine should be taken with food or immediately after meals or with milk or an antacid.

This medicine works best when there is a constant amount in the blood. *To help keep this amount constant, do not miss any doses. Also it is best to take the doses at evenly spaced times day and night.* For example, if you are to take 3 doses a day, the doses should be spaced about 8 hours apart. If this interferes with your sleep or other daily activities, or if you need help in planning the best times to take your medicine, check with your health care professional.

Dosing—The dose of mexiletine will be different for different patients. *Follow your doctor's orders or the directions on the label.* The following information includes only the average dose of mexiletine. *If your dose is different, do not change it* unless your doctor tells you to do so.

The number of capsules that you take depends on the strength of the medicine.

- For *oral* dosage form (capsules):
    - —For irregular heartbeat (arrhythmias):
        - Adults—At first, 200 milligrams (mg) every eight hours. Then, your doctor may raise or lower your dose as needed.
        - Children—Use and dose must be determined by your doctor.

Missed dose—If you miss a dose of this medicine and remember within 4 hours, take it as soon as possible. Then go back to your regular dosing schedule. However, if you do not remember until later, skip the missed dose and go back to your regular dosing schedule. Do not double doses.

Storage—To store this medicine:

- Keep out of the reach of children.
- Store away from heat and direct light.
- Do not store in the bathroom, near the kitchen sink, or in other damp places. Heat or moisture may cause the medicine to break down.
- Do not keep outdated medicine or medicine no longer needed. Be sure that any discarded medicine is out of the reach of children.

Precautions While Using This Medicine

It is important that your doctor check your progress at regular visits to make sure the medicine is working properly. This will allow for changes to be made in the amount of medicine you are taking, if necessary.

Your doctor may want you to carry a medical identification card or bracelet stating that you are using this medicine.

Before having any kind of surgery (including dental surgery) or emergency treatment, tell the medical doctor or dentist in charge that you are taking this medicine.

Mexiletine may cause some people to become dizzy, lightheaded, or less alert than they are normally. *Make sure you know how you react to this medicine before you drive, use machines, or do anything else that could be dangerous if you are dizzy or are not alert.*

Side Effects of This Medicine

Along with its needed effects, a medicine may cause some unwanted effects. Although not all of these side effects may occur, if they do occur they may need medical attention.

Check with your doctor as soon as possible if any of the
following side effects occur:

Less common

>   Chest pain; fast or irregular heartbeat; shortness of breath

Rare

>   Convulsions (seizures); fever or chills; unusual bleeding
>   or bruising

Other side effects may occur that usually do not need
medical attention. These side effects may go away during
treatment as your body adjusts to the medicine. However,
check with your doctor if any of the following side effects
continue or are bothersome:

More common

>   Dizziness or lightheadedness; heartburn; nausea and vom-
>   iting; nervousness; trembling or shaking of the hands;
>   unsteadiness or difficulty in walking

Less common

>   Blurred vision; confusion; constipation or diarrhea; head-
>   ache; numbness or tingling of fingers and toes; ringing
>   in the ears; skin rash; slurred speech; trouble in sleep-
>   ing; unusual tiredness or weakness

Other side effects not listed above may also occur in some
patients. If you notice any other effects, check with your
doctor.

MINOXIDIL   Systemic

A commonly used brand name in the U.S. and Canada is Loniten.
Generic name product may also be available in the U.S.

Description

Minoxidil (mi-NOX-i-dill) belongs to the general class of
medicines called antihypertensives. It is used to treat high
blood pressure (hypertension).

High blood pressure adds to the workload of the heart and

arteries. If it continues for a long time, the heart and arteries may not function properly. This can damage the blood vessels of the brain, heart, and kidneys, resulting in a stroke, heart failure, or kidney failure. High blood pressure may also increase the risk of heart attacks. These problems may be less likely to occur if blood pressure is controlled.

Minoxidil works by relaxing blood vessels so that blood passes through them more easily. This helps to lower blood pressure.

Minoxidil has other effects that could be bothersome for some patients. These include increased hair growth, weight gain, fast heartbeat, and chest pain. Before you take this medicine, be sure that you have discussed the use of it with your doctor.

Minoxidil is being applied to the scalp in liquid form by some balding men to stimulate hair growth. However, improper use of liquids made from minoxidil tablets can result in minoxidil being absorbed into the body, where it may cause unwanted effects on the heart and blood vessels.

Minoxidil is available only with your doctor's prescription, in the following dosage form:

Oral
- Tablets (U.S. and Canada)

Before Using This Medicine

In deciding to use a medicine, the risks of taking the medicine must be weighed against the good it will do. This is a decision you and your doctor will make. For minoxidil, the following should be considered:

Allergies—Tell your doctor if you have ever had any unusual or allergic reaction to minoxidil. Also tell your health care professional if you are allergic to any other substances, such as foods, preservatives, or dyes.

Pregnancy—Minoxidil has not been studied in pregnant women. However, there have been reports of babies born with extra thick or dark hair on their bodies after the mothers took minoxidil during pregnancy. Discuss this possible effect with your doctor.

Studies in rats found a decreased rate of conception, and studies in rabbits at 5 times the human dose have shown a decrease in successful pregnancies. Minoxidil did not cause birth defects in rats or rabbits.

Breast-feeding—Although minoxidil passes into breast milk, it has not been reported to cause problems in nursing babies.

Children—Although there is no specific information comparing use of minoxidil in children with use in other age groups, this medicine is not expected to cause different side effects or problems in children than it does in adults.

Older adults—Elderly patients may be more sensitive to the effects of minoxidil. In addition, minoxidil may reduce tolerance to cold temperatures in elderly patients.

Other medicines—Although certain medicines should not be used together at all, in other cases two different medicines may be used together even if an interaction might occur. In these cases, your doctor may want to change the dose, or other precautions may be necessary. When taking minoxidil it is especially important that your health care professional know if you are taking any of the following:

- Guanethidine (e.g., Ismelin) or
- Nitrates (medicine for angina)—Severe lowered blood pressure may occur

Other medical problems—The presence of other medical problems may affect the use of minoxidil. Make sure you tell your doctor if you have any other medical problems, especially:

- Angina (chest pain)—Minoxidil may make this condition worse

- Heart attack or stroke (recent)—Lowering blood pressure may make problems resulting from heart attack or stroke worse
- Heart or blood vessel disease—Minoxidil can cause fluid buildup, which can cause problems
- Kidney disease—Effects may be increased because of slower removal of minoxidil from the body
- Pheochromocytoma—Minoxidil may cause the tumor to be more active

---

Proper Use of This Medicine

In addition to the use of the medicine your doctor has prescribed, treatment for your high blood pressure may include weight control and care in the types of foods you eat, especially foods high in sodium. Your doctor will tell you which of these are most important for you. You should check with your doctor before changing your diet.

Many patients who have high blood pressure will not notice any signs of the problem. In fact, many may feel normal. It is very important that you *take your medicine exactly as directed* and that you keep your appointments with your doctor even if you feel well.

Remember that minoxidil will not cure your high blood pressure, but it does help control it. Therefore, you must continue to take it as directed if you expect to lower your blood pressure and keep it down. *You may have to take high blood pressure medicine for the rest of your life.* If high blood pressure is not treated, it can cause serious problems such as heart failure, blood vessel disease, stroke, or kidney disease.

To help you remember to take your medicine, try to get into the habit of taking it at the same time each day.

This medicine is usually given together with certain other medicines. If you are using a combination of drugs, make sure that you take each medicine at the proper time and do not mix them. Ask your health care professional to help you plan a way to remember to take your medicines at the right time.

Dosing—The dose of minoxidil will be different for different patients. *Follow your doctor's orders or the directions on the label.* The following information includes only the average doses of minoxidil. *If your dose is different, do not change it* unless your doctor tells you to do so:

- For *oral* dosage forms (tablets):

    —Adults and children over 12 years of age: 5 to 40 milligrams taken as a single dose or in divided doses.

    —Children up to 12 years of age: 200 micrograms to 1 milligram per kilogram of body weight a day to be taken as a single dose or in divided doses.

Missed dose—If you miss a dose of this medicine and remember it within a few hours, take it when you remember. However, if you do not remember until the next day, skip the missed dose and go back to your regular dosing schedule. Do not double doses.

Storage—To store this medicine:

- Keep out of the reach of children.
- Store away from heat and direct light.
- Do not store in the bathroom, near the kitchen sink, or in other damp places. Heat or moisture may cause the medicine to break down.
- Do not keep outdated medicine or medicine no longer needed. Be sure that any discarded medicine is out of the reach of children.

Precautions While Using This Medicine

It is important that your doctor check your progress at regular visits to make sure that this medicine is working properly.

Ask your doctor about checking your pulse rate before and after taking minoxidil. Then, while you are taking this medicine, *check your pulse regularly while you are resting*. If it increases by 20 beats or more a minute, check with your doctor right away.

While you are taking minoxidil, *weigh yourself every day*. A weight gain of 2 to 3 pounds (about 1 kg) in an adult is normal and should be lost with continued treatment. However, if you suddenly gain 5 pounds (2 kg) or more (for a child, 2 pounds [1 kg] or more) or if you notice swelling of your feet or lower legs, check with your doctor right away.

Do not take other medicines unless they have been discussed with your doctor. This especially includes over-the-counter (nonprescription) medicines for appetite control, asthma, colds, cough, hay fever, or sinus problems, since they may tend to increase your blood pressure.

Side Effects of This Medicine

Along with its needed effects, a medicine may cause some unwanted effects. Although not all of these side effects may occur, if they do occur they may need medical attention.

Check with your doctor immediately if any of the following side effects occur:

> *More common*
>> Fast or irregular heartbeat; weight gain (rapid) of more than 5 pounds (2 pounds in children)
>
> *Less common*
>> Chest pain; shortness of breath

Check with your doctor as soon as possible if any of the following side effects occur:

More common

> Bloating; flushing or redness of skin; swelling of feet or lower legs

Less common

> Numbness or tingling of hands, feet, or face

Rare

> Skin rash and itching

Other side effects may occur that usually do not need medical attention. These side effects may go away during treatment as your body adjusts to the medicine. However, check with your doctor if any of the following side effects continue or are bothersome:

More common

> Increase in hair growth, usually on face, arms, and back

Less common or rare

> Breast tenderness in males and females; headache

This medicine causes a temporary increase in hair growth in most people. Hair may grow longer and darker in both men and women. This may first be noticed on the face several weeks after you start taking minoxidil. Later, new hair growth may be noticed on the back, arms, legs, and scalp. Talk to your doctor about shaving or using a hair remover during this time. After treatment with minoxidil has ended, the hair will stop growing, although it may take several months for the new hair growth to go away.

Other side effects not listed above may also occur in some patients. If you notice any other effects, check with your doctor.

MORICIZINE   Systemic†

A commonly used brand name in the U.S. is Ethmozine.

†Not commercially available in Canada.

Description

Moricizine (mor-IH-siz-een) belongs to the group of medicines known as antiarrhythmics. It is used to correct irregular or rapid heartbeats to a normal rhythm by making the heart tissue less sensitive.

There is a chance that moricizine may cause new or make worse existing heart rhythm problems when it is used. Since other antiarrhythmic medicines have been shown to cause severe problems in some patients, moricizine is only used to treat serious heart rhythm problems. Discuss this possible effect with your doctor.

This medicine is available only with your doctor's prescription, in the following dosage form:

Oral
- Tablets (U.S.)

Before Using This Medicine

In deciding to use a medicine, the risks of taking the medicine must be weighed against the good it will do. This is a decision you and your doctor will make. For moricizine, the following should be considered:

Allergies—Tell your doctor if you have ever had any unusual or allergic reaction to moricizine. Also tell your health care professional if you are allergic to any other substances, such as foods, preservatives, or dyes.

Pregnancy—Moricizine has not been studied in pregnant women. However, this medicine has not been shown to cause birth defects or other problems in animal studies, although it affected weight gain in some animals. Before taking moricizine, make sure your doctor knows if you are pregnant or if you may become pregnant.

Breast-feeding—Moricizine passes into the milk of some animals and may also pass into the milk of humans. However, this medicine has not been reported to cause problems in nursing babies.

Children—Studies on this medicine have been done only in adult patients, and there is no specific information comparing use of moricizine in children with use in other age groups.

Older adults—Many medicines have not been studied specifically in older people. Therefore, it may not be known whether they work exactly the same way they do in younger adults or if they cause different side effects or problems in older people. There is no specific information comparing use of moricizine in the elderly with use in other age groups, although the risk of some unwanted effects may be increased.

Other medicines—Although certain medicines should not be used together at all, in other cases two different medicines may be used together even if an interaction might occur. In these cases, your doctor may want to change the dose, or other precautions may be necessary. Tell your health care professional if you are taking any other prescription or nonprescription (over-the-counter [OTC]) medicine.

Other medical problems—The presence of other medical problems may affect the use of moricizine. Make sure you tell your doctor if you have any other medical problems, especially:

- Kidney disease or
- Liver disease—Effects may be increased because of slower removal of moricizine from the body

- Heart disease or
- Recent heart attack or
- If you have a pacemaker—Risk of irregular heartbeats may be increased

Proper Use of This Medicine

Take moricizine exactly as directed by your doctor, even though you may feel well. Do not take more or less of it than your doctor ordered.

This medicine works best when there is a constant amount in the blood. *To help keep the amount constant, do not miss any doses. Also, it is best to take each dose at evenly spaced times day and night.* For example, if you are to take 3 doses a day, doses should be spaced about 8 hours apart. If you need help in planning the best times to take your medicine, check with your health care professional.

Dosing—The dose of moricizine will be different for different patients. *Follow your doctor's orders or the directions on the label.* The following information includes only the average doses of moricizine. *If your dose is different, do not change it* unless your doctor tells you to do so.

The number of tablets that you take depends on the strength of the medicine.

- For *oral* dosage form (tablets):
  - —For irregular heartbeat (arrhythmias):
    - Adults—600 to 900 milligrams (mg) a day. This is divided into three doses and taken every eight hours.
    - Children—Use and dose must be determined by your doctor.

Missed dose—If you miss a dose of moricizine and remember within 4 hours, take it as soon as possible. However, if you do not remember until later, skip the missed dose and go back to your regular dosing schedule. Do not double doses.

Storage—To store this medicine:
- Keep out of the reach of children.
- Store away from heat and direct light.

- Do not store in the bathroom, near the kitchen sink, or in other damp places. Heat or moisture may cause the medicine to break down.
- Do not keep outdated medicine or medicine no longer needed. Be sure that any discarded medicine is out of the reach of children.

Precautions While Using This Medicine

It is important that your doctor check your progress at regular visits to make sure the medicine is working properly. This will allow changes to be made in the amount of medicine you are taking, if necessary.

Your doctor may want you to carry a medical identification card or bracelet stating that you are using this medicine.

Before having any kind of surgery (including dental surgery) or emergency treatment, tell the medical doctor or dentist in charge that you are taking this medicine.

Moricizine may cause some people to become dizzy or lightheaded. Make sure you know how you react to this medicine before you drive, use machines, or do anything else that could be dangerous if you are dizzy.

Side Effects of This Medicine

Along with its needed effects, a medicine may cause some unwanted effects. Although not all of these side effects may occur, if they do occur they may need medical attention.

Check with your doctor as soon as possible if any of the following side effects occur:

Less common

Chest pain; fast or irregular heartbeat; shortness of breath; swelling of feet or lower legs

Rare
   Fever (sudden, high)

Other side effects may occur that usually do not need medical attention. These side effects may go away during treatment as your body adjusts to the medicine. However, check with your doctor if any of the following side effects continue or are bothersome:

More common
   Dizziness

Less common
   Blurred vision; diarrhea; dryness of mouth; headache; nausea or vomiting; nervousness; numbness or tingling in arms or legs or around mouth; pain in arms or legs; stomach pain; trouble in sleeping; unusual tiredness or weakness

Other side effects not listed above may also occur in some patients. If you notice any other effects, check with your doctor.

NIACIN—For High Cholesterol
Systemic

Some commonly used brand names are:

In the U.S.—

Endur-Acin	Nico-400
Nia-Bid	Nicobid Tempules
Niac	Nicolar
Niacels	Nicotinex Elixir
Niacor	Slo-Niacin

Generic name product may also be available.

In Canada—
   Novo-Niacin
   Generic name product may also be available.

Other commonly used names are nicotinic acid or vitamin B_3.

Description

Niacin (NYE-a-sin) is used to help lower high cholesterol and fat levels in the blood. This may help prevent medical problems caused by cholesterol and fat clogging the blood vessels.

Some strengths of niacin are available only with your doctor's prescription. Others are available without a prescription, since niacin is also a vitamin. However, it is best to take it only under your doctor's direction so that you can be sure you are taking the correct dose.

Niacin for use in the treatment of high cholesterol is available in the following dosage forms:

Oral

- Extended-release capsules (U.S.)
- Solution (U.S.)
- Tablets (U.S. and Canada)
- Extended-release tablets (U.S. and Canada)

Before Using This Medicine

If you are taking this medicine without a prescription, carefully read and follow any precautions on the label. For niacin, the following should be considered:

Allergies—Tell your doctor if you have ever had any unusual or allergic reaction to niacin. Also tell your health care professional if you are allergic to any other substances, such as foods, preservatives, or dyes.

Diet—Before prescribing medicine for your condition, your doctor will probably try to control your condition by prescribing a personal diet for you. Such a diet may be low in fats, sugars, and/or cholesterol. Many people are able to control their condition by carefully following their doctor's orders for proper diet and exercise. *Medicine is prescribed only when additional help is needed* and is effective only when a schedule of diet and exercise is properly followed.

Also, this medicine is less effective if you are greatly overweight. It may be very important for you to go on a reducing diet. However, check with your doctor before going on any diet.

Make certain your health care professional knows if you are on any special diet, such as a low-sodium or low-sugar diet.

Pregnancy—Studies have not been done in either humans or animals.

Breast-feeding—Niacin has not been reported to cause problems in nursing babies.

Children—There is no specific information comparing the use of niacin for high cholesterol in children with use in other age groups. However, use is not recommended in children under 2 years of age since cholesterol is needed for normal development.

Older adults—Many medicines have not been studied specifically in older people. Therefore, it may not be known whether they work exactly the same way they do in younger adults or if they cause different side effects or problems in older people. Although there is no specific information comparing the use of niacin for high cholesterol in the elderly with use in other age groups, it is not expected to cause different side effects or problems in older people than in younger adults.

Other medicines—Although certain medicines should not be used together at all, in other cases two different medicines may be used together even if an interaction might occur. In these cases, your doctor may want to change the dose, or other precautions may be necessary. Tell your health care professional if you are using any other prescription or nonprescription (over-the-counter [OTC]) medicine.

Other medical problems—The presence of other medical problems may affect the use of niacin. Make sure you tell your doctor if you have any other medical problems, especially:

- Bleeding problems or
- Diabetes mellitus (sugar diabetes) or
- Glaucoma or
- Gout or
- Liver disease or
- Low blood pressure or
- Stomach ulcer—Niacin may make these conditions worse

Proper Use of This Medicine

Use this medicine only as directed by your doctor. Do not use more or less of it, do not use it more often, and do not use it for a longer time than your doctor ordered. To do so may increase the chance of unwanted effects.

Remember that niacin will not cure your condition but it does help control it. Therefore, you must continue to take it as directed if you expect to keep your cholesterol levels down.

Follow carefully the special diet your doctor gave you. This is the most important part of controlling your condition, and is necessary if the medicine is to work properly.

If this medicine upsets your stomach, it may be taken with meals or milk. If stomach upset (nausea or diarrhea) continues, check with your doctor.

For patients taking the *extended-release capsule form* of this medicine:

- Swallow the capsule whole. Do not crush, break, or chew before swallowing. However, if the capsule is too large to swallow, you may mix the contents of the capsule with jam or jelly and swallow without chewing.

For patients taking the *extended-release tablet form* of this medicine:

- Swallow the tablet whole. If the tablet is scored, it

may be broken, but not crushed or chewed, before being swallowed.

Dosing—The dose of niacin will be different for different patients. *Follow your doctor's orders or the directions on the label.* The following information includes only the average doses of niacin. *If your dose is different, do not change it* unless your doctor tells you to do so.

The number of capsules or tablets or teaspoonfuls of solution that you take depends on the strength of the medicine.

- For *oral* dosage form (extended-release capsules, extended-release tablets, oral solution, or regular tablets):
  —For treatment of high cholesterol:
    - Adults and teenagers—1 to 2 grams three times a day.
    - Children—Use and dose must be determined by your doctor.

Missed dose—If you miss a dose of this medicine, take it as soon as possible. However, if it is almost time for your next dose, skip the missed dose and go back to your regular dosing schedule. Do not double doses.

Storage—To store this medicine:
- Keep out of the reach of children.
- Store away from heat and direct light.
- Do not store in the bathroom, near the kitchen sink, or in other damp places. Heat or moisture may cause the medicine to break down.
- Keep the liquid form of this medicine from freezing.
- Do not keep outdated medicine or medicine no longer needed. Be sure that any discarded medicine is out of the reach of children.

Precautions While Using This Medicine

It is very important that your doctor check your progress at regular visits. This will allow your doctor to see if the medicine is working properly to lower your cholesterol and triglyceride (fat) levels and if you should continue to take it.

Do not stop taking niacin without first checking with your doctor. When you stop taking this medicine, your blood cholesterol levels may increase again. Your doctor may want you to follow a special diet to help prevent this from happening.

This medicine may cause you to feel dizzy or faint, especially when you get up from a lying or sitting position. Getting up slowly may help. This effect should lessen after a week or two as your body gets used to the medicine. However, if the problem continues or gets worse, check with your doctor.

Side Effects of This Medicine

Along with its needed effects, a medicine may cause some unwanted effects. Although not all of these side effects may occur, if they do occur they may need medical attention. *Check with your doctor immediately* if any of the following side effects occur:

> *Less common*
>> *With prolonged use of extended-release niacin*
>>> Darkening of urine; light gray-colored stools; loss of appetite; severe stomach pain; yellow eyes or skin

Other side effects may occur that usually do not need medical attention. These side effects may go away during treatment as your body adjusts to the medicine. However, check with your doctor if any of the following side effects continue or are bothersome:

> *Less common*
>> Feeling of warmth; flushing or redness of skin, especially on face and neck; headache
> *With high doses*
>> Diarrhea; dizziness or faintness; dryness of skin; fever;

frequent urination; itching of skin; joint pain; muscle aching or cramping; nausea or vomiting; side, lower back, or stomach pain; swelling of feet or lower legs; unusual thirst; unusual tiredness or weakness; unusually fast, slow, or irregular heartbeat

Other side effects not listed above may also occur in some patients. If you notice any other effects, check with your health care professional.

NICOTINYL ALCOHOL Systemic*

A commonly used brand name in Canada is Roniacol.

*Not commercially available in the U.S.

Description

Nicotinyl (nik-oh-TIN-ill) alcohol belongs to the group of medicines called vasodilators. Vasodilators increase the size of blood vessels and are used to treat problems resulting from poor blood circulation.

Nicotinyl alcohol is available without a prescription, in the following dosage form:

Oral
- Extended-release tablets (Canada)

Before Using This Medicine

If you are taking this medicine without a prescription, carefully read and follow any precautions on the label. For nicotinyl alcohol, the following should be considered:

Allergies—Tell your doctor if you have ever had any unusual or allergic reaction to nicotinyl alcohol. Also tell your health care professional if you are allergic to any other substances, such as foods, preservatives, or dyes.

Pregnancy—Studies on effects in pregnancy have not been done in either humans or animals.

Breast-feeding—It is not known whether nicotinyl alcohol passes into breast milk. However, this medicine has not been reported to cause problems in nursing babies.

Older adults—Many medicines have not been studied specifically in older people. Therefore, it may not be known whether they work exactly the same way they do in younger adults or if they cause different side effects or problems in older people. There is no specific information comparing use of nicotinyl alcohol in the elderly with use in other age groups. However, nicotinyl alcohol may reduce tolerance to cold temperatures in elderly patients.

Other medicines—Although certain medicines should not be used together at all, in other cases two different medicines may be used together even if an interaction might occur. In these cases, your doctor may want to change the dose, or other precautions may be necessary. Tell your health care professional if you are taking any other prescription or nonprescription (over-the-counter [OTC]) medicine, or if you smoke.

Other medical problems—The presence of other medical problems may affect the use of nicotinyl alcohol. Make sure you tell your doctor if you have any other medical problems, especially:
- Angina (chest pain) or
- Diabetes mellitus (sugar diabetes) or
- Heart attack (recent) or
- Stomach ulcer or
- Stroke (recent)—Nicotinyl alcohol can make your condition worse
- Glaucoma or
- High cholesterol levels—The chance of side effects may be increased

Proper Use of This Medicine

Nicotinyl alcohol tablets should be swallowed whole. Do not break, crush, or chew the tablets before swallowing them.

Dosing—The dose of nicotinyl alcohol will be different for different patients. *Follow your doctor's orders or the directions on the label.* The following information includes only the average doses of nicotinyl alcohol. *If your dose is different, do not change it* unless your doctor tells you to do so:

• For *oral* dosage forms (tablets):
  —Adults: 150 to 300 milligrams two times a day, taken in the morning and evening.

Missed dose—If you miss a dose of this medicine, take it as soon as you remember. However, if it is almost time for your next dose, skip the missed dose and go back to your regular dosing schedule. Do not double doses.

Storage—To store this medicine:

• Keep out of the reach of children.
• Store away from heat and direct light.
• Do not store in the bathroom, near the kitchen sink, or in other damp places. Heat or moisture may cause the medicine to break down.
• Do not keep outdated medicine or medicine no longer needed. Be sure that any discarded medicine is out of the reach of children.

Precautions While Using This Medicine

It may take some time for this medicine to work. If you feel that the medicine is not working, do not stop taking it on your own. Instead, check with your doctor.

The helpful effects of this medicine may be decreased if you smoke.

Side Effects of This Medicine

Along with its needed effects, a medicine may cause some unwanted effects. Although not all of these side effects

may occur, if they do occur they may need medical attention.

Check with your doctor as soon as possible if any of the following side effects occur:

Rare

Swelling of feet or lower legs; yellow eyes or skin

Other side effects may occur that usually do not need medical attention. These side effects may go away during treatment as your body adjusts to the medicine. However, check with your doctor if any of the following side effects continue or are bothersome:

More common

Flushing; warmth or tingling

Less common or rare

Diarrhea; dizziness or faintness; increased hair loss; nausea and vomiting; skin rash

Other side effects not listed above may also occur in some patients. If you notice any other effects, check with your doctor.

NITRATES—Lingual Aerosol
Systemic

This information applies to nitroglycerin oral spray.
A commonly used brand name in the U.S. and Canada is Nitrolingual.
Another commonly used name is glyceryl trinitrate.

Description

Nitrates (NYE-trates) are used to treat the symptoms of angina (chest pain). Depending on the type of dosage form and how it is taken, nitrates are used to treat angina in three ways:

- to relieve an attack that is occurring by using the medicine when the attack begins;

- to prevent attacks from occurring by using the medicine just before an attack is expected to occur; or
- to reduce the number of attacks that occur by using the medicine regularly on a long-term basis.

When used as a lingual (in the mouth) spray, nitroglycerin is used either to relieve the pain of angina attacks or to prevent an expected angina attack.

Nitroglycerin works by relaxing blood vessels and increasing the supply of blood and oxygen to the heart while reducing its workload.

Nitroglycerin as discussed here is available only with your doctor's prescription, in the following dosage form:

Oral
- Lingual aerosol (U.S. and Canada)

Before Using This Medicine

In deciding to use a medicine, the risks of taking the medicine must be weighed against the good it will do. This is a decision you and your doctor will make. For nitroglycerin lingual aerosol, the following should be considered:

Allergies—Tell your doctor if you have ever had any unusual or allergic reaction to nitrates or nitrites. Also tell your health care professional if you are allergic to any other substances, such as certain foods, preservatives, or dyes.

Pregnancy—Studies on effects in pregnancy have not been done in either humans or animals.

Breast-feeding—It is not known whether this medicine passes into breast milk. Although most medicines pass into breast milk in small amounts, many of them may be used safely while breast-feeding. Mothers who are taking this medicine and who wish to breast-feed should discuss this with their doctor.

Children—Studies on this medicine have been done only in adult patients, and there is no specific information comparing use of nitroglycerin in children with use in other age groups.

Older adults—Dizziness or lightheadedness may be more likely to occur in the elderly, who may be more sensitive to the effects of nitrates.

Other medicines—Although certain medicines should not be used together at all, in other cases two different medicines may be used together even if an interaction might occur. In these cases, your doctor may want to change the dose, or other precautions may be necessary. When you are taking nitroglycerin, it is especially important that your health care professional know if you are taking any of the following:

- Antihypertensives (high blood pressure medicine) or
- Other heart medicine—May increase the effects of nitroglycerin on blood pressure

Other medical problems—The presence of other medical problems may affect the use of nitroglycerin. Make sure you tell your doctor if you have any other medical problems, especially:

- Anemia (severe)
- Glaucoma—May be worsened by nitroglycerin
- Head injury (recent) or
- Stroke (recent)—Nitroglycerin may increase pressure in the brain, which can make problems worse
- Heart attack (recent)—Nitroglycerin may lower blood pressure, which can aggravate problems associated with heart attack
- Kidney disease or
- Liver disease—Effects may be increased because of slower removal of nitroglycerin from the body
- Overactive thyroid

Proper Use of This Medicine

Use nitroglycerin spray exactly as directed by your doctor. It will work only if used correctly.

This medicine usually comes with patient instructions. Read them carefully before you actually need to use it. Then, if you need the medicine quickly, you will know how to use it.

To use nitroglycerin lingual spray:

- Remove the plastic cover. *Do not shake the container.*
- Hold the container upright. With the container held close to your mouth, press the button to spray onto or under your tongue. *Do not inhale the spray.*
- Release the button and close your mouth. Avoid swallowing immediately after using the spray.

For patients using nitroglycerin oral spray *to relieve the pain of an angina attack*:

- *When you begin to feel an attack of angina starting (chest pains or a tightness or squeezing in the chest), sit down. Then use 1 or 2 sprays as directed by your doctor.* This medicine works best when you are standing or sitting. However, since you may become dizzy, lightheaded, or faint soon after using a spray, it is safer to sit rather than stand while the medicine is working. If you become dizzy or faint while sitting, take several deep breaths and bend forward with your head between your knees.
- Remain calm and you should feel better in a few minutes.
- *This medicine usually gives relief in less than 5 minutes.* However, if the pain is not relieved, use a second spray. If the pain continues for another 5 minutes, a third spray may be used. *If you still have the chest pains after a total of 3 sprays in a 15-*

minute period, contact your doctor or go to a hospital emergency room immediately.

For patients using nitroglycerin oral spray *to prevent an expected angina attack*:

- You may prevent anginal chest pains for up to 1 hour by using a spray 5 to 10 minutes before expected emotional stress or physical exertion that in the past seemed to bring on an attack.

Dosing—The dose of nitroglycerin lingual spray will be different for different patients. *Follow your doctor's orders or the directions on the label.* The following information includes only the average doses of nitroglycerin lingual spray. *If your dose is different, do not change it* unless your doctor tells you to do so.

- For *oral* dosage form (lingual spray):
  —For chest pain:
    - Adults—One or two sprays on or under the tongue. The dose may be repeated every five minutes as needed. If the chest pain is not relieved after a total of three sprays in a fifteen-minute period, call your doctor or go to the emergency room right away.

Storage—To store this medicine:

- Keep out of the reach of children.
- Store away from heat and direct light.
- Keep the medicine from freezing.
- Do not puncture, break, or burn the aerosol container, even after it is empty.
- Do not keep outdated medicine or medicine no longer needed. Be sure that any discarded medicine is out of the reach of children.

Precautions While Using This Medicine

If you have been using this medicine regularly for several weeks, do not suddenly stop using it. Stopping suddenly may bring on attacks of angina. Check with your doctor for the best way to reduce gradually the amount you are using before stopping completely.

Dizziness, lightheadedness, or faintness may occur, especially when you get up quickly from a lying or sitting position. Getting up slowly may help. If you feel dizzy, sit or lie down.

The dizziness, lightheadedness, or fainting is also more likely to occur if you drink alcohol, stand for long periods of time, exercise, or if the weather is hot. *While you are taking this medicine, be careful to limit the amount of alcohol you drink. Also, use extra care during exercise or hot weather or if you must stand for long periods of time.*

After using a dose of this medicine you may get a headache that lasts for a short time. This is a common side effect, which should become less noticeable after you have used the medicine for a while. If this effect continues or if the headaches are severe, check with your doctor.

Side Effects of This Medicine

Along with its needed effects, a medicine may cause some unwanted effects. Although not all of these side effects may occur, if they do occur they may need medical attention.

Check with your doctor as soon as possible if any of the following side effects occur:

Rare

    Blurred vision; dryness of mouth; headache (severe or prolonged); skin rash

Signs and symptoms of overdose (in the order in which they may occur)

    Bluish-colored lips, fingernails, or palms of hands; dizziness (extreme) or fainting; feeling of extreme pressure in head; shortness of breath; unusual tiredness or weakness; weak and fast heartbeat; fever; convulsions (seizures)

Other side effects may occur that usually do not need medical attention. These side effects may go away during treatment as your body adjusts to the medicine. However, check with your doctor if any of the following side effects continue or are bothersome:

More common

Dizziness or lightheadedness, especially when getting up from a lying or sitting position; fast pulse; flushing of face and neck; headache; nausea or vomiting; restlessness

Other side effects not listed above may also occur in some patients. If you notice any other effects, check with your doctor.

NITRATES—Oral Systemic

Some commonly used brand names are:

In the U.S.—

Cardilate[1]	Nitrocap[4]
Dilatrate-SR[2]	Nitrocap T.D.[4]
Duotrate[5]	Nitroglyn[4]
IMDUR[3]	Nitrolin[4]
ISMO[3]	Nitronet[4]
Iso-Bid[2]	Nitrong[4]
Isonate[2]	Nitrospan[4]
Isorbid[2]	Pentylan[5]
Isordil[2]	Peritrate[5]
Isotrate[2]	Peritrate SA[5]
Klavikordal[4]	Sorbitrate[2]
Monoket[3]	Sorbitrate SA[2]
Niong[4]	

In Canada—

Apo-ISDN[2]	Nitrong SR[4]
Cardilate[1]	Novosorbide[2]
Cedocard-SR[2]	Peritrate[5]
Coronex[2]	Peritrate Forte[5]
Isordil[2]	Peritrate SA[5]

Other commonly used names are:

Eritrityl tetranitrate[1]   Pentaerithrityl tetranitrate[5]
Erythritol tetranitrate[1]   P.E.T.N.[5]
Glyceryl trinitrate[4]

Note: For quick reference, the following nitrates are numbered to match the corresponding brand names.

This information applies to the following medicines:

1. Erythrityl Tetranitrate (e-RI-thri-till tet-ra-NYE-trate)
2. Isosorbide Dinitrate (eye-soe-SOR-bide dye-NYE-trate)‡
3. Isosorbide Mononitrate (eye-soe-SOR-bide mon-oh-NYE-trate)†
4. Nitroglycerin (nye-troe-GLI-ser-in)‡
5. Pentaerythritol Tetranitrate (pen-ta-er-ITH-ri-tole tet-ra-NYE-trate)‡

Note: This information does *not* apply to amyl nitrite or mannitol hexanitrate.

---

†Not commercially available in Canada.
‡Generic name product may also be available in the U.S.

Description

Nitrates (NYE-trates) are used to treat the symptoms of angina (chest pain). Depending on the type of dosage form and how it is taken, nitrates are used to treat angina in three ways:

- to relieve an attack that is occurring by using the medicine when the attack begins;
- to prevent attacks from occurring by using the medicine just before an attack is expected to occur; or
- to reduce the number of attacks that occur by using the medicine regularly on a long-term basis.

When taken orally and swallowed, nitrates are used to reduce the number of angina attacks that occur. They do not act fast enough to relieve the pain of an angina attack.

Nitrates work by relaxing blood vessels and increasing the supply of blood and oxygen to the heart while reducing its workload.

Nitrates may also be used for other conditions as determined by your doctor.

The nitrates discussed here are available only with your doctor's prescription, in the following dosage forms:

Oral

Erythrityl tetranitrate
- Tablets (U.S. and Canada)

Isosorbide dinitrate
- Capsules (U.S.)
- Extended-release capsules (U.S.)
- Tablets (U.S. and Canada)
- Chewable tablets (U.S.)
- Extended-release tablets (U.S. and Canada)

Isosorbide mononitrate
- Extended-release tablets (U.S.)
- Tablets (U.S.)

Nitroglycerin
- Extended-release capsules (U.S.)
- Extended-release tablets (U.S. and Canada)

Pentaerythritol tetranitrate
- Extended-release capsules (U.S.)
- Tablets (U.S. and Canada)
- Extended-release tablets (U.S. and Canada)

Before Using This Medicine

In deciding to use a medicine, the risks of taking the medicine must be weighed against the good it will do. This is a decision you and your doctor will make. For nitrates, the following should be considered:

Allergies—Tell your doctor if you have ever had any unusual or allergic reaction to nitrates or nitrites. Also tell your health care professional if you are allergic to any other substances, such as certain foods, preservatives, or dyes.

Pregnancy—Nitrates have not been studied in pregnant women. However, studies in rabbits given large doses of isosorbide dinitrate have shown adverse effects on the fetus. Before taking these medicines, make sure your doctor knows if you are pregnant or if you may become pregnant.

Breast-feeding—It is not known whether these medicines pass into breast milk. Although most medicines pass into breast milk in small amounts, many of them may be used safely while breast-feeding. Mothers who are taking these medicines and who wish to breast-feed should discuss this with their doctor.

Children—Studies on these medicines have been done only in adult patients, and there is no specific information comparing use of nitrates in children with use in other age groups.

Older adults—Dizziness or lightheadedness may be more likely to occur in the elderly, who may be more sensitive to the effects of nitrates.

Other medicines—Although certain medicines should not be used together at all, in other cases two different medicines may be used together even if an interaction might occur. In these cases, your doctor may want to change the dose, or other precautions may be necessary. When you are taking nitrates, it is especially important that your health care professional know if you are taking any of the following:

- Antihypertensives (high blood pressure medicine) or
- Other heart medicine—May increase the effects of nitrates on blood pressure

Other medical problems—The presence of other medical problems may affect the use of nitrates. Make sure you tell your doctor if you have any other medical problems, especially:

- Anemia (severe)
- Glaucoma—May be worsened by nitrates
- Head injury (recent) or
- Stroke (recent)—Nitrates may increase pressure in the brain, which can make problems worse

- Heart attack (recent)—Nitrates may lower blood pressure, which can aggravate problems associated with heart attack
- Kidney disease or
- Liver disease—Effects may be increased because of slower removal of nitroglycerin from the body
- Overactive thyroid

Proper Use of This Medicine

Take this medicine exactly as directed by your doctor. It will work only if taken correctly.

This form of nitrate is used to reduce the number of angina attacks. In most cases, it will not relieve an attack that has already started, because it works too slowly (the extended-release form releases medicine gradually over a 6-hour period to provide its effect for 8 to 10 hours). Check with your doctor if you need a fast-acting medicine to relieve the pain of an angina attack.

Take this medicine with a full glass (8 ounces) of water on an empty stomach. If taken either 1 hour before or 2 hours after meals, it will start working sooner.

Extended-release capsules and tablets are not to be broken, crushed, or chewed before they are swallowed. If broken up, they will not release the medicine properly.

Dosing—The dose of nitrates will be different for different patients. *Follow your doctor's orders or the directions on the label.* The following information includes only the average doses of nitrates. *If your dose is different, do not change it* unless your doctor tells you to do so.

The number of capsules or tablets that you take depends on the strength of the medicine. Also, *the number of doses you take each day, the time allowed between doses, and the length of time you take the medicine depend on the medical problem for which you are taking nitrates.*

For erythrityl tetranitrate

- For angina (chest pain):

    —For *oral* dosage form (tablets):

    - Adults—5 to 10 milligrams (mg) three or four times a day.

    - Children—Dose must be determined by your doctor.

For isosorbide dinitrate

- For angina (chest pain):

    —For *regular (short-acting) oral* dosage forms (capsules or tablets):

    - Adults—5 to 40 mg four times a day.

    - Children—Dose must be determined by your doctor.

    —For *long-acting oral* dosage forms (extended-release capsules or tablets):

    - Adults—20 to 80 mg every eight to twelve hours.

    - Children—Dose must be determined by your doctor.

For isosorbide mononitrate

- For angina (chest pain):

    —For *regular (short-acting) oral* dosage form (tablets):

    - Adults—20 mg two times a day. The two doses should be taken seven hours apart.

    - Children—Use and dose must be determined by your doctor.

    —For *long-acting oral* dosage forms (extended-release tablets):

    - Adults—30 to 240 mg once a day.

    - Children—Use and dose must be determined by your doctor.

For nitroglycerin

- For angina (chest pain):

—For *long-acting oral* dosage forms (capsules or tablets):

- Adults—1.3 to 9.0 mg every eight to twelve hours.

- Children—Dose must be determined by your doctor.

For pentaerythritol tetranitrate

- For angina (chest pain):

—For *regular (short-acting) oral* dosage forms (tablets):

- Adults—10 to 20 mg four times a day.

- Children—Dose must be determined by your doctor.

—For *long-acting oral* dosage forms (capsules or tablets):

- Adults—30 to 80 mg two times a day.

- Children—Dose must be determined by your doctor.

Missed dose—If you are taking this medicine regularly and you miss a dose, take it as soon as possible. However, if the next scheduled dose is within 2 hours (or within 6 hours for extended-release capsules or tablets), skip the missed dose and go back to your regular dosing schedule. Do not double doses.

Storage—To store this medicine:

- Keep out of the reach of children.
- Store away from heat and direct light.
- Do not store in the bathroom, near the kitchen sink, or in other damp places. Heat or moisture may cause the medicine to break down.
- Do not keep outdated medicine or medicine no longer needed. Be sure that any discarded medicine is out of the reach of children.

Precautions While Using This Medicine

If you have been taking this medicine regularly for several weeks or more, do not suddenly stop using it. Stopping suddenly may bring on attacks of angina. Check with your doctor for the best way to reduce gradually the amount you are taking before stopping completely.

Dizziness, lightheadedness, or faintness may occur, especially when you get up quickly from a lying or sitting position. Getting up slowly may help. If you feel dizzy, sit or lie down.

The dizziness, lightheadedness, or fainting is also more likely to occur if you drink alcohol, stand for long periods of time, exercise, or if the weather is hot. *While you are taking this medicine, be careful to limit the amount of alcohol you drink. Also, use extra care during exercise or hot weather or if you must stand for long periods of time.*

After taking a dose of this medicine you may get a headache that lasts for a short time. This is a common side effect, which should become less noticeable after you have taken the medicine for a while. If this effect continues, or if the headaches are severe, check with your doctor.

For patients taking the *extended-release dosage forms of isosorbide dinitrate or pentaerythritol tetranitrate*:
- Partially dissolved tablets have been found in the stools of a few patients taking the extended-release tablets. Be alert to this possibility, especially if you have frequent bowel movements, diarrhea, or digestive problems. Notify your doctor if any such tablets are discovered. The tablets must be properly digested to provide the correct dose of medicine.

Side Effects of This Medicine

Along with its needed effects, a medicine may cause some unwanted effects. Although not all of these side effects

may occur, if they do occur they may need medical
attention.

Check with your doctor as soon as possible if any of the
following side effects occur:

Rare

Blurred vision; dryness of mouth; headache (severe or prolonged); skin rash

*Signs and symptoms of overdose (in the order in which
they may occur)*

Bluish-colored lips, fingernails, or palms of hands; dizziness (extreme) or fainting; feeling of extreme pressure
in head; shortness of breath; unusual tiredness or weakness; weak and fast heartbeat; fever; convulsions
(seizures)

Other side effects may occur that usually do not need
medical attention. These side effects may go away during
treatment as your body adjusts to the medicine. However,
check with your doctor if any of the following side effects
continue or are bothersome:

More common

Dizziness or lightheadedness, especially when getting up
from a lying or sitting position; fast pulse; flushing of
face and neck; headache; nausea or vomiting; restlessness

Other side effects not listed above may also occur in some
patients. If you notice any other effects, check with your
doctor.

NITRATES—Sublingual, Chewable, or Buccal   Systemic

Some commonly used brand names are:

In the U.S.—

Cardilate[1]	Nitrogard[3]
Isonate[2]	Nitrostat[3]
Isorbid[2]	Sorbitrate[2]
Isordil[2]	

In Canada—

Apo-ISDN[2]	Isordil[2]
Cardilate[1]	Nitrogard SR[3]
Coronex[2]	Nitrostat[3]

Other commonly used names are:

Eritrityl tetranitrate[1]	Glyceryl trinitrate[3]
Erythritol tetranitrate[1]	

Note: For quick reference, the following nitrates are numbered to match the corresponding brand names.

This information applies to the following medicines:

1. Erythrityl Tetranitrate (e-RI-thri-till tet-ra-NYE-trate)
2. Isosorbide Dinitrate (eye-soe-SOR-bide dye-NYE-trate)‡
3. Nitroglycerin (nye-troe-GLI-ser-in)‡§

Note: This information does *not* apply to amyl nitrite or pentaerythritol tetranitrate.

---

‡Generic name product may also be available in the U.S.
§Generic name product may also be available in Canada.

Description

Nitrates (NYE-trates) are used to treat the symptoms of angina (chest pain). Depending on the type of dosage form and how it is taken, nitrates are used to treat angina in three ways:

- to relieve an attack that is occurring by using the medicine when the attack begins;
- to prevent attacks from occurring by using the medicine just before an attack is expected to occur; or
- to reduce the number of attacks that occur by using the medicine regularly on a long-term basis.

Nitrates are available in different forms. Sublingual nitrates are generally placed under the tongue where they dissolve and are absorbed through the lining of the mouth. Some can also be used buccally, being placed under the lip or in the cheek. The chewable dosage forms, after being chewed and held in the mouth before swallowing, are absorbed in the same way. *It is important to remember that each dosage form is different and that the specific directions for each type must be followed if the medicine is to work properly.*

Nitrates that are used *to relieve the pain* of an angina attack include:

- sublingual nitroglycerin;
- buccal nitroglycerin;
- sublingual isosorbide dinitrate; and
- chewable isosorbide dinitrate.

Those that can be used *to prevent expected attacks* of angina include:

- sublingual nitroglycerin;
- buccal nitroglycerin;
- sublingual erythrityl tetranitrate;
- sublingual isosorbide dinitrate; and
- chewable isosorbide dinitrate.

Products that are used regularly on a long-term basis *to reduce the number of attacks* that occur include:

- buccal nitroglycerin;
- oral/sublingual erythrityl tetranitrate;
- chewable isosorbide dinitrate; and
- sublingual isosorbide dinitrate.

Nitrates work by relaxing blood vessels and increasing the supply of blood and oxygen to the heart while reducing its workload.

Nitrates may also be used for other conditions as determined by your doctor.

The nitrates discussed here are available only with your doctor's prescription, in the following dosage forms:

Buccal

Nitroglycerin
- Extended-release tablets (U.S. and Canada)

Chewable

Isosorbide dinitrate
- Tablets (U.S.)

Sublingual

Erythrityl tetranitrate
- Tablets (U.S. and Canada)

Isosorbide dinitrate
- Tablets (U.S. and Canada)

Nitroglycerin
- Tablets (U.S. and Canada)

Before Using This Medicine

In deciding to use a medicine, the risks of taking the medicine must be weighed against the good it will do. This is a decision you and your doctor will make. For nitrates, the following should be considered:

Allergies—Tell your doctor if you have ever had any unusual or allergic reaction to nitrates or nitrites. Also tell your health care professional if you are allergic to any other substances, such as certain foods, preservatives, or dyes.

Pregnancy—Nitrates have not been studied in pregnant women. However, studies in rabbits given large doses of isosorbide dinitrate have shown adverse effects on the fetus. Before taking these medicines, make sure your doctor knows if you are pregnant or if you may become pregnant.

Breast-feeding—It is not known whether these medicines pass into breast milk. Although most medicines pass into breast milk in small amounts, many of them may be used safely while breast-feeding. Mothers who are taking these medicines and who wish to breast-feed should discuss this with their doctor.

Children—Studies on these medicines have been done only in adult patients, and there is no specific information comparing use of nitrates in children with use in other age groups.

Older adults—Dizziness or lightheadedness may be more likely to occur in the elderly, who may be more sensitive to the effects of nitrates.

Other medicines—Although certain medicines should not be used together at all, in other cases two different medicines may be used together even if an interaction might occur. In these cases, your doctor may want to change the dose, or other precautions may be necessary. When you are taking nitrates, it is especially important that your health care professional know if you are taking any of the following:

- Antihypertensives (high blood pressure medicine) or
- Other heart medicine—May increase the effects of nitrates on blood pressure

Other medical problems—The presence of other medical problems may affect the use of nitrates. Make sure you tell your doctor if you have any other medical problems, especially:

- Anemia (severe)
- Glaucoma—May be worsened by nitrates
- Head injury (recent) or
- Stroke (recent)—Nitrates may increase pressure in the brain, which can make problems worse
- Heart attack (recent)—Nitrates may lower blood pressure, which can aggravate problems associated with heart attack
- Kidney disease or
- Liver disease—Effects may be increased because of slower removal of nitroglycerin from the body
- Overactive thyroid

Proper Use of This Medicine

Take this medicine exactly as directed by your doctor. It will work only if taken correctly.

Sublingual tablets should not be chewed, crushed, or swallowed. They work much faster when absorbed through the lining of the mouth. Place the tablet under the tongue, between the lip and gum, or between the cheek and gum and let it dissolve there. Do not eat, drink, smoke, or use chewing tobacco while a tablet is dissolving.

Buccal extended-release tablets should not be chewed, crushed, or swallowed. They are designed to release a dose of nitroglycerin over a period of hours, not all at once.

- Allow the tablet to dissolve slowly in place between the upper lip and gum (above the front teeth), or between the cheek and upper gum. If food or drink is to be taken during the 3 to 5 hours when the tablet is dissolving, place the tablet between the *upper* lip and gum, above the front teeth. If you have dentures, you may place the tablet anywhere between the cheek and gum.
- Touching the tablet with your tongue or drinking hot liquids may cause the tablet to dissolve faster.
- Do not go to sleep while a tablet is dissolving because it could slip down your throat and cause choking.
- If you accidentally swallow the tablet, replace it with another one.
- Do not use chewing tobacco while a tablet is in place.

Chewable tablets must be chewed well and held in the mouth for about 2 minutes before you swallow them. This will allow the medicine to be absorbed through the lining of the mouth.

For patients using *nitroglycerin or isosorbide dinitrate to relieve the pain of an angina attack*:

- *When you begin to feel an attack of angina starting (chest pains or a tightness or squeezing in the chest), sit down. Then place a tablet in your mouth, either sublingually or buccally, or chew a chewable tablet.* This medicine works best when you are standing or sitting. However, since you may become dizzy, lightheaded, or faint soon after using a tablet, it is safer to sit rather than stand while the medicine is working. If you become dizzy or faint while sitting, take several deep breaths and bend forward with your head between your knees.

- Remain calm and you should feel better in a few minutes.

- *This medicine usually gives relief in 1 to 5 minutes.* However, if the pain is not relieved, and you are using:

  —Sublingual tablets, either sublingually or buccally: Use a second tablet. If the pain continues for another 5 minutes, a third tablet may be used. *If you still have the chest pains after a total of 3 tablets in a 15-minute period, contact your doctor or go to a hospital emergency room immediately.*

  —Buccal extended-release tablets: *Use a sublingual (under the tongue) nitroglycerin tablet and check with your doctor.* Do not use another buccal tablet since the effects of a buccal tablet last for several hours.

For patients using *nitroglycerin, erythrityl tetranitrate, or isosorbide dinitrate to prevent an expected angina attack:*

- You may prevent anginal chest pains for up to 1 hour (6 hours for the extended-release nitroglycerin tablet) by using a buccal or sublingual tablet or chewing a chewable tablet 5 to 10 minutes before expected emotional stress or physical exertion that in the past seemed to bring on an attack.

For patients using *isosorbide dinitrate or extended-release buccal nitroglycerin regularly on a long-term basis to reduce the number of angina attacks that occur:*

- Chewable or sublingual isosorbide dinitrate and buccal extended-release nitroglycerin tablets can be used either to prevent angina attacks or to help relieve an attack that has already started.

Dosing—The dose of nitrates will be different for different patients. *Follow your doctor's orders or the directions on the label.* The following information includes only the average doses of nitrates. *If your dose is different, do not change it* unless your doctor tells you to do so.

For erythrityl tetranitrate

- For angina (chest pain):

  —For *buccal or sublingual* dosage form (tablets):

  - Adults—5 to 10 milligrams (mg) three or four times a day.

  - Children—Dose must be determined by your doctor.

For isosorbide dinitrate

- For angina (chest pain):

  —For *chewable* dosage form (tablets):

  - Adults—5 mg every two to three hours, chewed well and held in mouth for one or two minutes.

  - Children—Dose must be determined by your doctor.

  —For *buccal or sublingual* dosage form (tablets):

  - Adults—2.5 to 5 mg every two to three hours.

  - Children—Dose must be determined by your doctor.

For nitroglycerin

- For angina (chest pain):

  —For *buccal* dosage form (extended-release tablets):

  - Adults—1 mg every five hours while awake. Your doctor may increase your dose.

  - Children—Dose must be determined by your doctor.

  —For *sublingual* dosage form (tablets):

  - Adults—150 to 600 micrograms (mcg) (0.15 to 0.6 mg) every five minutes. If you still have chest pain after a total of three tablets in fifteen minutes, call your doctor or go to the emergency room right away.

• Children—Dose must be determined by your doctor.

Missed dose—For patients using isosorbide dinitrate or extended-release buccal nitroglycerin regularly on a long-term basis to reduce the number of angina attacks that occur:

• If you miss a dose of this medicine, use it as soon as possible. However, if the next scheduled dose is within 2 hours, skip the missed dose and go back to your regular dosing schedule. Do not double doses.

Stability and proper storage—

For sublingual nitroglycerin

• Sublingual nitroglycerin tablets may lose some of their strength if they are exposed to air, heat, or moisture for long periods of time. However, if you screw the cap on tightly after each use and you properly store the bottle, the tablets should retain their strength until the expiration date on the bottle.

• Some people think they should test the strength of their sublingual nitroglycerin tablets by looking for a tingling or burning sensation, a feeling of warmth or flushing, or a headache after a tablet has been dissolved under the tongue. This kind of testing is not completely reliable since some patients may be unable to detect these effects. In addition, newer, stabilized sublingual nitroglycerin tablets are less likely to produce these detectable effects.

• To help keep the nitroglycerin tablets at full strength:

—keep the medicine in the original glass, screw-cap bottle. For patients who wish to carry a small number of tablets with them for emergency use, a specially designed container is available. However, only containers specifically labeled as suitable for use with nitroglycerin sublingual tablets should be used.

—remove the cotton plug that comes in the bottle and *do not* put it back.

—*put the cap on the bottle quickly and tightly after each use.*

—to select a tablet for use, pour several into the bottle cap, take one, and pour the others back into the bottle. Try not to hold them in the palm of your hand because they may pick up moisture and crumble.

—do not keep other medicines in the same bottle with the nitroglycerin since they will weaken the nitroglycerin effect.

—keep the medicine handy at all times but try not to carry the bottle close to the body. Medicine may lose strength because of body warmth. Instead, carry the tightly closed bottle in your purse or the pocket of a jacket or other loose-fitting clothing whenever possible.

—store the bottle of nitroglycerin tablets in a cool, dry place. Storage at average room temperature away from direct heat or direct sunlight is best. Do not store in the refrigerator or in a bathroom medicine cabinet because the moisture usually present in these areas may cause the tablets to crumble if the container is not tightly closed. Do not keep the tablets in your automobile glove compartment.

- Keep out of the reach of children.
- Do not keep outdated medicine or medicine no longer needed. Be sure that any discarded medicine is out of the reach of children.

For erythrityl tetranitrate, isosorbide dinitrate, and buccal extended-release nitroglycerin

- These forms of nitrates are more stable than sublingual nitroglycerin.
- Keep out of the reach of children.
- Store away from heat and direct light.

- Do not store in the bathroom, near the kitchen sink, or in other damp places. Heat or moisture may cause the medicine to break down.

- Do not keep outdated medicine or medicine no longer needed. Be sure that any discarded medicine is out of the reach of children.

Precautions While Using This Medicine

If you have been taking this medicine regularly for several weeks, do not suddenly stop using it. Stopping suddenly may bring on attacks of angina. Check with your doctor for the best way to reduce gradually the amount you are taking before stopping completely.

Dizziness, lightheadedness, or faintness may occur, especially when you get up quickly from a lying or sitting position. Getting up slowly may help. If you feel dizzy, sit or lie down.

The dizziness, lightheadedness, or fainting is also more likely to occur if you drink alcohol, stand for long periods of time, exercise, or if the weather is hot. *While you are taking this medicine, be careful to limit the amount of alcohol you drink. Also, use extra care during exercise or hot weather or if you must stand for long periods of time.*

After taking a dose of this medicine you may get a headache that lasts for a short time. This is a common side effect, which should become less noticeable after you have taken the medicine for a while. If this effect continues or if the headaches are severe, check with your doctor.

Side Effects of This Medicine

Along with its needed effects, a medicine may cause some unwanted effects. Although not all of these side effects may occur, if they do occur they may need medical attention.

Check with your doctor as soon as possible if any of the following side effects occur:

Rare

Blurred vision; dryness of mouth; headache (severe or prolonged); skin rash

Signs and symptoms of overdose (in the order in which they may occur)

Bluish-colored lips, fingernails, or palms of hands; dizziness (extreme) or fainting; feeling of extreme pressure in head; shortness of breath; unusual tiredness or weakness; weak and fast heartbeat; fever; convulsions (seizures)

Other side effects may occur that usually do not need medical attention. These side effects may go away during treatment as your body adjusts to the medicine. However, check with your doctor if any of the following side effects continue or are bothersome:

More common

Dizziness or lightheadedness, especially when getting up from a lying or sitting position; fast pulse; flushing of face and neck; headache; nausea or vomiting; restlessness

Other side effects not listed above may also occur in some patients. If you notice any other effects, check with your doctor.

NITRATES—Topical Systemic

Some commonly used brand names are:

In the U.S.—

Deponit[2]	Nitrol[1]
Nitro-Bid[1]	Nitrong[1]
Nitrodisc[2]	Nitrostat[1]
Nitro-Dur[2]	NTS[2]
Nitro-Dur II[2]	Transderm-Nitro[2]

In Canada—

Nitro-Bid[1]	Nitrong[1]
Nitrol[1]	Transderm-Nitro[2]

Another commonly used name for nitroglycerin is glyceryl trinitrate.

Note: For quick reference, the following nitrates are numbered to match the corresponding brand names.

This information applies to the following medicines:

1. Nitroglycerin Ointment‡
2. Nitroglycerin Transdermal Patches‡

---

‡Generic name product may also be available in the U.S.

Description

Nitrates (NYE-trates) are used to treat the symptoms of angina (chest pain). Depending on the type of dosage form and how it is taken, nitrates are used to treat angina in three ways:

- to relieve an attack that is occurring by using the medicine when the attack begins;
- to prevent attacks from occurring by using the medicine just before an attack is expected to occur; or
- to reduce the number of attacks that occur by using the medicine regularly on a long-term basis.

When applied to the skin, nitrates are used to reduce the number of angina attacks that occur. The only nitrate available for this purpose is topical nitroglycerin (nye-troe-GLI-ser-in).

Topical nitroglycerin is absorbed through the skin. It works by relaxing blood vessels and increasing the supply of blood and oxygen to the heart while reducing its workload. This helps prevent future angina attacks from occurring.

Topical nitroglycerin may also be used for other conditions as determined by your doctor.

Nitroglycerin as discussed here is available only with your doctor's prescription, in the following dosage forms:

Topical

- Ointment (U.S. and Canada)
- Transdermal (stick-on) patch (U.S. and Canada)

Before Using This Medicine

In deciding to use a medicine, the risks of taking the medicine must be weighed against the good it will do. This is a decision you and your doctor will make. For nitroglycerin applied to the skin, the following should be considered:

Allergies—Tell your doctor if you have ever had any unusual or allergic reaction to nitrates or nitrites. Also tell your health care professional if you are allergic to any other substances, such as certain foods, preservatives, or dyes.

Pregnancy—Nitrates have not been studied in pregnant women. Before taking these medicines, make sure your doctor knows if you are pregnant or if you may become pregnant.

Breast-feeding—It is not known whether this medicine passes into breast milk. Although most medicines pass into breast milk in small amounts, many of them may be used safely while breast-feeding. Mothers who are taking these medicines and who wish to breast-feed should discuss this with their doctor.

Children—Studies on these medicines have been done only in adult patients, and there is no specific information comparing use of nitrates in children with use in other age groups.

Older adults—Dizziness or lightheadedness may be more likely to occur in the elderly, who may be more sensitive to the effects of nitrates.

Other medicines—Although certain medicines should not be used together at all, in other cases two different medicines may be used together even if an interaction might occur. In these cases, your doctor may want to change the dose, or other precautions may be necessary. When you are using nitroglycerin, it is especially important that your

health care professional know if you are taking any of
the following:

- Antihypertensives (high blood pressure medicine) or
- Other heart medicine—May increase the effects of nitroglycerin on blood pressure

Other medical problems—The presence of other medical
problems may affect the use of nitroglycerin. Make sure
you tell your doctor if you have any other medical problems, especially:

- Anemia (severe)
- Glaucoma—May be worsened by nitroglycerin
- Head injury (recent) or
- Stroke (recent)—Nitroglycerin may increase pressure in the
  brain, which can make problems worse
- Heart attack (recent)—Nitroglycerin may lower blood pres-
  sure, which can aggravate problems associated with heart
  attack
- Kidney disease or
- Liver disease—Effects may be increased because of slower
  removal of nitroglycerin from the body
- Overactive thyroid

Proper Use of This Medicine

Use nitroglycerin exactly as directed by your doctor. It
will work only if applied correctly.

*The ointment and transdermal forms of nitroglycerin are
used to reduce the number of angina attacks. They will
not relieve an attack that has already started* because they
work too slowly. Check with your doctor if you need a
fast-acting medicine to relieve the pain of an angina attack.

*This medicine usually comes with patient instructions.
Read them carefully before using.*

For patients using the *ointment* form of this medicine:

- Before applying a new dose of ointment, remove any

ointment remaining on the skin from a previous dose. This will allow the fresh ointment to release the nitroglycerin properly.

- This medicine comes with dose-measuring papers. Use them to measure the length of ointment squeezed from the tube and to apply the ointment to the skin. *Do not rub or massage the ointment into the skin; just spread in a thin, even layer, covering an area of the same size each time it is applied.*

- Apply the ointment to skin that has little or no hair.

- Apply each dose of ointment to a different area of skin to prevent irritation or other skin problems.

- If your doctor has ordered an occlusive dressing (airtight covering, such as kitchen plastic wrap) to be applied over this medicine, make sure you know how to apply it. Since occlusive dressings increase the amount of medicine absorbed through the skin and the possibility of side effects, use them only as directed. If you have any questions about this, check with your health care professional.

For patients using the *transdermal (stick-on patch) system:*

- Do not try to trim or cut the adhesive patch to adjust the dosage. Check with your doctor if you think the medicine is not working as it should.

- Apply the patch to a clean, dry skin area with little or no hair and free of scars, cuts, or irritation. Remove the previous patch before applying a new one.

- Apply a new patch if the first one becomes loose or falls off.

- Apply each dose to a different area of skin to prevent skin irritation or other problems.

Dosing—The dose of nitroglycerin will be different for different patients. *Follow your doctor's orders or the directions on the label.* The following information includes only the average doses of nitrates. *If your dose is different, do not change it* unless your doctor tells you to do so.

For nitroglycerin
- For angina (chest pain):
  —For *ointment* dosage form:
  - Adults—15 to 30 milligrams (mg) (about one to two inches of ointment squeezed from tube) every six to eight hours.
  - Children—Use and dose must be determined by your doctor.

  —For *transdermal system (skin patch)* dosage form:
  - Adults—Apply one transdermal dosage system (skin patch) to intact skin once a day. The patch is usually left on for 12 to 14 hours a day and then taken off. Follow your doctor's instructions for when to put on and take off the skin patch.
  - Children—Use and dose must be determined by your doctor.

Missed dose—
- For patients using the *ointment* form of this medicine: If you miss a dose of this medicine, apply it as soon as possible unless the next scheduled dose is within 2 hours. Then go back to your regular dosing schedule. Do not increase the amount used.
- For patients using the *transdermal (stick-on patch) system*: If you miss a dose of this medicine, apply it as soon as possible. Then go back to your regular dosing schedule.

Storage—
- To store the *ointment* form of this medicine:
  —Keep out of the reach of children.
  —Store the tube of nitroglycerin ointment in a cool place and keep it tightly closed.
  —Do not keep outdated medicine or medicine no longer needed. Be sure that any discarded medicine is out of the reach of children.
- To store the *transdermal (stick-on patch) system*:

—Keep out of the reach of children.

—Store away from heat and direct light.

—Do not store in the bathroom, near the kitchen sink, or in other damp places. Heat or moisture may cause the medicine to break down.

—Do not keep outdated medicine or medicine no longer needed. Be sure that any discarded medicine is out of the reach of children.

Precautions While Using This Medicine

If you have been using nitroglycerin regularly for several weeks or more, do not suddenly stop using it. Stopping suddenly may bring on attacks of angina. Check with your doctor for the best way to reduce gradually the amount you are using before stopping completely.

Dizziness, lightheadedness, or faintness may occur, especially when you get up quickly from a lying or sitting position. Getting up slowly may help. If you feel dizzy, sit or lie down.

The dizziness, lightheadedness, or fainting is also more likely to occur if you drink alcohol, stand for long periods of time, exercise, or if the weather is hot. *While you are taking this medicine, be careful to limit the amount of alcohol you drink. Also, use extra care during exercise or hot weather or if you must stand for long periods of time.*

After using a dose of this medicine you may get a headache that lasts for a short time. This is a common side effect, which should become less noticeable after you have used the medicine for a while. If this effect continues, or if the headaches are severe, check with your doctor.

Side Effects of This Medicine

Along with its needed effects, a medicine may cause some unwanted effects. Although not all of these side effects

may occur, if they do occur they may need medical attention.

Check with your doctor as soon as possible if any of the following side effects occur:

Rare

Blurred vision; dryness of mouth; headache (severe or prolonged)

Signs and symptoms of overdose (in the order in which they may occur)

Bluish-colored lips, fingernails, or palms of hands; dizziness (extreme) or fainting; feeling of extreme pressure in head; shortness of breath; unusual tiredness or weakness; weak and fast heartbeat; fever; convulsions (seizures)

Other side effects may occur that usually do not need medical attention. These side effects may go away during treatment as your body adjusts to the medicine. However, check with your doctor if any of the following side effects continue or are bothersome:

More common

Dizziness or lightheadedness, especially when getting up from a lying or sitting position; fast pulse; flushing of face and neck; headache; nausea or vomiting; restlessness

Less common

Sore, reddened skin

Other side effects not listed above may also occur in some patients. If you notice any other effects, check with your doctor.

PENTOXIFYLLINE Systemic

A commonly used brand name in the U.S. and Canada is Trental.
Another commonly used name is oxypentifylline.

Description

Pentoxifylline (pen-tox-IF-i-lin) improves the flow of blood through blood vessels. It is used to reduce leg pain caused by poor blood circulation. Pentoxifylline makes it possible to walk farther before having to rest because of leg cramps.

Pentoxifylline is available only with your doctor's prescription, in the following dosage form:

Oral
- Extended-release tablets (U.S. and Canada)

Before Using This Medicine

In deciding to use a medicine, the risks of taking the medicine must be weighed against the good it will do. This is a decision you and your doctor will make. For pentoxifylline, the following should be considered:

Allergies—Tell your doctor if you have ever had any unusual or allergic reaction to pentoxifylline or to other xanthines such as aminophylline, caffeine, dyphylline, ethylenediamine (contained in aminophylline), oxtriphylline, theobromine, or theophylline. Also tell your health care professional if you are allergic to any other substances, such as foods, preservatives, or dyes.

Pregnancy—Pentoxifylline has not been studied in pregnant women. Studies in animals have not shown that it causes birth defects. However, at very high doses it has caused other harmful effects. Before taking this medicine, make sure your doctor knows if you are pregnant or if you may become pregnant.

Breast-feeding—Pentoxifylline passes into breast milk. The medicine has not been reported to cause problems in nursing babies. However, pentoxifylline has caused noncancerous tumors in animals when given for a long time in doses much larger than those used in humans. Therefore, your doctor may not want you to breast-feed while taking it. Be sure that you discuss the risks and benefits of this medicine with your doctor.

Children—Studies on this medicine have been done only in adult patients, and there is no specific information comparing use of pentoxifylline in children with use in other age groups.

Older adults—Side effects may be more likely to occur in the elderly, who are usually more sensitive than younger adults to the effects of pentoxifylline.

Other medicines—Although certain medicines should not be used together at all, in other cases two different medicines may be used together even if an interaction might occur. In these cases, your doctor may want to change the dose, or other precautions may be necessary. When you are taking pentoxifylline, it is important that your health care professional know if you are taking any other prescription or nonprescription (over-the-counter [OTC]) medicine, or if you smoke tobacco.

Other medical problems—The presence of other medical problems may affect the use of pentoxifylline. Make sure you tell your doctor if you have any other medical problems, especially:

- Any condition in which there is a risk of bleeding (e.g., recent stroke)—Pentoxifylline may make the condition worse
- Kidney disease or
- Liver disease—The chance of side effects may be increased

Proper Use of This Medicine

Swallow the tablet whole. Do not crush, break, or chew it before swallowing.

Pentoxifylline should be taken with meals to lessen the chance of stomach upset. Taking an antacid with the medicine may also help.

Dosing—The dose of pentoxifylline will be different for different patients. *Follow your doctor's orders or the directions on the label.* The following information includes only the average doses of pentoxifylline. *If your dose is different, do not change it* unless your doctor tells you to do so.

- For *oral* dosage form (extended-release tablets):

  —For peripheral vascular disease (circulation problems):

  - Adults—400 milligrams (mg) two to three times a day, taken with meals.
  - Children—Use must be determined by your doctor.

Missed dose—If you miss a dose of this medicine, take it as soon as possible. However, if it is almost time for your next dose, skip the missed dose and go back to your regular dosing schedule. Do not double doses.

Storage—To store this medicine:

- Keep out of the reach of children.
- Store away from heat and direct light.
- Do not store in the bathroom, near the kitchen sink, or in other damp places. Heat or moisture may cause the medicine to break down.
- Do not keep outdated medicine or medicine no longer needed. Be sure that any discarded medicine is out of the reach of children.

Precautions While Using This Medicine

It may take several weeks for this medicine to work. If you feel that pentoxifylline is not working, do not stop taking it on your own. Instead, check with your doctor.

Smoking tobacco may worsen your condition since nicotine may further narrow your blood vessels. Therefore, it is best to avoid smoking.

Side Effects of This Medicine

Along with its needed effects, a medicine may cause some unwanted effects. Although not all of these side effects may occur, if they do occur they may need medical attention.

Check with your doctor as soon as possible if any of the following side effects occur:

Rare

Chest pain; irregular heartbeat

Signs and symptoms of overdose (in the order in which they may occur)

Drowsiness; flushing; faintness; unusual excitement; convulsions (seizures)

Other side effects may occur that usually do not need medical attention. These side effects may go away during treatment as your body adjusts to the medicine. However, check with your doctor if any of the following side effects continue or are bothersome:

Less common

Dizziness; headache; nausea or vomiting; stomach discomfort

Other side effects not listed above may also occur in some patients. If you notice any other effects, check with your doctor.

PHENOXYBENZAMINE   Systemic

A commonly used brand name in the U.S. is Dibenzyline.

Description

Phenoxybenzamine (fen-ox-ee-BEN-za-meen) belongs to the general class of medicines called antihypertensives. It is used to treat high blood pressure (hypertension) due to a disease called pheochromocytoma.

Phenoxybenzamine blocks the effects of certain chemicals in the body. When these chemicals are present in large amounts, they cause high blood pressure.

Phenoxybenzamine may also be used for other conditions as determined by your doctor.

Phenoxybenzamine is available only with your doctor's prescription, in the following dosage form:

Oral
- Capsules (U.S.)

Before Using This Medicine

In deciding to use a medicine, the risks of taking the medicine must be weighed against the good it will do. This is a decision you and your doctor will make. For phenoxybenzamine, the following should be considered:

Allergies—Tell your doctor if you have ever had any unusual or allergic reaction to phenoxybenzamine. Also, tell your health care professional if you are allergic to any other substances, such as foods, preservatives, or dyes.

Pregnancy—Phenoxybenzamine has not been studied in pregnant women or animals. Make sure your doctor knows if you are pregnant or if you may become pregnant before taking phenoxybenzamine.

Breast-feeding—It is not known whether phenoxybenzamine passes into breast milk. However, this medicine has not been reported to cause problems in nursing babies.

Children—Although there is no specific information about the use of phenoxybenzamine in children, it is not expected to cause different side effects or problems in children than it does in adults.

Older adults—Dizziness or lightheadedness may be more likely to occur in the elderly, who are more sensitive to the effects of phenoxybenzamine. In addition, phenoxybenzamine may reduce tolerance to cold temperatures in elderly patients.

Other medicines—Although certain medicines should not be used together at all, in other cases two different medicines may be used together even if an interaction might occur. In these cases, your doctor may want to change the dose, or other precautions may be necessary. Tell your health care professional if you are taking any other prescription or nonprescription (over-the-counter [OTC]) medicine.

Other medical problems—The presence of other medical problems may affect the use of phenoxybenzamine. Make sure you tell your doctor if you have any other medical problems, especially:

- Angina (chest pain) or
- Heart or blood vessel disease—Some kinds may be worsened by phenoxybenzamine
- Kidney disease—Effects may be increased
- Lung infection—Symptoms such as stuffy nose may be worsened
- Recent heart attack or stroke—Lowering blood pressure may make problems resulting from stroke or heart attack worse

---

Proper Use of This Medicine

To help you remember to take your medicine, try to get into the habit of taking it at the same time each day.

Dosing—The dose of phenoxybenzamine will be different for different patients. *Follow your doctor's orders or the* *directions on the label.* The following information includes only the average doses of phenoxybenzamine. *If your dose is different, do not change it* unless your doctor tells you to do so.

- For *oral* dosage form (capsules):

  —For high blood pressure caused by pheo-chromocytoma:

  - Adults—At first, 10 milligrams (mg) two times a day. Then, your doctor may increase your dose to 20 to 40 mg two or three times a day.
  - Children—Dose is based on body weight and must be determined by your doctor. The usual starting dose is 0.2 mg per kilogram (kg) (0.09 mg per pound) of body weight taken once a day. Then, your doctor may increase your dose to 0.4 to 1.2 mg per kg (0.18 to 0.55 mg per pound) of body weight a day. This is divided into three or four doses.

Missed dose—If you miss a dose of this medicine, take it as soon as you remember. However, if it is almost time for your next dose, skip the missed dose and go back to your regular dosing schedule. Do not double doses.

Storage—To store this medicine:

- Keep out of the reach of children.
- Store away from heat and direct light.
- Do not store in the bathroom, near the kitchen sink, or in other damp places. Heat or moisture may cause the medicine to break down.
- Do not keep outdated medicine or medicine no longer needed. Be sure that any discarded medicine is out of the reach of children.

Precautions While Using This Medicine

It is important that your doctor check your progress at regular visits to make sure that this medicine is working properly and to check for unwanted effects.

Do not take other medicines unless they have been discussed with your doctor. This especially includes over-the-counter (nonprescription) medicines for appetite control, asthma, colds, cough, hay fever, or sinus problems, since they may interfere with the effects of this medicine.

Phenoxybenzamine may cause some people to become dizzy, drowsy, or less alert than they are normally. This is more likely to happen when you begin to take it or when you increase the amount of medicine you are taking. *Make sure you know how you react to this medicine before you drive, use machines, or do anything else that could be dangerous if you are dizzy or not alert.*

Dizziness, lightheadedness, or fainting may occur, especially when you get up from a lying or sitting position. Getting up slowly may help, but if the problem continues or gets worse, check with your doctor.

The dizziness, lightheadedness, or fainting is also more likely to occur if you drink alcohol, stand for a long time, exercise, or if the weather is hot. *While you are taking this medicine, be careful in the amount of alcohol you drink. Also, use extra care during exercise or hot weather or if you must stand for a long time.*

Before having any kind of surgery (including dental surgery) or emergency treatment, *tell the medical doctor or dentist in charge that you are using this medicine.*

Phenoxybenzamine may cause dryness of the mouth, nose, and throat. For temporary relief of mouth dryness, use sugarless candy or gum, melt bits of ice in your mouth, or use a saliva substitute. However, if dry mouth continues for more than 2 weeks, check with your medical doctor or dentist. Continuing dryness of the mouth may increase the chance of dental disease, including tooth decay, gum disease, and fungus infections.

Side Effects of This Medicine

In rats and mice, phenoxybenzamine has been found to increase the risk of development of malignant tumors. It is not known if phenoxybenzamine increases the chance of tumors in humans.

Along with its needed effects, a medicine may cause some unwanted effects. The following side effects may go away as your body adjusts to the medicine. However, check with your doctor if any of these effects continue or are bothersome:

More common

Dizziness or lightheadedness, especially when getting up from a lying or sitting position; fast heartbeat; pinpoint pupils; stuffy nose

Less common

Confusion; drowsiness; dryness of mouth; headache; lack of energy; sexual problems in males; unusual tiredness or weakness

Other side effects not listed above may also occur in some patients. If you notice any other effects, check with your doctor.

Additional Information

Once a medicine has been approved for marketing for a certain use, experience may show that it is also useful for other medical problems. Although this use is not included in product labeling, phenoxybenzamine is used in certain patients with the following medical condition:

• Benign prostatic hypertrophy

Other than the above information, there is no additional information relating to proper use, precautions, or side effects for this use.

PRAZOSIN   Systemic

A commonly used brand name in the U.S. and Canada is Minipress.
Generic name product may also be available.

Description

Prazosin (PRA-zoe-sin) belongs to the general class of
medicines called antihypertensives. It is used to treat high
blood pressure (hypertension).

High blood pressure adds to the workload of the heart and
arteries. If it continues for a long time, the heart and arteries may not function properly. This can damage the blood
vessels of the brain, heart, and kidneys, resulting in a
stroke, heart failure, or kidney failure. High blood pressure
may also increase the risk of heart attacks. These problems
may be less likely to occur if blood pressure is controlled.

Prazosin works by relaxing blood vessels so that blood
passes through them more easily. This helps to lower
blood pressure.

Prazosin may also be used for other conditions as determined by your doctor.

Prazosin is available only with your doctor's prescription,
in the following dosage forms:

Oral

- Capsules (U.S.)
- Tablets (Canada)

Before Using This Medicine

In deciding to use a medicine, the risks of taking the
medicine must be weighed against the good it will do.
This is a decision you and your doctor will make. For
prazosin, the following should be considered:

Allergies—Tell your doctor if you have ever had any un-usual or allergic reaction to prazosin, doxazosin, or tera-zosin. Also tell your health care professional if you are allergic to any other substance, such as foods, preservatives, or dyes.

Pregnancy—Limited use of prazosin to control high blood pressure in pregnant women has not shown that prazosin causes birth defects or other problems. Studies in animals given many times the highest recommended human dose of prazosin also have not shown that prazosin causes birth defects. However, in rats given many times the highest recommended human dose, lower birth weights were seen.

Breast-feeding—Prazosin passes into breast milk in small amounts. However, it has not been reported to cause problems in nursing babies.

Children—Studies on this medicine have been done only in adult patients, and there is no specific information comparing use of prazosin in children with use in other age groups.

Older adults—Dizziness, lightheadedness, or fainting (especially when getting up from a lying or sitting position) may be more likely to occur in the elderly, who are more sensitive to the effects of prazosin. In addition, prazosin may reduce tolerance to cold temperatures in elderly patients.

Other medicines—Although certain medicines should not be used together at all, in other cases two different medicines may be used together even if an interaction might occur. In these cases, your doctor may want to change the dose, or other precautions may be necessary. Tell your health care professional if you are taking any other prescription or nonprescription (over-the-counter [OTC]) medicine.

Other medical problems—The presence of other medical problems may affect the use of prazosin. Make sure you tell your doctor if you have any other medical problems, especially:

- Angina (chest pain) or
- Heart disease (severe)—Prazosin may make these conditions worse
- Kidney disease—Possible increased sensitivity to the effects of prazosin

---

Proper Use of This Medicine

For patients *taking this medicine for high blood pressure:*

- In addition to the use of the medicine your doctor has prescribed, treatment for your high blood pressure may include weight control and care in the types of foods you eat, especially foods high in sodium. Your doctor will tell you which of these are most important for you. You should check with your doctor before changing your diet.

- Many patients who have high blood pressure will not notice any signs of the problem. In fact, many may feel normal. It is very important that you *take your medicine exactly as directed* and that you keep your appointments with your doctor even if you feel well.

- Remember that prazosin will not cure your high blood pressure, but it does help control it. Therefore, you must continue to take it as directed if you expect to lower your blood pressure and keep it down. *You may have to take high blood pressure medicine for the rest of your life.* If high blood pressure is not treated, it can cause serious problems such as heart failure, blood vessel disease, stroke, or kidney disease.

To help you remember to take your medicine, try to get into the habit of taking it at the same time each day.

Dosing—The dose of prazosin will be different for different patients. *Follow your doctor's orders or the directions on the label.* The following information includes only the average doses of prazosin. *If your dose is different, do not change it* unless your doctor tells you to do so.

The number of capsules or tablets that you take depends on the strength of the medicine.

- For *oral* dosage form (capsules or tablets):
  —For high blood pressure:
    - Adults—At first, 0.5 or 1 milligram (mg) two or three times a day. Then, your doctor will slowly increase your dose to 6 to 15 mg a day. This is divided into two or three doses.
    - Children—Dose is based on body weight and must be determined by your doctor. The usual dose is 50 to 400 micrograms (mcg) (0.05 to 0.4 mg) per kilogram of body weight (22.73 to 181.2 mcg per pound [0.023 to 0.18 mg per pound]) a day. This is divided into two or three doses.

Missed dose—If you miss a dose of this medicine, take it as soon as possible. However, if it is almost time for your next dose, skip the missed dose and go back to your regular dosing schedule. Do not double doses.

Storage—To store this medicine:
- Keep out of the reach of children.
- Store away from heat and direct light.
- Do not store in the bathroom, near the kitchen sink, or in other damp places. Heat or moisture may cause the medicine to break down.
- Do not keep outdated medicine or medicine no longer needed. Be sure that any discarded medicine is out of the reach of children.

Precautions While Using This Medicine

It is important that your doctor check your progress at regular visits to make sure that this medicine is working properly.

For patients *taking this medicine for high blood pressure:*

- *Do not take other medicines unless they have been discussed with your doctor.* This especially includes over-the-counter (nonprescription) medicines for appetite control, asthma, colds, cough, hay fever, or sinus problems, since they may tend to make prazosin less effective.

Dizziness, lightheadedness, or sudden fainting may occur after you take this medicine, especially when you get up from a lying or sitting position. These effects are more likely to occur when you take the first dose of this medicine. Taking the first dose at bedtime may prevent problems. However, *be especially careful if you need to get up during the night.* These effects may also occur with any doses you take after the first dose. Getting up slowly may help lessen this problem. *If you feel dizzy, lie down so that you do not faint.* Then sit for a few moments before standing to prevent the dizziness from returning.

The dizziness, lightheadedness, or fainting is more likely to occur if you drink alcohol, stand for a long time, exercise, or if the weather is hot. *While you are taking this medicine, be careful to limit the amount of alcohol you drink. Also, use extra care during exercise or hot weather or if you must stand for a long time.*

Prazosin may cause some people to become drowsy or less alert than they are normally. *Make sure you know how you react to this medicine before you drive, use machines, or do anything else that could be dangerous if you are dizzy, drowsy, or are not alert.* After you have taken several doses of this medicine, these effects should lessen.

Side Effects of This Medicine

Along with its needed effects, a medicine may cause some unwanted effects. Although not all of these side effects

may occur, if they do occur they may need medical attention.

Check with your doctor as soon as possible if any of the following side effects occur:

More common

Dizziness or lightheadedness, especially when getting up from a lying or sitting position; fainting (sudden)

Less common

Loss of bladder control; pounding heartbeat; swelling of feet or lower legs

Rare

Chest pain; painful inappropriate erection of penis (continuing); shortness of breath

Other side effects may occur that usually do not need medical attention. These side effects may go away during treatment as your body adjusts to the medicine. However, check with your doctor if any of the following side effects continue or are bothersome:

More common

Drowsiness; headache; lack of energy

Less common

Dryness of mouth; nervousness; unusual tiredness or weakness

Rare

Frequent urge to urinate; nausea

Other side effects not listed above may also occur in some patients. If you notice any other effects, check with your doctor.

Additional Information

Once a medicine has been approved for marketing for a certain use, experience may show that it is also useful for other medical problems. Although these uses are not included in product labeling, prazosin is used in certain patients with the following medical conditions:

- Congestive heart failure
- Ergot alkaloid poisoning
- Pheochromocytoma
- Raynaud's disease
- Benign enlargement of the prostate

For patients taking this medicine for *benign enlargement of the prostate*:

- Prazosin will not shrink the size of your prostate, but it does help to relieve the symptoms.

Other than the above information, there is no additional information relating to proper use, precautions, or side effects for these uses.

PRAZOSIN AND POLYTHIAZIDE Systemic†

A commonly used brand name in the U.S. is Minizide.

†Not commercially available in Canada.

Description

Prazosin (PRA-zoe-sin) and polythiazide (pol-i-THYE-a-zide) combination is used in the treatment of high blood pressure (hypertension).

High blood pressure adds to the workload of the heart and arteries. If it continues for a long time, the heart and arteries may not function properly. This can damage the blood vessels of the brain, heart, and kidneys, resulting in a stroke, heart failure, or kidney failure. High blood pressure may also increase the risk of heart attacks. These problems may be less likely to occur if blood pressure is controlled.

Prazosin works by relaxing blood vessels so that blood

passes through them more easily. The polythiazide in this combination is a thiazide diuretic (water pill) that helps to reduce the amount of water in the body by increasing the flow of urine. Both of these actions help to lower blood pressure.

This medicine is available only with your doctor's prescription, in the following dosage form:

Oral

• Capsules (U.S.)

Before Using This Medicine

In deciding to use a medicine, the risks of taking the medicine must be weighed against the good it will do. This is a decision you and your doctor will make. For prazosin and polythiazide, the following should be considered:

Allergies—Tell your doctor if you have ever had any unusual or allergic reaction to prazosin, sulfonamides (sulfa drugs), bumetanide, furosemide, acetazolamide, dichlorphenamide, methazolamide, or any of the thiazide diuretics. Also tell your health care professional if you are allergic to any other substance, such as foods, preservatives, or dyes.

Pregnancy—When polythiazide (contained in this combination medicine) is used during pregnancy, it may cause side effects including jaundice, blood problems, and low potassium in the newborn infant. The combination of prazosin and polythiazide has not been shown to cause birth defects.

Breast-feeding—Polythiazide passes into breast milk. Prazosin passes into breast milk in small amounts. However, prazosin and polythiazide combination has not been reported to cause problems in nursing babies.

Children—Although there is no specific information about the use of this medicine in children, it is not expected to cause different side effects or problems in children than it does in adults. However, extra caution may be necessary in infants with jaundice, because these medicines can make the condition worse.

Older adults—Dizziness, lightheadedness, or fainting or symptoms of too much potassium loss may be more likely to occur in the elderly, who are more sensitive to the effects of prazosin and polythiazide. In addition, this medicine may reduce tolerance to cold temperatures in elderly patients.

Other medicines—Although certain medicines should not be used together at all, in other cases two different medicines may be used together even if an interaction might occur. In these cases, your doctor may want to change the dose, or other precautions may be necessary. When you are taking prazosin and polythiazide, it is especially important that your health care professional know if you are taking any of the following:

- Cholestyramine or
- Colestipol—Use with thiazide diuretics may prevent the diuretic from working properly; take the diuretic at least 1 hour before or 4 hours after cholestyramine or colestipol
- Digitalis glycosides (heart medicine)—Polythiazide may cause low potassium in the blood, which can lead to symptoms of digitalis toxicity
- Lithium (e.g., Lithane)—Risk of lithium overdose, even at usual doses, may be increased

Other medical problems—The presence of other medical problems may affect the use of prazosin and polythiazide. Make sure you tell your doctor if you have any other medical problems, especially:

- Angina (chest pain) or
- Heart disease (severe)—Prazosin may make these conditions worse

- Diabetes mellitus (sugar diabetes)—Polythiazide may increase the amount of sugar in the blood
- Gout (history of) or
- Lupus erythematosus (history of) or
- Pancreatitis (inflammation of the pancreas)—Thiazide diuretics may make these conditions worse
- Kidney disease—Effects of this combination medicine may be increased because of increased sensitivity to the effects of prazosin and slower removal of polythiazide from the body. If kidney disease is severe, polythiazide may not work
- Liver disease—If polythiazide causes loss of too much water from the body, liver disease can become much worse

---

Proper Use of This Medicine

In addition to the use of the medicine your doctor has prescribed, treatment for your high blood pressure may include weight control and care in the types of foods you eat, especially foods high in sodium. Your doctor will tell you which of these are most important for you. You should check with your doctor before changing your diet.

Many patients who have high blood pressure will not notice any signs of the problem. In fact, many may feel normal. It is very important that you *take your medicine exactly as directed* and that you keep your appointments with your doctor even if you feel well.

Remember that this medicine will not cure your high blood pressure but it does help control it. Therefore, you must continue to take it as directed if you expect to lower your blood pressure and keep it down. *You may have to take high blood pressure medicine for the rest of your life.* If high blood pressure is not treated, it can cause serious problems such as heart failure, blood vessel disease, stroke, or kidney disease.

This medicine may cause you to have an unusual feeling of tiredness when you begin to take it. You may also notice an increase in the amount of urine or in your frequency of urination. After taking the medicine for a while, these effects should lessen.

It is best to plan your dose or doses according to a schedule that will least affect your personal activities and sleep. Ask your health care professional to help you plan the best time to take this medicine.

To help you remember to take your medicine, try to get into the habit of taking it at the same time each day.

Dosing—The dose of prazosin and polythiazide combination will be different for different patients. *Follow your doctor's orders or the directions on the label.* The following information includes only the average doses of prazosin and polythiazide combination. *If your dose is different, do not change it* unless your doctor tells you to do so.

The number of capsules that you take depends on the strength of the medicine.

- For *oral* dosage form (capsules):
  —For high blood pressure:
    - Adults—1 capsule two or three times a day.
    - Children—Dose must be determined by your doctor.

Missed dose—If you miss a dose of this medicine, take it as soon as possible. However, if it is almost time for your next dose, skip the missed dose and go back to your regular dosing schedule. Do not double doses.

Storage—To store this medicine:
- Keep out of the reach of children.
- Store away from heat and direct light.
- Do not store in the bathroom, near the kitchen sink, or in other damp places. Heat or moisture may cause the medicine to break down.
- Do not keep outdated medicine or medicine no longer

needed. Be sure that any discarded medicine is out of the reach of children.

Precautions While Using This Medicine

It is important that your doctor check your progress at regular visits to make sure this medicine is working properly.

Do not take other medicines unless they have been discussed with your doctor. This especially includes over-the-counter (nonprescription) medicine for appetite control, asthma, colds, cough, hay fever, or sinus problems, since they may tend to increase your blood pressure.

This medicine may cause a loss of potassium from your body.

- To help prevent this, your doctor may want you to:
    —eat or drink foods that have a high potassium content (for example, orange or other citrus fruit juices), or

    —take a potassium supplement, or

    —take another medicine to help prevent the loss of the potassium in the first place.

- It is very important to follow these directions. Also, it is important not to change your diet on your own. This is more important if you are already on a special diet (as for diabetes), or if you are taking a potassium supplement or a medicine to reduce potassium loss. Extra potassium may not be necessary, and in some cases, too much potassium could be harmful.

Check with your doctor if you become sick and have severe or continuing vomiting or diarrhea. These problems may cause you to lose additional water and potassium.

Dizziness, lightheadedness, or sudden fainting may occur after you take this medicine, especially when you get up from a lying or sitting position. These effects are more likely to occur when you take the first dose of this medicine. Taking the first dose at bedtime may prevent problems. However, *be especially careful if you need to get up during the night.* These effects may also occur with any doses you take after the first dose. Getting up slowly may help lessen this problem. *If you feel dizzy, lie down so that you do not faint.* Then sit for a few moments before standing to prevent the dizziness from returning.

Make sure you know how you react to this medicine before you drive, use machines, or do anything else that could be dangerous if you are dizzy or are not alert. After you have taken several doses of this medicine, these effects should lessen.

The dizziness, lightheadedness, or fainting is also more likely to occur if you drink alcohol, stand for a long time, exercise, or if the weather is hot. *While you are taking this medicine, be careful to limit the amount of alcohol you drink. Also, use extra care during exercise or hot weather or if you must stand for a long time.*

For *diabetic patients*:

• Polythiazide (contained in this combination medicine) may raise blood sugar levels. While you are using this medicine, be especially careful in testing for sugar in your blood or urine. If you have any questions about this, check with your doctor.

Some people who take this medicine may become more sensitive to sunlight than they are normally. Exposure to sunlight, even for brief periods of time, may cause a skin rash, itching, redness or other discoloration of the skin, or a severe sunburn. When you begin taking this medicine:

• Stay out of direct sunlight, especially between the hours of 10:00 a.m. and 3:00 p.m., if possible.

• Wear protective clothing, including a hat and sunglasses.

• Apply a sun block product that has a skin protection

factor (SPF) of at least 15. Some patients may require a product with a higher SPF number, especially if they have a fair complexion. If you have any questions about this, check with your health care professional.

• Do not use a sunlamp or tanning bed or booth.

• Apply a sun block lipstick that has an SPF of at least 15 to protect your lips.

If you have a severe reaction from the sun, check with your doctor.

Side Effects of This Medicine

Along with its needed effects, a medicine may cause some unwanted effects. Although not all of these side effects may occur, if they do occur they may need medical attention.

Check with your doctor as soon as possible if any of the following side effects occur, especially since some of them may mean that your body is losing too much potassium:

Signs and symptoms of too much potassium loss

Dryness of mouth (severe); increased thirst; irregular heartbeat (continuing); mood or mental changes; muscle cramps or pain; nausea or vomiting; unusual tiredness or weakness; weak pulse

Signs and symptoms of too much sodium loss

Confusion; convulsions; decreased mental activity; irritability; muscle cramps; unusual tiredness or weakness

More common

Dizziness or lightheadedness, especially when getting up from a lying or sitting position; sudden fainting

Less common

Inability to control urination; irregular heartbeat; pounding heartbeat; swelling of feet or lower legs; weight gain

Rare

Black, tarry stools; blood in urine or stools; chest pain;

cough or hoarseness; fever or chills; joint pain; lower
back or side pain; painful or difficult urination; painful,
inappropriate erection of penis, continuing; pinpoint red
spots on skin; shortness of breath; skin rash or hives;
stomach pain (severe) with nausea and vomiting; unusual bleeding or bruising; yellow eyes or skin

Other side effects may occur that usually do not need
medical attention. These side effects may go away during
treatment as your body adjusts to the medicine. However,
check with your doctor if any of the following side effects
continue or are bothersome:

Less common

Decreased sexual ability; diarrhea; drowsiness; headache;
increased sensitivity of skin to sunlight; lack of energy;
loss of appetite; nervousness; stomach upset or pain

Rare

Frequent urge to urinate; nausea

Other side effects not listed above may also occur in some
patients. If you notice any other effects, check with your
doctor.

PROBUCOL   Systemic

Some commonly used brand names are:

In the U.S.—
Lorelco

In Canada—
Lorelco

Other—

Bifenabid	Panesclerina
Lesterol	Superlipid
Lurselle	

Description

Probucol (PROE-byoo-kole) is used to lower levels of cholesterol (a fat-like substance) in the blood. This may help

prevent medical problems caused by cholesterol clogging the blood vessels.

Probucol is available only with your doctor's prescription, in the following dosage form:

Oral
- Tablets (U.S. and Canada)

Before Using This Medicine

In deciding to use a medicine, the risks of taking the medicine must be weighed against the good it will do. This is a decision you and your doctor will make. For probucol, the following should be considered:

Allergies—Tell your doctor if you have ever had any unusual or allergic reaction to probucol. Also tell your health care professional if you are allergic to any other substances, such as foods, preservatives, or dyes.

Diet—Before prescribing medicine for your condition, your doctor will probably try to control your condition by prescribing a personal diet for you. Such a diet may be low in fats, sugars, and/or cholesterol. Many people are able to control their condition by carefully following their doctor's orders for proper diet and exercise. Medicine is prescribed only when additional help is needed and is effective only when a schedule of diet and exercise is properly followed.

Also, this medicine is less effective if you are greatly overweight. It may be very important for you to go on a reducing diet. However, check with your doctor before going on any diet.

Make certain your health care professional knows if you are on a low-sodium, low-sugar, or any other special diet.

Pregnancy—Probucol has not been studied in pregnant women. However, it has not been shown to cause birth defects or other problems in rats or rabbits.

Breast-feeding—It is not known whether probucol passes into the breast milk. However, this medicine is not recommended for use during breast-feeding because it may cause unwanted effects in nursing babies.

Children—There is no specific information about the use of probucol in children. However, use is not recommended in children under 2 years of age since cholesterol is needed for normal development.

Older adults—Many medicines have not been studied specifically in older people. Therefore, it may not be known whether they work exactly the same way they do in younger adults or if they cause different side effects or problems in older people. There is no specific information comparing use of probucol in the elderly with use in other age groups.

Other medicines—Although certain medicines should not be used together at all, in other cases two different medicines may be used together even if an interaction might occur. In these cases, your doctor may want to change the dose, or other precautions may be necessary. Tell your health care professional if you are taking any other prescription or nonprescription (over-the-counter [OTC]) medicine.

Other medical problems—The presence of other medical problems may affect the use of probucol. Make sure you tell your doctor if you have any other medical problems, especially:

- Gallbladder disease or gallstones or
- Heart disease—Probucol may make these conditions worse
- Liver disease—Higher blood levels of probucol may result, which may increase the chance of side effects

Proper Use of This Medicine

Many patients who have high cholesterol levels will not notice any signs of the problem. In fact, many may feel normal. *Take this medicine exactly as directed by your doctor, even though you may feel well.* Try not to miss any doses and do not take more medicine than your doctor ordered.

Remember that this medicine will not cure your condition, but it does help control it. Therefore, you must continue to take it as directed if you expect to keep your cholesterol levels down.

Follow carefully the special diet your doctor gave you. This is the most important part of controlling your condition, and is necessary if the medicine is to work properly.

This medicine works better when taken with meals.

Dosing—The dose of probucol will be different for different patients. *Follow your doctor's orders or the directions on the label.* The following information includes only the average doses of probucol. *If your dose is different, do not change it* unless your doctor tells you to do so:

- The number of tablets that you take depends on the strength of the medicine.
- For *oral* dosage form (tablets):
  —Adults: 500 milligrams two times a day taken with the morning and evening meals.
  —Children:
    - Up to 2 years of age—Use is not recommended.
    - 2 years of age and over—Dose must be determined by your doctor.

Missed dose—If you miss a dose of this medicine, take it as soon as possible. However, if it is almost time for your next dose, skip the missed dose and go back to your regular dosing schedule. Do not double doses.

Storage—To store this medicine:

- Keep out of the reach of children.
- Store away from heat and direct light.
- Do not store in the bathroom, near the kitchen sink,

or in other damp places. Heat or moisture may cause
the medicine to break down.

- Do not keep outdated medicine or medicine no longer
  needed. Be sure that any discarded medicine is out
  of the reach of children.

Precautions While Using This Medicine

*It is very important that your doctor check your progress
at regular visits.* This will allow your doctor to see if the
medicine is working properly to lower your cholesterol
levels and to decide if you should continue to take it.

*Do not stop taking this medicine without first checking
with your doctor.* When you stop taking this medicine,
your blood fat levels may increase again. Your doctor may
want you to follow a special diet to help prevent this.

Side Effects of This Medicine

Along with its needed effects, a medicine may cause some
unwanted effects. Although not all of these side effects may
occur, if they do occur they may need medical attention.

Check with your doctor as soon as possible if any of the
following side effects occur:

More common

Dizziness or fainting; fast or irregular heartbeat

Rare

Swellings on face, hands, or feet, or in mouth; unusual
bleeding or bruising; unusual tiredness or weakness

Other side effects may occur that usually do not need
medical attention. These side effects may go away during
treatment as your body adjusts to the medicine. However,
check with your doctor if any of the following side effects
continue or are bothersome:

More common

Bloating; diarrhea; nausea and vomiting; stomach pain

Less common

Headache; numbness or tingling of fingers, toes, or face

Other side effects not listed above may also occur in some patients. If you notice any other effects, check with your doctor.

PROCAINAMIDE   Systemic

Some commonly used brand names are:

In the U.S.—

Procan SR	Pronestyl
Promine	Pronestyl-SR

Generic name product may also be available.

In Canada—

Procan SR	Pronestyl-SR
Pronestyl	

Generic name product may also be available.

Description

Procainamide (proe-KANE-a-mide) is used to correct irregular heartbeats to a normal rhythm and to slow an overactive heart. This allows the heart to work more efficiently. Procainamide produces its beneficial effects by slowing nerve impulses in the heart and reducing sensitivity of heart tissues.

Procainamide is available only with your doctor's prescription, in the following dosage forms:

Oral

- Capsules (U.S. and Canada)
- Tablets (U.S.)
- Extended-release tablets (U.S. and Canada)

Parenteral

- Injection (U.S. and Canada)

Before Using This Medicine

In deciding to use a medicine, the risks of taking the medicine must be weighed against the good it will do. This is a decision you and your doctor will make. For procainamide, the following should be considered:

Allergies—Tell your doctor if you have ever had any unusual or allergic reaction to procainamide, procaine, or any other "caine-type" medicine. Also tell your health care professional if you are allergic to any other substance, such as foods, preservatives, or dyes.

Pregnancy—Procainamide has not been studied in pregnant women. However, it has been used in some pregnant women and has not been shown to cause problems. Before taking this medicine, make sure your doctor knows if you are pregnant or if you may become pregnant.

Breast-feeding—Procainamide passes into breast milk.

Children—Procainamide has been used in a limited number of children. In effective doses, the medicine has not been shown to cause different side effects or problems than it does in adults.

Older adults—Dizziness or lightheadedness is more likely to occur in the elderly, who are usually more sensitive to the effects of this medicine.

Other medicines—Although certain medicines should not be used together at all, in other cases two different medicines may be used together even if an interaction might occur. In these cases, your doctor may want to change the dose, or other precautions may be necessary. When you are taking procainamide, it is especially important that your health care professional know if you are taking any of the following:

- Antiarrhythmics (medicines for heart rhythm problems), other—Effects on the heart may be increased

- Antihypertensives (high blood pressure medicine)—Effects on blood pressure may be increased
- Antimyasthenics (ambenonium [e.g., Mytelase], neostigmine [e.g., Prostigmin], pyridostigmine [e.g., Mestinon])—Effects may be blocked by procainamide
- Pimozide (e.g., Orap)—May increase the risk of heart rhythm problems

Other medical problems—The presence of other medical problems may affect the use of procainamide. Make sure you tell your doctor if you have any other medical problems, especially:

- Asthma—Possible allergic reaction
- Kidney disease or
- Liver disease—Effects may be increased because of slower removal of procainamide from the body
- Lupus erythematosus (history of)—Procainamide may cause the condition to become active
- Myasthenia gravis—Procainamide may increase muscle weakness

---

Proper Use of This Medicine

Take procainamide exactly as directed by your doctor, even though you may feel well. Do not take more medicine than ordered.

Procainamide should be taken with a glass of water on an empty stomach 1 hour before or 2 hours after meals so that it will be absorbed more quickly. However, to lessen stomach upset, your doctor may want you to take the medicine with food or milk.

For patients taking the *extended-release tablets:*

- Swallow the tablet whole without breaking, crushing, or chewing it.

This medicine works best when there is a constant amount in the blood. *To help keep the amount constant, do not miss any doses. Also, it is best to take the doses at evenly spaced times day and night.* For example, if you are to take 6 doses a day, the doses should be spaced about 4 hours apart. If this interferes with your sleep or other daily activities, or if you need help in planning the best times to take your medicine, check with your health care professional.

Dosing—The dose of procainamide will be different for different patients. *Follow your doctor's orders or the directions on the label.* The following information includes only the average doses of procainamide. *If your dose is different, do not change it* unless your doctor tells you to do so.

The number of capsules or tablets that you take depends on the strength of the medicine.

- For *regular (short-acting) oral* dosage forms (capsules or tablets):
    —For atrial arrhythmias (fast or irregular heartbeat):
      - Adults—500 milligrams (mg) to 1000 mg (1 gram) every four to six hours.
      - Children—12.5 mg per kilogram (5.68 mg per pound) of body weight four times a day.
    —For ventricular arrhythmias (fast or irregular heartbeat):
      - Adults—50 mg per kilogram (22.73 mg per pound) of body weight per day divided into eight doses taken every three hours.
      - Children—12.5 mg per kilogram (5.68 mg per pound) of body weight four times a day.
- For *long-acting oral* dosage form (extended-release tablets):
    —For atrial arrhythmias (fast or irregular heartbeat):
      - Adults—1000 mg (1 gram) every six hours.
      - Children—Use is not recommended.
    —For ventricular arrhythmias (fast or irregular heartbeat):

- • Adults—50 mg per kilogram (22.73 mg per pound) of body weight per day divided into four doses taken every six hours.
- • For *injection* dosage form:
  - —For arrhythmias (fast or irregular heartbeat):
    - • Adults—
      - —*First few doses:* May be given intramuscularly (into the muscle) at 50 mg per kilogram (22.73 mg per pound) of body weight per day in divided doses every three hours; or may be given intravenously (into the vein) by slowly injecting 100 mg (mixed in fluid) every five minutes or infusing 500 to 600 mg (mixed in fluid) over a twenty-five- to thirty-minute period.
      - —*Doses after the first few doses:* 2 to 6 mg (mixed in fluid) per minute infused into the vein.
    - • Children—Dose must be determined by your doctor.

Missed dose—If you miss a dose of this medicine and remember within 2 hours (4 hours if you are taking the long-acting tablets), take it as soon as possible. However, if you do not remember until later, skip the missed dose and go back to your regular dosing schedule. Do not double doses.

Storage—To store this medicine:

- • Keep out of the reach of children.
- • Store away from heat and direct light.
- • Do not store in the bathroom, refrigerator, near the kitchen sink, or in other damp places. Moisture usually present in these areas may cause the medicine to break down. Keep the container tightly closed and store in a dry place.
- • Do not keep outdated medicine or medicine no longer

needed. Be sure that any discarded medicine is out of the reach of children.

Precautions While Using This Medicine

It is important that your doctor check your progress at regular visits to make sure the medicine is working properly. This will allow necessary changes in the amount of medicine you are taking, which also may help reduce side effects.

Do not stop taking this medicine without first checking with your doctor. Stopping it suddenly may cause a serious change in the activity of your heart. Your doctor may want you to reduce gradually the amount you are taking before stopping completely.

Before having any kind of surgery (including dental surgery) or emergency treatment, tell the medical doctor or dentist in charge that you are taking this medicine.

Your doctor may want you to carry a medical identification card or bracelet stating that you are taking this medicine.

Dizziness or lightheadedness may occur, especially in elderly patients and when large doses are used. *Elderly patients should use extra care to avoid falling. Make sure you know how you react to this medicine before you drive, use machines, or do anything else that could be dangerous if you are dizzy or are not alert.*

Tell the doctor in charge that you are taking this medicine before you have any medical tests. The results of some tests may be affected by this medicine.

Side Effects of This Medicine

Along with its needed effects, a medicine may cause some unwanted effects. Although not all of these side effects

may occur, if they do occur they may need medical attention.

Check with your doctor as soon as possible if any of the following side effects occur:

Less common

> Fever and chills; joint pain or swelling; pains with breathing; skin rash or itching

Rare

> Confusion; fever or sore mouth, gums, or throat; hallucinations (seeing, hearing, or feeling things that are not there); mental depression; unusual bleeding or bruising; unusual tiredness or weakness

Signs and symptoms of overdose

> Confusion; decrease in urination; dizziness (severe) or fainting; drowsiness; fast or irregular heartbeat; nausea and vomiting

Other side effects may occur that usually do not need medical attention. These side effects may go away during treatment as your body adjusts to the medicine. However, check with your doctor if any of the following side effects continue or are bothersome:

More common

> Diarrhea; loss of appetite

Less common

> Dizziness or lightheadedness

The medicine in the extended-release tablets is contained in a special wax form (matrix). The medicine is slowly released, after which the wax matrix passes out of the body. Sometimes it may be seen in the stool. This is normal and is no cause for concern.

Other side effects not listed above may also occur in some patients. If you notice any other effects, check with your doctor.

PROPAFENONE Systemic

A commonly used brand name in the U.S. and Canada is Rythmol.

Description

Propafenone (proe-pa-FEEN-none) belongs to the group of medicines known as antiarrhythmics. It is used to correct irregular heartbeats to a normal rhythm.

Propafenone produces its helpful effects by slowing nerve impulses in the heart and making the heart tissue less sensitive.

There is a chance that propafenone may cause new or make worse existing heart rhythm problems when it is used. Since similar medicines have been shown to cause severe problems in some patients, propafenone is only used to treat serious heart rhythm problems. Discuss this possible effect with your doctor.

This medicine is available only with your doctor's prescription, in the following dosage form:

Oral
- Tablets (U.S. and Canada)

Before Using This Medicine

In deciding to use a medicine, the risks of taking the medicine must be weighed against the good it will do. This is a decision you and your doctor will make. For propafenone, the following should be considered:

Allergies—Tell your doctor if you have ever had any unusual or allergic reaction to propafenone. Also tell your health care professional if you are allergic to any other substances, such as foods, preservatives, or dyes.

Pregnancy—Propafenone has not been studied in pregnant women. Although this medicine has not been shown to cause birth defects in animal studies, it has been shown to reduce fertility in monkeys, dogs, and rabbits. In addition, in rats it caused decreased growth in the infant and deaths of mothers and infants. Before taking propafenone, make sure your doctor knows if you are pregnant or if you may become pregnant.

Breast-feeding—Propafenone passes into breast milk. However, this medicine has not been reported to cause problems in nursing babies.

Children—Propafenone can cause serious side effects in any patient. Therefore, it is especially important that you discuss with the child's doctor the good that this medicine may do as well as the risks of using it.

Older adults—Many medicines have not been studied specifically in older people. Therefore, it may not be known whether they work exactly the same way they do in younger adults or if they cause different side effects or problems in older people. There is no specific information comparing use of propafenone in the elderly with use in other age groups.

Other medicines—Although certain medicines should not be used together at all, in other cases two different medicines may be used together even if an interaction might occur. In these cases, your doctor may want to change the dose, or other precautions may be necessary. When you are taking propafenone it is especially important that your health care professional know if you are taking either of the following:

- Digoxin (e.g., Lanoxin) or
- Warfarin (e.g., Coumadin)—Effects of these medicines may be increased when used with propafenone

Other medical problems—The presence of other medical problems may affect the use of propafenone. Make sure

you tell your doctor if you have any other medical problems, especially:

- Asthma or
- Bronchitis or
- Emphysema—Propafenone can increase trouble in breathing
- Bradycardia (unusually slow heartbeat)—There is a risk of further decreased heart function
- Congestive heart failure—Propafenone may make this condition worse
- Kidney disease or
- Liver disease—Effects of propafenone may be increased because of slower removal from the body
- Recent heart attack—Risk of irregular heartbeat may be increased
- If you have a pacemaker—Propafenone may interfere with the pacemaker and require more careful follow-up by the doctor

---

Proper Use of This Medicine

Take propafenone exactly as directed by your doctor, even though you may feel well. Do not take more or less of it than your doctor ordered.

This medicine works best when there is a constant amount in the blood. *To help keep the amount constant, do not miss any doses. Also, it is best to take each dose at evenly spaced times day and night.* For example, if you are to take 3 doses a day, doses should be spaced about 8 hours apart. If you need help in planning the best times to take your medicine, check with your health care professional.

Dosing—The dose of propafenone will be different for different patients. *Follow your doctor's orders or the directions on the label.* The following information includes only the average doses of propafenone. *If your dose is different, do not change it* unless your doctor tells you to do so:

- The number of tablets that you take depends on the strength of the medicine.
- For *oral* dosage forms (tablets):

  —Adults: 150 milligrams every eight hours; may be increased to 225 milligrams every eight hours or 300 mg every twelve hours; up to 300 mg every eight hours.

Missed dose—If you miss a dose of propafenone and remember within 4 hours, take it as soon as possible. However, if you do not remember until later, skip the missed dose and go back to your regular dosing schedule. Do not double doses.

Storage—To store this medicine:

- Keep out of the reach of children.
- Store away from heat and direct light.
- Do not store in the bathroom, near the kitchen sink, or in other damp places. Heat or moisture may cause the medicine to break down.
- Do not keep outdated medicine or medicine no longer needed. Be sure that any discarded medicine is out of the reach of children.

Precautions While Using This Medicine

It is important that your doctor check your progress at regular visits to make sure the medicine is working properly. This will allow changes to be made in the amount of medicine you are taking, if necessary.

Your doctor may want you to carry a medical identification card or bracelet stating that you are using this medicine.

Before having any kind of surgery (including dental surgery) or emergency treatment, tell the medical doctor or dentist in charge that you are taking this medicine.

Propafenone may cause some people to become dizzy or lightheaded. Make sure you know how you react to this medicine before you drive, use machines, or do anything else that could be dangerous if you are dizzy.

Side Effects of This Medicine

Along with its needed effects, a medicine may cause some unwanted effects. Although not all of these side effects may occur, if they do occur they may need medical attention.

Check with your doctor as soon as possible if any of the following side effects occur:

More common

Fast or irregular heartbeat

Less common

Chest pain; shortness of breath; swelling of feet or lower legs

Rare

Fever or chills; joint pain; low blood pressure; slow heartbeat; trembling or shaking

Other side effects may occur that usually do not need medical attention. These side effects may go away during treatment as your body adjusts to the medicine. However, check with your doctor if any of the following side effects continue or are bothersome:

More common

Change in taste or bitter or metallic taste; dizziness

Less common

Blurred vision; constipation or diarrhea; dryness of mouth; headache; nausea and/or vomiting; skin rash; unusual tiredness or weakness

Other side effects not listed above may also occur in some patients. If you notice any other effects, check with your doctor.

QUINIDINE   Systemic

Some commonly used brand names are:

In the U.S.—

Cardioquin   Quinalan
Cin-Quin   Quinidex Extentabs
Duraquin   Quinora
Quinaglute Dura-tabs

Generic name product may also be available.

In Canada—

Apo-Quinidine   Quinaglute Dura-tabs
Cardioquin   Quinate
Novoquinidin   Quinidex Extentabs

Generic name product may also be available.

Description

Quinidine (KWIN-i-deen) is used to correct certain irregular heartbeats to a normal rhythm and to slow an overactive heart. The injection dosage form is also used to treat malaria.

Quinidine acts directly on the heart tissues to make them less responsive. It also slows impulses along special nerve networks to the heart. This allows the heart to work more efficiently.

Do not confuse this medicine with *quinine*, which, although related, has different medical uses.

Quinidine is available only with your doctor's prescription, in the following dosage forms:

Oral

- Capsules (U.S.)
- Tablets (U.S. and Canada)
- Extended-release tablets (U.S. and Canada)

Parenteral

- Injection (U.S. and Canada)

Before Using This Medicine

In deciding to use a medicine, the risks of taking the medicine must be weighed against the good it will do. This is a decision you and your doctor will make. For quinidine, the following should be considered:

Allergies—Tell your doctor if you have ever had any unusual or allergic reaction to quinidine or quinine. Also tell your health care professional if you are allergic to any other substance, such as foods, preservatives, or dyes.

Pregnancy—Studies on effects in pregnancy have not been done in either humans or animals. However, a closely related medicine, quinine, has been shown to cause birth defects of the nervous system, fingers, and toes, and decreased hearing in the infant. Quinine also may cause contractions of the uterus.

Breast-feeding—Quinidine passes into breast milk. However, it has not been reported to cause problems in nursing babies.

Children—Studies on this medicine have been done only in adult patients, and there is no specific information comparing use of quinidine in children with use in other age groups. Use of the extended-release tablets in children is not recommended.

Older adults—Many medicines have not been studied specifically in older people. Therefore, it may not be known whether they work exactly the same way they do in younger adults. Although there is no specific information comparing use of quinidine in the elderly with use in other age groups, this medicine is not expected to cause different side effects or problems in older people than it does in younger adults.

Other medicines—Although certain medicines should not be used together at all, in other cases two different medicines may be used together even if an interaction might occur. In these cases, your doctor may want to change the dose, or other precautions may be necessary. When you are taking quinidine, it is especially important that your health care professional knows if you are taking any of the following:

- Anticoagulants (blood thinners)—Risk of bleeding may be increased
- Other heart medicine (especially digoxin)—Effects on the heart may be increased
- Pimozide (e.g., Orap)—Risk of heart rhythm problems may be increased
- Urinary alkalizers (medicine that makes the urine less acid, such as acetazolamide [e.g., Diamox], calcium- and/or magnesium-containing antacids, dichlorphenamide [e.g., Daranide], methazolamide [e.g., Neptazane], potassium or sodium citrate and/or citric acid, sodium bicarbonate [baking soda])—Effects may be increased because levels of quinidine in the body may be increased

Other medical problems—The presence of other medical problems may affect the use of quinidine. Make sure you tell your doctor if you have any other medical problems, especially:

- Asthma or emphysema—Possible allergic reaction
- Blood disease
- Infection
- Kidney disease or
- Liver disease—Effects may be increased because of slower removal of quinidine from the body
- Myasthenia gravis—Muscle weakness may be increased
- Overactive thyroid
- Psoriasis

Proper Use of This Medicine

Take quinidine with a full glass (8 ounces) of water on an empty stomach 1 hour before or 2 hours after meals so that it will be absorbed more quickly. However, to lessen stomach upset, your doctor may want you to take the medicine with food or milk.

For patients taking the *extended-release tablet* form of this medicine:

- Swallow the tablets whole.
- Do not break, crush, or chew before swallowing.

Take quinidine exactly as directed by your doctor even though you may feel well. Do not take more medicine than ordered and do not miss any doses.

Dosing—The dose of quinidine will be different for different patients. *Follow your doctor's orders or the directions on the label.* The following information includes only the average doses of quinidine. *If your dose is different, do not change it* unless your doctor tells you to do so.

The number of capsules or tablets that you take depends on the strength of the medicine. Also, *the number of doses you take each day, the time allowed between doses, and the length of time you take the medicine depend on the medical problem for which you are taking quinidine.* When you first begin to take quinidine for irregular heartbeat, you may need to take a higher number of doses each day. This depends on what type of irregular heartbeat you have and will be determined by your doctor.

- For *regular (short-acting) oral* dosage forms (capsules and tablets):

    —For irregular heartbeat:

    - Adults—200 to 650 milligrams (mg) two to four times a day.
    - Children—6 to 8.25 mg per kilogram (kg) (2.73 to 3.75 mg per pound) of body weight five times a day.

- For *long-acting oral* dosage forms (tablets):

    —For irregular heartbeat:

    - Adults—300 to 660 mg every six to twelve hours.
    - Children—Use is not recommended.

- For *injection* dosage form:

—For irregular heartbeat:

• Adults—400 to 600 mg injected into the muscle every two hours. Or, 600 to 800 mg in a solution and injected into a vein.

• Children—Dose must be determined by your doctor.

—For malaria:

• Adults—10 mg per kg (4.54 mg per pound) of body weight in a solution and injected slowly into a vein over one to two hours. Then, 0.02 mg per kg (0.009 mg per pound) of body weight per minute is given. Or, 12 to 24 mg per kg (5.45 to 10.91 mg per pound) of body weight in a solution and injected slowly into a vein over a four-hour period every eight hours.

• Children—Dose must be determined by your doctor.

Missed dose—If you miss a dose of this medicine and remember within 2 hours of the missed dose, take it as soon as possible. However, if you do not remember until later, skip the missed dose and go back to your regular dosing schedule. Do not double doses.

Storage—To store this medicine:

• Keep out of the reach of children.

• Store away from heat and direct light.

• Do not store in the bathroom, near the kitchen sink, or in other damp places. Heat or moisture may cause the medicine to break down.

• Do not keep outdated medicine or medicine no longer needed. Be sure that any discarded medicine is out of the reach of children.

Precautions While Using This Medicine

It is very important that your doctor check your progress at regular visits to make sure that the quinidine is working properly and does not cause unwanted effects.

Do not stop taking this medicine without first checking with your doctor, to avoid possible worsening of your condition.

Before having any kind of surgery (including dental surgery) or emergency treatment, tell the medical doctor or dentist in charge that you are taking this medicine.

Your doctor may want you to carry a medical identification card or bracelet stating that you are using this medicine.

Some people who are unusually sensitive to this medicine may have side effects after the first dose or first few doses. Check with your doctor right away if the following side effects occur: breathing difficulty, changes in vision, dizziness, fever, headache, ringing in ears, or skin rash.

Side Effects of This Medicine

Along with its needed effects, a medicine may cause some unwanted effects. Although not all of these side effects may occur, if they do occur they may need medical attention.

Check with your doctor immediately if any of the following side effects occur:

  Less common
    Blurred vision or any change in vision; dizziness, lightheadedness, or fainting; fever; headache (severe); ringing or buzzing in the ears or any loss of hearing; skin rash, hives, or itching; wheezing, shortness of breath, or troubled breathing

  Rare
    Fast heartbeat; unusual bleeding or bruising; unusual tiredness or weakness

Other side effects may occur that usually do not need medical attention. These side effects may go away during treatment as your body adjusts to the medicine. However, check with your doctor if any of the following side effects continue or are bothersome:

More common

Bitter taste; diarrhea; flushing of skin with itching; loss of appetite; nausea or vomiting; stomach pain or cramping

Less common

Confusion

Other side effects not listed above may also occur in some patients. If you notice any other effects, check with your doctor.

RAUWOLFIA ALKALOIDS Systemic

Some commonly used brand names are:

In the U.S.—

Harmonyl[1]	Rauverid[2]
Raudixin[2]	Serpalan[3]
Rauval[2]	Wolfina[2]

In Canada—

Novoreserpine[3]	Serpasil[3]
Reserfia[3]	

Note: For quick reference, the following rauwolfia alkaloids are numbered to match the corresponding brand names.

This information applies to the following medicines:

1. Deserpidine (de-SER-pi-deen)†
2. Rauwolfia Serpentina (rah-WOOL-fee-a ser-pen-TEE-na)†‡
3. Reserpine (re-SER-peen)‡

---

†Not commercially available in Canada.
‡Generic product may also be available in the U.S.

Description

Rauwolfia alkaloids belong to the general class of medicines called antihypertensives. They are used to treat high blood pressure (hypertension).

High blood pressure adds to the workload of the heart and arteries. If it continues for a long time, the heart and arteries may not function properly. This can damage the blood vessels of the brain, heart, and kidneys, resulting in a stroke, heart failure, or kidney failure. High blood pressure may also increase the risk of heart attacks. These problems may be less likely to occur if blood pressure is controlled.

Rauwolfia alkaloids work by controlling nerve impulses along certain nerve pathways. As a result, they act on the heart and blood vessels to lower blood pressure.

Rauwolfia alkaloids may also be used to treat other conditions as determined by your doctor.

These medicines are available only with your doctor's prescription, in the following dosage forms:

Oral

Deserpidine
- Tablets (U.S.)
Rauwolfia Serpentina
- Tablets (U.S.)
Reserpine
- Tablets (U.S. and Canada)

Before Using This Medicine

In deciding to use a medicine, the risks of taking the medicine must be weighed against the good it will do. This is a decision you and your doctor will make. For rauwolfia alkaloids, the following should be considered:

Allergies—Tell your doctor if you have ever had any unusual or allergic reaction to rauwolfia alkaloids. Also tell your health care professional if you are allergic to any other substance, such as foods, preservatives, or dyes.

Pregnancy—Rauwolfia alkaloids have not been studied in pregnant women. However, too much use of rauwolfia alkaloids during pregnancy may cause unwanted effects (difficult breathing, low temperature, loss of appetite) in the baby. In rats, use of rauwolfia alkaloids during pregnancy causes birth defects, and in guinea pigs, it decreases newborn survival rates. Before taking this medicine, make sure your doctor knows if you are pregnant or if you may become pregnant.

Breast-feeding—Rauwolfia alkaloids pass into breast milk and may cause unwanted effects (difficult breathing, low temperature, loss of appetite) in infants of mothers taking large doses of this medicine. Be sure you have discussed this with your doctor before taking this medicine.

Children—Although there is no specific information comparing use of rauwolfia alkaloids in children with use in other age groups, rauwolfia alkaloids are not expected to cause different side effects or problems in children than they do in adults.

Older adults—Many medicines have not been studied specifically in older people. Therefore, it may not be known whether they work exactly the same way they do in younger adults. Although there is no specific information comparing use of rauwolfia alkaloids in the elderly with use in other age groups, dizziness or drowsiness may be more likely to occur in the elderly, who are more sensitive to the effects of rauwolfia alkaloids.

Other medicines—Although certain medicines should not be used together at all, in other cases two different medicines may be used together even if an interaction might occur. In these cases, your doctor may want to change the dose, or other precautions may be necessary. When you are taking rauwolfia alkaloids, it is especially important that your health care professional know if you are taking any of the following:

- Monoamine oxidase (MAO) inhibitors (furazolidone [e.g., Furoxone], isocarboxazid [e.g., Marplan], phenelzine [e.g., Nardil], procarbazine [e.g., Matulane], selegiline [e.g., Eldepryl], tranylcypromine [e.g., Parnate])—Taking a rauwolfia alkaloid while you are taking or within 2 weeks of

taking MAO inhibitors may increase the risk of central
nervous system depression or may cause a severe high
blood pressure reaction

Other medical problems—The presence of other medical
problems may affect the use of rauwolfia alkaloids. Make
sure you tell your doctor if you have any other medical
problems, especially:

- Allergies or other breathing problems such as asthma—Rau-
  wolfia alkaloids can cause breathing problems
- Epilepsy
- Gallstones or
- Stomach ulcer or
- Ulcerative colitis—Rauwolfia alkaloids increase activity of
  the stomach, which may make the condition worse
- Heart disease—Rauwolfia alkaloids can cause heart rhythm
  problems or slow heartbeat
- Kidney disease—Some patients may not do well when
  blood pressure is lowered by rauwolfia alkaloids
- Mental depression (or history of)—Rauwolfia alkaloids
  cause mental depression
- Parkinson's disease—Rauwolfia alkaloids can cause parkin-
  sonism-like effects
- Pheochromocytoma

Proper Use of This Medicine

For patients taking this medicine *for high blood pressure*:

- In addition to the use of the medicine your doctor
  has prescribed, treatment for your high blood pressure
  may include weight control and care in the types of
  foods you eat, especially foods high in sodium. Your
  doctor will tell you which of these are most important
  for you. You should check with your doctor before
  changing your diet.
- Many patients who have high blood pressure will not
  notice any signs of the problem. In fact, many may
  feel normal. It is very important that you *take your*

medicine exactly as directed and that you keep your appointments with your doctor even if you feel well.

- Remember that this medicine will not cure your high blood pressure, but it does help control it. Therefore, you must continue to take it as directed if you expect to lower your blood pressure and keep it down. *You may have to take high blood pressure medicine for the rest of your life.* If high blood pressure is not treated, it can cause serious problems such as heart failure, blood vessel disease, stroke, or kidney disease.

To help you remember to take your medicine, try to get into the habit of taking it at the same time each day.

This medicine is sometimes given together with certain other medicines. If you are using a combination of drugs, make sure that you take each medicine at the proper time and do not mix them. Ask your health care professional to help you plan a way to remember to take your medicines at the right times.

If this medicine upsets your stomach, it may be taken with meals or milk. If stomach upset (nausea, vomiting, stomach cramps or pain) continues or gets worse, check with your doctor.

Dosing—The dose of these medicines will be different for different patients. *Follow your doctor's orders or the directions on the label.* The following information includes only the average doses of these medicines. *If your dose is different, do not change it* unless your doctor tells you to do so.

The number of tablets that you take depends on the strength of the medicine.

For deserpidine

- For *oral* dosage form (tablets):
  —For high blood pressure:
  - Adults—250 to 500 micrograms (mcg) a day.

This may be taken as a single dose or divided into two doses.

• Children—Dose must be determined by your doctor.

For rauwolfia serpentina
• For *oral* dosage form (tablets):
—For high blood pressure:

• Adults—50 to 200 milligrams (mg) a day. This may be taken as a single dose or divided into two doses.

• Children—Dose must be determined by your doctor.

For reserpine
• For *oral* dosage form (tablets):
—For high blood pressure:

• Adults—100 to 250 micrograms (mcg) a day.

• Children—Dose is based on body weight and must be determined by your doctor. The usual dose is 5 to 20 mcg per kilogram (kg) (2.27 to 9.1 mcg per pound) of body weight a day. This may be taken as a single dose or divided into two doses.

Missed dose—If you miss a dose of this medicine, do not take the missed dose at all and do not double the next one. Instead, go back to your regular dosing schedule.

Storage—To store this medicine:
• Keep out of the reach of children.
• Store away from heat and direct light.
• Do not store in the bathroom, near the kitchen sink, or in other damp places. Heat or moisture may cause the medicine to break down.
• Do not keep outdated medicine or medicine no longer needed. Be sure that any discarded medicine is out of the reach of children.

Precautions While Using This Medicine

It is important that your doctor check your progress at regular visits to make sure that this medicine is working properly.

For patients taking this medicine *for high blood pressure*:

- *Do not take other medicines unless they have been discussed with your doctor.* This especially includes over-the-counter (nonprescription) medicines for appetite control, asthma, colds, cough, hay fever, or sinus problems, since they may tend to increase your blood pressure.

Before having any kind of surgery (including dental surgery) or emergency treatment, *tell the medical doctor or dentist in charge that you are taking this medicine.*

In some patients, this medicine may cause mental depression. *Tell your doctor right away:*

- if you or anyone else notices unusual changes in your mood.
- if you start having early-morning sleeplessness or unusually vivid dreams or nightmares.

This medicine will add to the effects of alcohol and other CNS depressants (medicines that slow down the nervous system, possibly causing drowsiness). Some examples of CNS depressants are antihistamines or medicine for hay fever, other allergies, or colds; sedatives, tranquilizers, or sleeping medicine; prescription pain medicine or narcotics; barbiturates; medicine for seizures; muscle relaxants; or anesthetics, including some dental anesthetics. *Check with your doctor before taking any of the above while you are using this medicine.*

This medicine may cause some people to become drowsy or less alert than they are normally. This is more likely to happen when you begin to take it or when you increase the amount of medicine you are taking. *Make sure you know how you react to this medicine before you drive, use machines, or do anything else that could be dangerous if you are not alert.*

This medicine may cause dryness of the mouth. For temporary relief, use sugarless candy or gum, melt bits of ice in your mouth, or use a saliva substitute. However, if dry mouth continues for more than 2 weeks, check with your medical doctor or dentist. Continuing dryness of the mouth may increase the chance of dental disease, including tooth decay, gum disease, and fungus infections.

This medicine often causes stuffiness in the nose. However, do not use nasal decongestant medicines without first checking with your health care professional.

Side Effects of This Medicine

Suggestions that rauwolfia alkaloids may increase the risk of breast cancer occurring later have not been proven. However, rats and mice given 100 to 300 times the human dose had an increased number of tumors.

Along with its needed effects, a medicine may cause some unwanted effects. Although not all of these side effects may occur, if they do occur they may need medical attention.

Check with your doctor immediately if any of the following side effects occur:

Less common

Drowsiness or faintness; impotence or decreased sexual interest; lack of energy or weakness; mental depression or inability to concentrate; nervousness or anxiety; vivid dreams or nightmares or early-morning sleeplessness

Check with your doctor as soon as possible if any of the following side effects occur:

More common

Dizziness

Less common

Black, tarry stools; bloody vomit; chest pain; headache; irregular heartbeat; shortness of breath; slow heartbeat; stomach cramps or pain

Rare

Painful or difficult urination; skin rash or itching; stiffness; trembling and shaking of hands and fingers; unusual bleeding or bruising

Signs and symptoms of overdose

Dizziness or drowsiness (severe); flushing of skin; pinpoint pupils of eyes; slow pulse

Other side effects may occur that usually do not need medical attention. These side effects may go away during treatment as your body adjusts to the medicine. However, check with your doctor if any of the following side effects continue or are bothersome:

More common

Diarrhea; dryness of mouth; loss of appetite; nausea and vomiting; stuffy nose

Less common

Swelling of feet and lower legs

After you stop using this medicine, it may still produce some side effects that need attention. During this period of time *check with your doctor immediately* if you notice any of the following side effects:

Drowsiness or faintness; impotence or decreased sexual interest; irregular or slow heartbeat; lack of energy or weakness; mental depression or inability to concentrate; nervousness or anxiety; vivid dreams or nightmares or early-morning sleeplessness

Other side effects not listed above may also occur in some patients. If you notice any other effects, check with your doctor.

Additional Information

Once a medicine has been approved for marketing for a certain use, experience may show that it is also useful for other medical problems. Although this use is not included in product labeling, reserpine is used in certain patients with the following medical condition:

- Raynaud's disease

Other than the above information, there is no additional information relating to proper use, precautions, or side effects for this use.

RAUWOLFIA ALKALOIDS AND THIAZIDE DIURETICS Systemic

Some commonly used brand names are:

In the U.S.—

Demi-Regroton[5]	Mallopres[6]
Diupres[4]	Metatensin[10]
Diurese-R[10]	Naquival[10]
Diurigen with Reserpine[4]	Oreticyl[1]
Diutensen-R[8]	Oreticyl Forte[1]
Enduronyl[2]	Rauzide[3]
Enduronyl Forte[2]	Regroton[5]
Hydropine[7]	Renese-R[9]
Hydropine H.P.[7]	Salazide[7]
Hydropres[6]	Salutensin[7]
Hydrosine[6]	Salutensin-Demi[7]
Hydrotensin[6]	

In Canada—

Dureticyl[2]	Salutensin[7]
Hydropres[6]	

Note: For quick reference, the following rauwolfia alkaloids and thiazide diuretics are numbered to match the corresponding brand names.

This information applies to the following medicines:

1. Deserpidine (de-SER-pi-deen) and Hydrochlorothiazide (hye-droe-klor-oh-THYE-a-zide)†
2. Deserpidine and Methyclothiazide (meth-i-kloe-THYE-a-zide)‡

3. Rauwolfia Serpentina (rah-WOOL-fee-a ser-pen-TEE-na) and Bendroflumethiazide (ben-droe-floo-meth-EYE-a-zide)†
4. Reserpine (re-SER-peen) and Chlorothiazide (klor-oh-THYE-a-zide)†‡
5. Reserpine and Chlorthalidone (klor-THAL-i-done)†
6. Reserpine and Hydrochlorothiazide‡
7. Reserpine and Hydroflumethiazide (hye-droe-floo-meth-EYE-a-zide)‡
8. Reserpine and Methyclothiazide†
9. Reserpine and Polythiazide (pol-i-THYE-a-zide)†
10. Reserpine and Trichlormethiazide (trye-klor-meth-EYE-a-zide)†‡

---

†Not commercially available in Canada.
‡Generic name product may also be available in the U.S.

Description

Rauwolfia alkaloid and thiazide diuretic combinations are used in the treatment of high blood pressure (hypertension).

High blood pressure adds to the workload of the heart and arteries. If it continues for a long time, the heart and arteries may not function properly. This can damage the blood vessels of the brain, heart, and kidneys, resulting in a stroke, heart failure, or kidney failure. High blood pressure may also increase the risk of heart attacks. These problems may be less likely to occur if blood pressure is controlled.

Rauwolfia alkaloids work by controlling nerve impulses along certain nerve pathways. As a result, they act on the heart and blood vessels to lower blood pressure. Thiazide diuretics help to reduce the amount of water in the body by increasing the flow of urine. This also helps to lower blood pressure.

These medicines are available only with your doctor's prescription, in the following dosage forms:

Oral

Deserpidine and Hydrochlorothiazide
• Tablets (U.S.)
Deserpidine and Methyclothiazide
• Tablets (U.S. and Canada)

Rauwolfia Serpentina and Bendroflumethiazide
- Tablets (U.S.)

Reserpine and Chlorothiazide
- Tablets (U.S.)

Reserpine and Chlorthalidone
- Tablets (U.S.)

Reserpine and Hydrochlorothiazide
- Tablets (U.S. and Canada)

Reserpine and Hydroflumethiazide
- Tablets (U.S. and Canada)

Reserpine and Methyclothiazide
- Tablets (U.S.)

Reserpine and Polythiazide
- Tablets (U.S.)

Reserpine and Trichlormethiazide
- Tablets (U.S.)

Before Using This Medicine

In deciding to use a medicine, the risks of taking the medicine must be weighed against the good it will do. This is a decision you and your doctor will make. For rauwolfia alkaloids and thiazide diuretics, the following should be considered:

Allergies—Tell your doctor if you have ever had any unusual or allergic reaction to sulfonamides (sulfa drugs), thiazide diuretics (water pills), or rauwolfia alkaloids. Also tell your health care professional if you are allergic to any other substance, such as foods, preservatives, or dyes.

Pregnancy—Too much use of thiazide diuretics (contained in this combination medicine) during pregnancy may cause unwanted effects including jaundice, blood problems, and low potassium in the baby. Too much use of rauwolfia alkaloids may cause difficult breathing, low temperature, and loss of appetite in the baby. This medicine has not been shown to cause birth defects in humans. In rats, use of rauwolfia alkaloids during pregnancy decreases newborn survival rates. Be sure that you have discussed this with your doctor before taking this medicine.

Breast-feeding—Rauwolfia alkaloids pass into breast milk and may cause unwanted effects (difficult breathing, low temperature, loss of appetite) in infants of mothers taking it in large doses. Thiazide diuretics also pass into breast milk. Be sure you have discussed this with your doctor before taking this medicine.

Children—Although there is no specific information comparing use of these medicines in children with use in other age groups, these medicines are not expected to cause different side effects or problems in children than they do in adults.

Older adults—Many medicines have not been studied specifically in older people. Therefore, it may not be known whether they work exactly the same way they do in younger adults. Although there is no specific information comparing use of rauwolfia alkaloid and thiazide diuretic combinations in the elderly with use in other age groups, this medicine is not expected to cause different side effects or problems in older people than it does in younger adults. However, drowsiness, dizziness, or faintness or symptoms of too much potassium loss may be more likely to occur in the elderly, who are more sensitive to the effects of rauwolfia alkaloids and thiazide diuretics.

Other medicines—Although certain medicines should not be used together at all, in other cases two different medicines may be used together even if an interaction might occur. In these cases, your doctor may want to change the dose, or other precautions may be necessary. When you are taking rauwolfia alkaloids and thiazide diuretics, it is especially important that your health care professional know if you are taking any of the following:

- Cholestyramine or
- Colestipol—Use with thiazide diuretics may prevent the diuretic from working properly; take the diuretic at least 1 hour before or 4 hours after cholestyramine or colestipol

- Digitalis glycosides (heart medicine)—Thiazide diuretics may cause low potassium in the blood, which can lead to symptoms of digitalis toxicity
- Lithium (e.g., Lithane)—Risk of lithium overdose, even at usual doses, may be increased
- Monoamine oxidase (MAO) inhibitors (furazolidone [e.g., Furoxone], isocarboxazid [e.g., Marplan], phenelzine [e.g., Nardil], procarbazine [e.g., Matulane], selegiline [e.g., Eldepryl], tranylcypromine [e.g., Parnate])—Taking a rauwolfia alkaloid while you are taking or within 2 weeks of taking MAO inhibitors may increase the risk of central nervous system depression or may cause a severe high blood pressure reaction

Other medical problems—The presence of other medical problems may affect the use of rauwolfia alkaloids and thiazide diuretics. Make sure you tell your doctor if you have any other medical problems, especially:

- Allergies or other breathing problems such as asthma—Rauwolfia alkaloids can cause breathing problems
- Diabetes mellitus (sugar diabetes)—Thiazide diuretics may change the amount of diabetes medicine needed
- Epilepsy
- Gallstones or
- Stomach ulcer or
- Ulcerative colitis—Rauwolfia alkaloids increase activity of the stomach, which may make the condition worse
- Gout (history of)—Thiazide diuretics may increase the amount of uric acid in the blood, which can lead to gout
- Heart disease—Rauwolfia alkaloids can cause heart rhythm problems or slow heartbeat
- Kidney disease—Some patients may not do well when blood pressure is lowered by this medicine. If kidney disease is severe, thiazide diuretics may not work
- Liver disease—If thiazide diuretics cause loss of too much water from the body, liver disease can become much worse
- Lupus erythematosus (history of)—Thiazide diuretics may worsen the condition
- Mental depression (or history of)—Rauwolfia alkaloids cause mental depression

- Pancreatitis (inflammation of pancreas)
- Parkinson's disease—Rauwolfia alkaloids can cause parkinsonism-like effects
- Pheochromocytoma

Proper Use of This Medicine

In addition to the use of the medicine your doctor has prescribed, treatment for your high blood pressure may include weight control and care in the types of foods you eat, especially foods high in sodium. Your doctor will tell you which of these are most important for you. You should check with your doctor before changing your diet.

Many patients who have high blood pressure will not notice any signs of the problem. In fact, many may feel normal. It is very important that you *take your medicine exactly as directed* and that you keep your appointments with your doctor even if you feel well.

Remember that this medicine will not cure your high blood pressure, but it does help control it. Therefore, you must continue to take it as directed if you expect to lower your blood pressure and keep it down. *You may have to take high blood pressure medicine for the rest of your life.* If high blood pressure is not treated, it can cause serious problems such as heart failure, blood vessel disease, stroke, or kidney disease.

This medicine may cause you to have an unusual feeling of tiredness when you begin to take it. You may also notice an increase in the amount of urine or in your frequency of urination. After you have taken the medicine for a while, these effects should lessen. In general, to keep the increase in urine from affecting your sleep:

- If you are to take a single dose a day, take it in the morning after breakfast.
- If you are to take more than one dose a day, take the

last dose no later than 6 p.m., unless otherwise directed by your doctor.

However, it is best to plan your dose or doses according to a schedule that will least affect your personal activities and sleep. Ask your health care professional to help you plan the best time to take this medicine.

To help you remember to take your medicine, try to get into the habit of taking it at the same time each day.

If this medicine upsets your stomach, it may be taken with meals or milk. If stomach upset (nausea, vomiting, stomach pain or cramps) continues, check with your doctor.

Dosing—The dose of these medicines will be different for different patients. *Follow your doctor's orders or the directions on the label.* The following information includes only the average doses of these medicines. *If your dose is different, do not change it* unless your doctor tells you to do so.

For deserpidine and hydrochlorothiazide combination

- For *oral* dosage form (tablets):
  - —For high blood pressure:
    - Adults—1 tablet two times a day.
    - Children—Dose must be determined by your doctor.

For deserpidine and methyclothiazide combination

- For *oral* dosage form (tablets):
  - —For high blood pressure:
    - Adults—One-half to 1 tablet a day.
    - Children—Dose must be determined by your doctor.

For rauwolfia serpentina and bendroflumethiazide combination

- For *oral* dosage form (tablets):
  - —For high blood pressure:
    - Adults—1 to 4 tablets a day.

• Children—Dose must be determined by your doctor.

For reserpine and chlorothiazide combination
  • For *oral* dosage form (tablets):
    —For high blood pressure:
      • Adults—1 or 2 tablets one or two times a day.
      • Children—Dose must be determined by your doctor.

For reserpine and chlorthalidone combination
  • For *oral* dosage form (tablets):
    —For high blood pressure:
      • Adults—1 or 2 tablets once a day.
      • Children—Dose must be determined by your doctor.

For reserpine and hydrochlorothiazide combination
  • For *oral* dosage form (tablets):
    —For high blood pressure:
      • Adults—1 tablet one to four times a day.
      • Children—Dose must be determined by your doctor.

For reserpine and hydroflumethiazide combination
  • For *oral* dosage form (tablets):
    —For high blood pressure:
      • Adults—1 tablet one or two times a day.
      • Children—Dose must be determined by your doctor.

For reserpine and methyclothiazide combination
  • For *oral* dosage form (tablets):
    —For high blood pressure:
      • Adults—1 to 4 tablets a day.
      • Children—Dose must be determined by your doctor.

For reserpine and polythiazide combination
  • For *oral* dosage form (tablets):

—For high blood pressure:

- Adults—One-half to 2 tablets a day.

- Children—Dose must be determined by your doctor.

For reserpine and trichlormethiazide combination

- For *oral* dosage form (tablets):

   —For high blood pressure:

   - Adults—1 or 2 tablets a day. This may be taken as a single dose or divided into smaller doses.

   - Children—Dose must be determined by your doctor.

Missed dose—If you miss a dose of this medicine, take it as soon as possible. However, if it is almost time for your next dose, skip the missed dose and go back to your regular dosing schedule. Do not double doses.

Storage—To store this medicine:

- Keep out of the reach of children.

- Store away from heat and direct light.

- Do not store in the bathroom, near the kitchen sink, or in other damp places. Heat or moisture may cause the medicine to break down.

- Do not keep outdated medicine or medicine no longer needed. Be sure that any discarded medicine is out of the reach of children.

Precautions While Using This Medicine

It is important that your doctor check your progress at regular visits to make sure that this medicine is working properly.

Do not take other medicines unless they have been discussed with your doctor. This especially includes over-the-counter (nonprescription) medicines for appetite control, asthma, colds, cough, hay fever, or sinus problems, since they may tend to increase your blood pressure.

Before having any kind of surgery (including dental surgery), or emergency treatment, *tell the medical doctor or dentist in charge that you are taking this medicine.*

This medicine may cause a loss of potassium from your body.

- To help prevent this, your doctor may want you to:
  —eat or drink foods that have a high potassium content (for example, orange or other citrus fruit juices), or
  —take a potassium supplement, or
  —take another medicine to help prevent the loss of the potassium in the first place.
- It is very important to follow these directions. Also, it is important not to change your diet on your own. This is more important if you are already on a special diet (as for diabetes), or if you are taking a potassium supplement or a medicine to reduce potassium loss. Extra potassium may not be necessary and, in some cases, too much potassium could be harmful.

Check with your doctor if you become sick and have severe or continuing vomiting or diarrhea. These problems may cause you to lose additional water and potassium.

This medicine may cause some people to become drowsy or less alert than they are normally. This is more likely to happen when you begin to take it or when you increase the amount of medicine you are taking. *Make sure you know how you react to this medicine before you drive, use machines, or do anything else that could be dangerous if you are not alert.*

Dizziness, lightheadedness, or fainting may occur, especially when you get up from a lying or sitting position. This is more likely to occur in the morning. Getting up slowly may help. When you get up from lying down, sit on the edge of the bed with your feet dangling for 1 or 2 minutes. Then stand up slowly. If the problem continues or gets worse, check with your doctor.

The dizziness, lightheadedness, or fainting is also more likely to occur if you drink alcohol, stand for a long time, exercise, or if the weather is hot. *While you are taking this medicine, be careful to limit the amount of alcohol you drink. Also, use extra care during exercise or hot weather or if you must stand for a long time.*

In some patients, this medicine may cause mental depression. *Tell your doctor right away:*

- if you or anyone else notices unusual changes in your moods.
- if you start having early-morning sleeplessness or unusually vivid dreams or nightmares.

This medicine will add to the effects of alcohol and other CNS depressants (medicines that slow down the nervous system, possibly causing drowsiness). Some examples of CNS depressants are antihistamines or medicine for hay fever, other allergies, or colds; sedatives, tranquilizers, or sleeping medicine; prescription pain medicine or narcotics; barbiturates; medicine for seizures; muscle relaxants; or anesthetics, including dental anesthetics. *Check with your doctor before taking any of the above while you are taking this medicine.*

For *diabetic patients*:

- This medicine may raise blood sugar levels. While you are using this medicine, be especially careful in testing for sugar in your urine. If you have any questions about this, check with your doctor.

Some people who take this medicine may become more sensitive to sunlight than they are normally. Exposure to sunlight, even for brief periods of time, may cause severe sunburn; skin rash, redness, itching, or discoloration; or vision changes. When you begin taking this medicine:

- Stay out of direct sunlight, especially between the hours of 10:00 a.m. and 3:00 p.m., if possible.
- Wear protective clothing, including a hat and sunglasses.
- Apply a sun block product that has a skin protection factor (SPF) of at least 15. Some patients may require a product with a higher SPF number, especially if they have a fair complexion. If you have any questions about this, check with your health care professional.
- Do not use a sunlamp or tanning bed or booth.

If you have a severe reaction from the sun, check with your doctor.

This medicine often causes stuffiness in the nose. However, do not use nasal decongestant medicines without first checking with your health care professional.

This medicine may cause dryness of the mouth. For temporary relief, use sugarless candy or gum, melt bits of ice in your mouth, or use a saliva substitute. However, if dry mouth continues for more than 2 weeks, check with your medical doctor or dentist. Continuing dryness of the mouth may increase the chance of dental disease, including tooth decay, gum disease, and fungus infections.

Side Effects of This Medicine

Suggestions that rauwolfia alkaloids may increase the risk of breast cancer occurring later have not been proven. However, rats and mice given 100 to 300 times the human dose had an increased risk of tumors.

Along with its needed effects, a medicine may cause some unwanted effects. Although not all of these side effects may occur, if they do occur they may need medical attention.

Check with your doctor immediately if any of the following side effects occur:

Less common

Drowsiness or faintness; impotence or decreased sexual interest; lack of energy or weakness; mental depression or inability to concentrate; nervousness or anxiety; vivid dreams or nightmares or early-morning sleeplessness

Check with your doctor as soon as possible if any of the following side effects occur:

Less common

Black, tarry stools; bloody vomit; chest pain; headache; irregular or slow heartbeat; joint pain; shortness of breath

Rare

Painful or difficult urination; skin rash or itching; sore throat and fever; stiffness; stomach pain (severe) with nausea and vomiting; trembling and shaking of hands and fingers; unusual bleeding or bruising; yellow eyes or skin

Symptoms of too much potassium loss or overdose

Dry mouth; increased thirst; muscle cramps or pain; nausea or vomiting

Other signs and symptoms of overdose

Dizziness or drowsiness, severe; flushing of skin; pinpoint pupils of eyes; slow pulse

Other side effects may occur that usually do not need medical attention. These side effects may go away during treatment as your body adjusts to the medicine. However, check with your doctor if any of the following side effects continue or are bothersome:

More common

Diarrhea; dizziness, especially when getting up from a lying or sitting position; loss of appetite; stuffy nose

After you stop using this medicine, it may still produce some side effects that need attention. During this period of time *check with your doctor immediately* if you notice any of the following side effects:

Drowsiness or faintness; impotence or decreased sexual interest; irregular or slow heartbeat; lack of energy or weakness; mental depression or inability to concentrate; nervousness or anxiety; vivid dreams or nightmares or early-morning sleeplessness

Other side effects not listed above may also occur in some patients. If you notice any other effects, check with your doctor.

RESERPINE, HYDRALAZINE, AND HYDROCHLOROTHIAZIDE Systemic

Some commonly used brand names are:

In the U.S.—

Cam-Ap-Es	Ser-Ap-Es
Cherapas	Serpazide
Ser-A-Gen	Tri-Hydroserpine
Seralazide	Unipres

Generic name product may also be available.

In Canada—
Ser-Ap-Es

Description

Reserpine (re-SER-peen), hydralazine (hye-DRAL-a-zeen), and hydrochlorothiazide (hye-droe-KLOR-oh-THYE-a-zide) combinations are used to treat high blood pressure (hypertension).

High blood pressure adds to the workload of the heart and arteries. If it continues for a long time, the heart and arteries may not function properly. This can damage the blood vessels of the brain, heart, and kidneys, resulting in a stroke, heart failure, or kidney failure. High blood pressure may also increase the risk of heart attacks. These problems may be less likely to occur if blood pressure is controlled.

Reserpine works by controlling nerve impulses along certain nerve pathways. As a result, it acts on the heart and blood vessels to lower blood pressure. Hydralazine works by relaxing blood vessels and increasing the supply of blood to the heart while reducing its workload. Hydrochlorothiazide is a thiazide diuretic (water pill) that helps to reduce the amount of water in the body by increasing the flow of urine. This also helps to lower blood pressure.

This medicine is available only with your doctor's prescription, in the following dosage form:

Oral

- Tablets (U.S. and Canada)

Before Using This Medicine

In deciding to use a medicine, the risks of taking the medicine must be weighed against the good it will do. This is a decision you and your doctor will make. For reserpine, hydralazine, and hydrochlorothiazide, the following should be considered:

Allergies—Tell your doctor if you have ever had any unusual or allergic reaction to hydralazine, sulfonamides (sulfa drugs), thiazide diuretics (water pills), or rauwolfia alkaloids. Also tell your health care professional if you are allergic to any other substances, such as foods, preservatives, or dyes.

Pregnancy—Too much use of reserpine and hydrochlorothiazide during pregnancy may cause unwanted effects (jaundice, blood problems, low potassium, difficult breathing, low temperatures, and loss of appetite) in the baby. In rats, rauwolfia alkaloids (like reserpine) decrease newborn survival rates.

Studies with hydralazine have not been done in humans. However, studies in mice have shown that hydralazine causes birth defects (cleft palate, defects in head and face bones); these birth defects may also occur in rabbits, but do not occur in rats. Be sure that you have discussed this with your doctor before taking this medicine.

Breast-feeding—Reserpine passes into breast milk and may cause unwanted effects (difficult breathing, low temperature, loss of appetite) in infants of mothers taking large doses of it. Hydrochlorothiazide also passes into breast milk. Be sure you have discussed this with your doctor before taking this medicine.

Children—Although there is no specific information comparing use of this medicine in children with use in other age groups, this medicine is not expected to cause different side effects or problems in children than it does in adults.

Older adults—Many medicines have not been studied specifically in older people. Therefore, it may not be known whether they work exactly the same way they do in younger adults. Although there is no specific information comparing use of reserpine, hydralazine, and hydrochlorothiazide combination in the elderly with use in other age groups, this medicine is not expected to cause different side effects or problems in older people than it does in younger adults. However, drowsiness, dizziness, or faintness, or symptoms of too much potassium loss may be more likely to occur in the elderly, who are usually more sensitive to the effects of this medicine. Also, this medicine may reduce tolerance to cold temperatures in elderly patients.

Other medicines—Although certain medicines should not be used together at all, in other cases two different medicines may be used together even if an interaction might occur. In these cases, your doctor may want to change the dose, or other precautions may be necessary. When you are taking this medicine, it is especially important that your health care professional know if you are taking any of the following:

- Cholestyramine or

- Colestipol—Use with thiazide diuretics may prevent the diuretic from working properly; take the diuretic at least 1 hour before or 4 hours after cholestyramine or colestipol
- Diazoxide (e.g., Proglycem)—Effect on blood pressure may be increased
- Digitalis glycosides (heart medicine)—Hydrochlorothiazide may cause low potassium in the blood, which can lead to symptoms of digitalis toxicity
- Lithium (e.g., Lithane)—Risk of lithium overdose, even at usual doses, may be increased
- Monoamine oxidase (MAO) inhibitors (furazolidone [e.g., Furoxone], isocarboxazid [e.g., Marplan], phenelzine [e.g., Nardil], procarbazine [e.g., Matulane], selegiline [e.g., Eldepryl], tranylcypromine [e.g., Parnate])—Taking a rauwolfia alkaloid while you are taking or within 2 weeks of taking MAO inhibitors may increase the risk of central nervous system depression or may cause a severe high blood pressure reaction

Other medical problems—The presence of other medical problems may affect the use of this medicine. Make sure you tell your doctor if you have any other medical problems, especially:

- Allergies or other breathing problems such as asthma—Reserpine can cause breathing problems
- Diabetes mellitus (sugar diabetes)—Hydrochlorothiazide may change the amount of diabetes medicine needed
- Epilepsy
- Gallstones or
- Stomach ulcer or
- Ulcerative colitis—Reserpine increases activity of the stomach, which may make the condition worse
- Gout (history of)—Hydrochlorothiazide may increase the amount of uric acid in the blood, which can lead to gout
- Heart disease—Reserpine can cause heart rhythm problems or slow heartbeat. Lowering blood pressure may worsen some conditions
- Kidney disease—Some patients may not do well when blood pressure is lowered by this medicine. Effects of hydralazine may be increased because of slower removal

from the body. If kidney disease is severe, hydrochlorothiazide may not work

- Liver disease—If hydrochlorothiazide causes loss of too much water from the body, liver disease can become much worse
- Lupus erythematosus (history of)—Hydrochlorothiazide may worsen the condition
- Mental depression (or history of)—Reserpine causes mental depression
- Pancreatitis (inflammation of pancreas)
- Parkinson's disease—Reserpine can cause parkinsonism-like effects
- Pheochromocytoma
- Stroke (recent)—Lowering blood pressure may make problems resulting from this condition worse

---

Proper Use of This Medicine

In addition to the use of the medicine your doctor has prescribed, treatment for your high blood pressure may include weight control and care in the types of foods you eat, especially foods high in sodium. Your doctor will tell you which of these are most important for you. You should check with your doctor before changing your diet.

Many patients who have high blood pressure will not notice any signs of the problem. In fact, many may feel normal. It is very important that you *take your medicine exactly as directed* and that you keep your appointments with your doctor even if you feel well.

Remember that this medicine will not cure your high blood pressure, but it does help control it. Therefore, you must continue to take it as directed if you expect to lower your blood pressure and keep it down. *You may have to take high blood pressure medicine for the rest of your life.* If high blood pressure is not treated, it can cause serious problems such as heart failure, blood vessel disease, stroke, or kidney disease.

This medicine may cause you to have an unusual feeling of tiredness when you begin to take it. You may also notice an increase in the amount of urine or in your frequency of urination. After you have taken the medicine for a while, these effects should lessen. In general, to keep the increase in urine from affecting your sleep:

- If you are to take a single dose a day, take it in the morning after breakfast.
- If you are to take more than one dose a day, take the last dose no later than 6 p.m., unless otherwise directed by your doctor.

However, it is best to plan your dose or doses according to a schedule that will least affect your personal activities and sleep. Ask your health care professional to help you plan the best time to take this medicine.

To help you remember to take your medicine, try to get into the habit of taking it at the same time each day.

If this medicine upsets your stomach, it may be taken with meals or milk. If stomach upset (nausea, vomiting, stomach pain or cramps) continues, check with your doctor.

Dosing—The dose of reserpine, hydralazine, and hydrochlorothiazide combination will be different for different patients. *Follow your doctor's orders or the directions on the label.* The following information includes only the average doses of reserpine, hydralazine, and hydrochlorothiazide combination. *If your dose is different, do not change it* unless your doctor tells you to do so.

- For *oral* dosage form (tablets):
    —For high blood pressure:
        - Adults—1 or 2 tablets three times a day.
        - Children—Use and dose must be determined by your doctor.

Missed dose—If you miss a dose of this medicine, take it as soon as possible. However, if it is almost time for

your next dose, skip the missed dose and go back to your regular dosing schedule. Do not double doses.

Storage—To store this medicine:

- Keep out of the reach of children.
- Store away from heat and direct light.
- Do not store in the bathroom, near the kitchen sink, or in other damp places. Heat or moisture may cause the medicine to break down.
- Do not keep outdated medicine or medicine no longer needed. Be sure that any discarded medicine is out of the reach of children.

Precautions While Using This Medicine

It is important that your doctor check your progress at regular visits to make sure that this medicine is working properly.

Do not take other medicines unless they have been discussed with your doctor. This especially includes over-the-counter (nonprescription) medicines for appetite control, asthma, colds, cough, hay fever, or sinus problems, since they may tend to increase your blood pressure.

Before having any kind of surgery (including dental surgery), or emergency treatment, *make sure the medical doctor or dentist in charge knows that you are taking this medicine.*

This medicine may cause some people to have headaches or to feel dizzy or drowsy. *Make sure you know how you react to this medicine before you drive, use machines, or do anything else that could be dangerous if you are dizzy or are not alert.*

Dizziness, lightheadedness, or fainting may occur, especially when you get up from a lying or sitting position. This is more likely to occur in the morning. *Getting up*

slowly may help. When you get up from lying down, sit on the edge of the bed with your feet dangling for 1 or 2 minutes. Then stand up slowly. If the problem continues or gets worse, check with your doctor.

The dizziness, lightheadedness, or fainting is also more likely to occur if you drink alcohol, stand for a long time, exercise, or if the weather is hot. *While you are taking this medicine, be careful to limit the amount of alcohol you drink. Also, use extra care during exercise or hot weather or if you must stand for a long time.*

In some patients, this medicine may cause mental depression. *Tell your doctor right away:*

- if you or anyone else notices unusual changes in your mood.
- if you start having early-morning sleeplessness or unusually vivid dreams or nightmares.

This medicine will add to the effects of alcohol and other CNS depressants (medicines that slow down the nervous system, possibly causing drowsiness). Some examples of CNS depressants are antihistamines or medicine for hay fever, other allergies, or colds; sedatives, tranquilizers, or sleeping medicine; prescription pain medicine or narcotics; barbiturates; medicine for seizures; muscle relaxants; or anesthetics, including dental anesthetics. *Check with your doctor before taking any of the above while you are taking this medicine.*

This medicine may cause a loss of potassium from your body.

- To help prevent this, your doctor may want you to:

  —eat or drink foods that have a high potassium content (for example, orange or other citrus fruit juices), or

  —take a potassium supplement, or

  —take another medicine to help prevent the loss of the potassium in the first place.

- It is very important to follow these directions. Also, it is important not to change your diet on your own. This is more important if you are already on a special diet (as for diabetes), or if you are taking a potassium supplement or a medicine to reduce potassium loss. Extra potassium may not be necessary and, in some cases, too much potassium could be harmful.

Check with your doctor if you become sick and have severe or continuing nausea, vomiting, or diarrhea. These problems may cause you to lose additional water and potassium.

For *diabetic patients:*

- This medicine may raise blood sugar levels. While you are using this medicine, be especially careful in testing for sugar in your urine. If you have any questions about this, check with your doctor.

Some people who take this medicine may become more sensitive to sunlight than they are normally. Exposure to sunlight, even for brief periods of time, may cause severe sunburn; skin rash, redness, itching, or discoloration; or vision changes. When you begin taking this medicine:

- Stay out of direct sunlight, especially between the hours of 10:00 a.m. and 3:00 p.m., if possible.
- Wear protective clothing, including a hat and sunglasses.
- Apply a sun block product that has a skin protection factor (SPF) of at least 15. Some patients may require a product with a higher SPF number, especially if they have a fair complexion. If you have any questions about this, check with your health care professional.
- Do not use a sunlamp or tanning bed or booth.

If you have a severe reaction from the sun, check with your doctor.

This medicine often causes stuffiness in the nose. However, do not use nasal decongestant medicines without first checking with your health care professional.

This medicine may cause dryness of the mouth. For temporary relief, use sugarless candy or gum, melt bits of ice in your mouth, or use a saliva substitute. However, if dry mouth continues for more than 2 weeks, check with your medical doctor or dentist. Continuing dryness of the mouth may increase the chance of dental disease, including tooth decay, gum disease, and fungus infections.

Side Effects of This Medicine

Suggestions that this medicine may increase the risk of breast cancer occurring later have not been proven. However, rats and mice given 100 to 300 times the human dose had an increased number of tumors.

Along with its needed effects, a medicine may cause some unwanted effects. Although not all of these side effects may occur, if they do occur they may need medical attention.

Check with your doctor immediately if any of the following side effects occur:

More common

General feeling of discomfort or illness or weakness

Less common

Drowsiness or faintness; impotence or decreased sexual interest; lack of energy or weakness; mental depression or inability to concentrate; nervousness or anxiety; vivid dreams or nightmares or early-morning sleeplessness

Check with your doctor as soon as possible if any of the following side effects occur:

Signs and symptoms of too much potassium loss

Dryness of mouth; increased thirst; irregular heartbeat;

mood or mental changes; muscle cramps or pain; weak pulse

Signs and symptoms of too much sodium loss

Confusion; convulsions; decreased mental activity; irritability; muscle cramps; unusual tiredness or weakness

Less common

Black, tarry stools; blisters on skin; bloody vomit; chest pain; fever and sore throat; headache; irregular heartbeat; joint pain; numbness, tingling, pain, or weakness in hands or feet; shortness of breath; skin rash or itching; slow heartbeat; stomach cramps or pain; swelling of lymph glands

Rare

Lower back or side pain; painful or difficult urination; stiffness; stomach pain (severe) with nausea and vomiting; trembling and shaking of hands and fingers; unusual bleeding or bruising; yellow eyes or skin

Signs and symptoms of overdose

Dizziness or drowsiness (severe); dryness of mouth; flushing of skin; increased thirst; muscle cramps or pain; nausea or vomiting (severe); pinpoint pupils of eyes; slow pulse

Other side effects may occur that usually do not need medical attention. These side effects may go away during treatment as your body adjusts to the medicine. However, check with your doctor if any of the following side effects continue or are bothersome:

More common

Diarrhea; dizziness, especially when getting up from a lying or sitting position; loss of appetite; nausea or vomiting; stuffy nose

Less common

Constipation; flushing or redness of skin; increased sensitivity of skin to sunlight; swelling of feet and lower legs; watering or irritated eyes

After you stop using this medicine, it may still produce some side effects that need attention. During this period

of time *check with your doctor immediately* if you notice
any of the following side effects:

> Drowsiness or faintness; general feeling of discomfort or ill-
> ness or weakness; impotence or decreased sexual interest;
> irregular heartbeat; mental depression or inability to con-
> centrate; nervousness or anxiety; vivid dreams or night-
> mares or early-morning sleeplessness

Other side effects not listed above may also occur in some
patients. If you notice any other effects, check with your
doctor.

TERAZOSIN　Systemic

A commonly used brand name in the U.S. and Canada is Hytrin.

Description

Terazosin (ter-AY-zoe-sin) is used to treat high blood pressure (hypertension).

High blood pressure adds to the workload of the heart and
arteries. If it continues for a long time, the heart and arteries may not function properly. This can damage the blood
vessels of the brain, heart, and kidneys, resulting in a
stroke, heart failure, or kidney failure. High blood pressure
may also increase the risk of heart attacks. These problems
may be less likely to occur if blood pressure is controlled.

Terazosin helps to lower blood pressure by relaxing blood
vessels so that blood passes through them more easily.

Terazosin is also used to treat benign enlargement of the
prostate (benign prostatic hyperplasia [BPH]). Benign enlargement of the prostate is a problem that can occur in
men as they get older. The prostate gland is located below
the bladder. As the prostate gland enlarges, certain muscles
in the gland may become tight and get in the way of the
tube that drains urine from the bladder. This can cause

problems in urinating, such as a need to urinate often, a weak stream when urinating, or a feeling of not being able to empty the bladder completely.

Terazosin helps relax the muscles in the prostate and the opening of the bladder. This may help increase the flow of urine and/or decrease the symptoms. However, terazosin will not help shrink the prostate. The prostate may continue to grow. This may cause the symptoms to become worse over time. Therefore, even though terazosin may lessen the problems caused by enlarged prostate now, surgery still may be needed in the future.

Terazosin is available only with your doctor's prescription, in the following dosage form:

Oral

- Tablets (U.S. and Canada)

Before Using This Medicine

In deciding to use a medicine, the risks of taking the medicine must be weighed against the good it will do. This is a decision you and your doctor will make. For terazosin, the following should be considered:

Allergies—Tell your doctor if you have ever had any unusual or allergic reaction to terazosin, prazosin, or doxazosin. Also tell your health care professional if you are allergic to any other substances, such as foods, preservatives, or dyes.

Pregnancy—Studies have not been done in humans. Studies in animals given many times the highest recommended human dose have not shown that terazosin causes birth defects. However, these studies have shown a decrease in successful pregnancies.

Breast-feeding—It is not known whether terazosin passes into breast milk. Although most medicines pass into breast milk in small amounts, many of them may be used safely while breast-feeding. Mothers who are taking this medicine and who wish to breast-feed should discuss this with their doctor.

Children—Studies of this medicine have been done only in adult patients, and there is no specific information comparing use of terazosin in children with use in other age groups.

Older adults—Dizziness, lightheadedness, or fainting (especially when getting up from a lying or sitting position) may be more likely to occur in the elderly, who are more sensitive to the effects of terazosin.

Other medicines—Although certain medicines should not be used together at all, in other cases two different medicines may be used together even if an interaction might occur. In these cases, your doctor may want to change the dose, or other precautions may be necessary. Tell your health care professional if you are taking any other prescription or nonprescription (over-the-counter [OTC]) medicine.

Other medical problems—The presence of other medical problems may affect the use of terazosin. Make sure you tell your doctor if you have any other medical problems, especially:

- Angina (chest pain)—Terazosin may make this condition worse
- Heart disease (severe)—Terazosin may make this condition worse
- Kidney disease—Possible increased sensitivity to the effects of terazosin

Proper Use of This Medicine

For patients *taking this medicine for high blood pressure:*
- In addition to the use of the medicine your doctor

has prescribed, treatment for your high blood pressure may include weight control and care in the types of foods you eat, especially foods high in sodium. Your doctor will tell you which of these are most important for you. You should check with your doctor before changing your diet.

- Many patients who have high blood pressure will not notice any signs of the problem. In fact, many may feel normal. It is very important that you *take your medicine exactly as directed* and that you keep your appointments with your doctor even if you feel well.

- Remember that terazosin will not cure your high blood pressure but it does help control it. Therefore, you must continue to take it as directed if you expect to lower your blood pressure and keep it down. *You may have to take high blood pressure medicine for the rest of your life.* If high blood pressure is not treated, it can cause serious problems such as heart failure, blood vessel disease, stroke, or kidney disease.

For patients *taking this medicine for benign enlargement of the prostate:*

- Remember that terazosin will not shrink the size of your prostate but it does help to relieve the symptoms.

- It may take up to 6 weeks before your symptoms get better.

To help you remember to take your medicine, try to get into the habit of taking it at the same time each day.

Dosing—The dose of terazosin will be different for different patients. *Follow your doctor's orders or the directions on the label.* The following information includes only the average doses of terazosin. *If your dose is different, do not change it* unless your doctor tells you to do so.

The number of tablets that you take depends on the strength of the medicine.

- For *oral* dosage form (tablets):
  - —For benign enlargement of the prostate:
    - Adults—At first, 1 milligram (mg) taken at bedtime. Then, 5 to 10 mg once a day.
  - —For high blood pressure:
    - Adults—At first, 1 mg taken at bedtime. Then, 1 to 5 mg once a day.
    - Children—Use and dose must be determined by your doctor.

Missed dose—If you miss a dose of this medicine, take it as soon as possible the same day. However, if you do not remember the missed dose until the next day, skip the missed dose and go back to your regular dosing schedule. Do not double doses.

Storage—To store this medicine:

- Keep out of the reach of children.
- Store away from heat and direct light.
- Do not store in the bathroom, near the kitchen sink, or in other damp places. Heat or moisture may cause the medicine to break down.
- Do not keep outdated medicine or medicine no longer needed. Be sure that any discarded medicine is out of the reach of children.

Precautions While Using This Medicine

It is important that your doctor check your progress at regular visits to make sure that this medicine is working properly.

For patients *taking this medicine for high blood pressure:*

- *Do not take other medicines unless they have been discussed with your doctor.* This especially includes over-the-counter (nonprescription) medicines for appetite control, asthma, colds, cough, hay fever, or sinus problems, since they may tend to increase your blood pressure.

Dizziness, lightheadedness, or sudden fainting may occur after you take this medicine, especially when you get up from a lying or sitting position. These effects are more likely to occur when you take the first dose of this medicine. Taking the first dose at bedtime may prevent problems. However, *be especially careful if you need to get up during the night*. These effects may also occur with any doses you take after the first dose. Getting up slowly may help lessen this problem. *If you feel dizzy, lie down so that you do not faint*. Then sit for a few moments before standing to prevent the dizziness from returning.

The dizziness, lightheadedness, or fainting is more likely to occur if you drink alcohol, stand for long periods of time, exercise, or if the weather is hot. *While you are taking this medicine, be careful to limit the amount of alcohol you drink. Also, use extra care during exercise or hot weather or if you must stand for long periods of time.*

Terazosin may cause some people to become drowsy or less alert than they are normally. *Make sure you know how you react to this medicine before you drive, use machines, or do anything else that could be dangerous if you are dizzy, drowsy, or are not alert.* After you have taken several doses of this medicine, these effects should lessen.

Side Effects of This Medicine

Along with its needed effects, a medicine may cause some unwanted effects. Although not all of these side effects may occur, if they do occur they may need medical attention.

Check with your doctor as soon as possible if any of the following side effects occur:

More common
  Dizziness

Less common
  Chest pain; dizziness or lightheadedness when getting up
    from a lying or sitting position; fainting (sudden); fast
    or irregular heartbeat; pounding heartbeat; shortness of
    breath; swelling of feet or lower legs

Rare
  Weight gain

Other side effects may occur that usually do not need
medical attention. These side effects may go away during
treatment as your body adjusts to the medicine. However,
check with your doctor if any of the following side effects
continue or are bothersome:

More common
  Headache; unusual tiredness or weakness

Less common
  Back or joint pain; blurred vision; drowsiness; nausea and
    vomiting; stuffy nose

Other side effects not listed above may also occur in some
patients. If you notice any other effects, check with your
doctor.

THROMBOLYTIC AGENTS   Systemic

Some commonly used brand names are:

In the U.S.—
  Abbokinase[4]   Eminase[2]
  Abbokinase Open-Cath[4]   Kabikinase[3]
  Activase[1]   Streptase[3]

In Canada—
  Abbokinase[4]   Lysatec rt-PA[1]
  Abbokinase Open-Cath[4]   Streptase[3]
  Activase rt-PA[1]

Other commonly used names are:

| Anisoylated plasminogen-
streptokinase activator
complex[2]
APSAC[2] | Tissue-type plasminogen
activator (recombinant)[1]
t-PA[1]
rt-PA[1] |

Note: For quick reference, the following thrombolytic agents are numbered to match the corresponding brand names.

This information applies to the following medicines:

1. Alteplase, Recombinant (AL-ti-plase)
2. Anistreplase (an-EYE-strep-lase)†
3. Streptokinase (strep-toe-KYE-nase)
4. Urokinase (yoor-oh-KYE-nase)

———————————————————————

†Not commercially available in Canada.

———————————————————————

Description

Thrombolytic agents are used to dissolve blood clots that
have formed in certain blood vessels. These medicines are
usually used when a blood clot seriously lessens the flow
of blood to certain parts of the body.

Thrombolytic agents are also used to dissolve blood clots
that form in tubes that are placed into the body. The tubes
allow treatments (such as dialysis or injections into a vein)
to be given over a long period of time.

These medicines are to be given only by or under the
direct supervision of a doctor.

These medicines are available in the following dosage forms:

Parenteral
    Alteplase, Recombinant
        • Injection (U.S. and Canada)
    Anistreplase
        • Injection (U.S.)
    Streptokinase
        • Injection (U.S. and Canada)
    Urokinase
        • Injection (U.S. and Canada)

———————————————————————

Before Receiving This Medicine

In deciding to use a medicine, the risks of using the medicine must be weighed against the good it will do. This is

a decision you and your doctor will make. For thrombolytic agents, the following should be considered:

Allergies—Tell your doctor if you have ever had any unusual or allergic reaction to alteplase, anistreplase, streptokinase, or urokinase. Also tell your health care professional if you are allergic to any other substances, such as foods, preservatives, or dyes.

Pregnancy—Tell your doctor if you are pregnant or if you have recently delivered a baby.

There is a slight chance that use of a thrombolytic agent during the first five months of pregnancy may cause a miscarriage. However, both streptokinase and urokinase have been used in pregnant women and have not been reported to cause this problem. Also, studies in pregnant women (for streptokinase) and studies in animals (for urokinase) have not shown that these medicines cause either miscarriage or harm to the fetus (including birth defects). Studies on birth defects with alteplase and anistreplase have not been done in either pregnant women or animals.

Breast-feeding—It is not known whether thrombolytic agents pass into the breast milk. Although most medicines pass into breast milk in small amounts, many of them may be used safely while breast-feeding. Mothers who are taking any of these medicines and who wish to breast-feed should discuss this with their doctor.

Children—These medicines have been tested in children and, in effective doses, have not been shown to cause different side effects or problems than they do in adults.

Older adults—The need for treatment with a thrombolytic agent (instead of other kinds of treatment) may be increased in elderly patients with blood clots. However, the chance of bleeding may also be increased. It is especially important that you discuss the use of this medicine with your doctor.

Other medicines—Although certain medicines should not be used together at all, in other cases two different medicines may be used together even if an interaction might occur. In these cases, your doctor may want to change the dose, or other precautions may be necessary. Before you receive a thrombolytic agent, it is especially important that your doctor know if you are taking any of the following:

- Anticoagulants (blood thinners) or
- Aspirin or
- Cefamandole (e.g., Mandol) or
- Cefoperazone (e.g., Cefobid) or
- Cefotetan (e.g., Cefotan) or
- Divalproex (e.g., Depakote) or
- Enoxaparin (e.g., Lovenox) or
- Heparin or
- Indomethacin (e.g., Indocin) or
- Inflammation or pain medicine (except narcotics) or
- Phenylbutazone (e.g., Butazolidin) or
- Plicamycin (e.g., Mithracin) or
- Sulfinpyrazone (e.g., Anturane) or
- Ticlopidine (e.g., Ticlid) or
- Valproic acid (e.g., Depakene)—The chance of bleeding may be increased

Also, tell your doctor if you have had an injection of anistreplase or streptokinase within the past year. If you have, these medicines may not work properly if they are given to you again. Your doctor may decide to use alteplase or urokinase instead.

Other medical problems or recent childbirth—The presence of other medical problems or recent delivery of a child may affect the use of thrombolytic agents. Make sure you tell your doctor if you have any other medical problems, especially:

- Blood disease, bleeding problems, or a history of bleeding in any part of the body or
- Brain disease or tumor or
- Colitis or stomach ulcer (or history of) or
- Heart or blood vessel disease or
- High blood pressure or

- Liver disease (severe) or
- Stroke (or history of) or
- Tuberculosis (TB) (active)—The chance of serious bleeding may be increased
- Streptococcal ("strep") infection (recent)—Anistreplase or streptokinase may not work properly after a streptococcal infection; your doctor may decide to use a different thrombolytic agent

Also, tell your doctor if you have recently had any of the following conditions:

- Falls or blows to the body or head or any other injury or
- Injections into a blood vessel or
- Placement of any tube into the body or
- Surgery, including dental surgery—The chance of serious bleeding may be increased

If you have recently delivered a baby, use of these medicines may cause serious bleeding.

Proper Use of This Medicine

Dosing—The dose of these medicines will be different for different patients. The dose you receive will depend on the medicine you receive and will be based on the condition for which you are receiving the medicine. In some cases, the dose will also depend on your body weight.

Precautions While Receiving This Medicine

Thrombolytic agents can cause bleeding that usually is not serious. However, serious bleeding may occur in some people. *To help prevent serious bleeding, carefully follow any instructions given by your health care professional. Also, move around as little as possible, and do not get out of bed on your own, unless your health care professional tells you it is all right to do so.*

Side Effects of This Medicine

Along with its needed effects, a medicine may cause some unwanted effects. Although not all of these side effects may occur, if they do occur they may need medical attention.

Tell your health care professional immediately if any of the following side effects occur:

More common

Bleeding or oozing from cuts, gums, or around the place of injection; fever

Less common or rare

Bruising; changes in facial skin color; confusion; double vision; fast or irregular breathing; flushing or redness of skin; headache (mild); muscle pain (mild); nausea; shortness of breath, troubled breathing, tightness in chest, and/or wheezing; skin rash, hives, or itching; swelling of eyes, face, lips, or tongue; trouble in speaking; weakness in arms or legs

Symptoms of bleeding inside the body

Abdominal or stomach pain or swelling; back pain or backaches; blood in urine; bloody or black, tarry stools; constipation; coughing up blood; dizziness; headaches (sudden, severe, or continuing); joint pain, stiffness, or swelling; muscle pain or stiffness (severe or continuing); nosebleeds; unexpected or unusually heavy bleeding from vagina; vomiting of blood or material that looks like coffee grounds

Other side effects not listed above may also occur in some patients. If you notice any other effects, check with your doctor.

TOCAINIDE   Systemic

A commonly used brand name in the U.S. and Canada is Tonocard.

Description

Tocainide (toe-KAY-nide) belongs to the group of medicines known as antiarrhythmics. It is used to correct irregular heartbeats to a normal rhythm.

Tocainide produces its helpful effects by slowing nerve impulses in the heart and making the heart tissue less sensitive.

Tocainide is available only with your doctor's prescription, in the following dosage form:

Oral
  • Tablets (U.S. and Canada)

Before Using This Medicine

In deciding to use a medicine, the risks of taking the medicine must be weighed against the good it will do. This is a decision you and your doctor will make. For tocainide, the following should be considered:

Allergies—Tell your doctor if you have ever had any unusual or allergic reaction to tocainide or anesthetics. Also tell your health care professional if you are allergic to any other substances, such as foods, preservatives, or dyes.

Pregnancy—Tocainide has not been shown to cause birth defects or other problems in humans. Studies in animals have shown that high doses of tocainide may increase the possibility of death in the animal fetus, although it has not been shown to cause birth defects.

Breast-feeding—It is not known whether tocainide passes into breast milk. However, this medicine has not been reported to cause problems in nursing babies.

Children—Studies on this medicine have been done only in adult patients and there is no specific information comparing use of tocainide in children with use in other age groups.

Older adults—Dizziness or lightheadedness may be more likely to occur in the elderly, who are usually more sensitive to the effects of tocainide.

Other medicines—Although certain medicines should not be used together at all, in other cases two different medicines may be used together even if an interaction might occur. In these cases, your doctor may want to change the dose, or other precautions may be necessary. Tell your health care professional if you are taking any other prescription or nonprescription (over-the-counter [OTC]) medicine.

Other medical problems—The presence of other medical problems may affect the use of tocainide. Make sure you tell your doctor if you have any other medical problems, especially:

- Congestive heart failure—Tocainide may make this condition worse
- Kidney disease or
- Liver disease—Effects may be increased because of slower removal of tocainide from the body

---

Proper Use of This Medicine

Take tocainide exactly as directed by your doctor, even though you may feel well. Do not take more medicine than ordered.

If tocainide upsets your stomach, your doctor may advise you to take it with food or milk.

This medicine works best when there is a constant amount in the blood. *To help keep the amount constant, do not miss any doses. Also, it is best to take the doses at evenly spaced times day and night.* For example, if you are to take 3 doses a day, the doses should be spaced about 8 hours apart. If this interferes with your sleep or other daily activities, or if you need help in planning the best times to take your medicine, check with your health care professional.

Dosing—The dose of tocainide will be different for different patients. *Follow your doctor's orders or the directions on the label.* The following information includes only the average doses of tocainide. *If your dose is different, do not change it* unless your doctor tells you to do so.

The number of tablets that you take depends on the strength of the medicine.

- For *oral* dosage form (tablets):
    - —For irregular heartbeat:
        - Adults—At first, 400 milligrams (mg) every eight hours. Then, your doctor may increase your dose up to 600 mg three times a day.
        - Children—Use and dose must be determined by your doctor.

Missed dose—If you miss a dose of tocainide and remember within 4 hours, take it as soon as possible. Then go back to your regular dosing schedule. However, if you do not remember until later, skip the missed dose and go back to your regular dosing schedule. Do not double doses.

Storage—To store this medicine:

- Keep out of the reach of children.
- Store away from heat and direct light.
- Do not store in the bathroom, near the kitchen sink, or in other damp places. Heat or moisture may cause the medicine to break down.
- Do not keep outdated medicine or medicine no longer needed. Be sure that any discarded medicine is out of the reach of children.

Precautions While Using This Medicine

It is important that your doctor check your progress at regular visits to make sure the medicine is working properly. This will allow changes to be made in the amount of medicine you are taking, if necessary.

Your doctor may want you to carry a medical identification card or bracelet stating that you are using this medicine.

Tocainide may cause some people to become dizzy, lightheaded, or less alert than they are normally. *Make sure you know how you react to this medicine before you drive, use machines, or do anything else that could be dangerous if you are dizzy or are not alert.*

Before having any kind of surgery (including dental surgery) or emergency treatment, tell the medical doctor or dentist in charge that you are taking this medicine.

Side Effects of This Medicine

Along with its needed effects, a medicine may cause some unwanted effects. Although not all of these side effects may occur, if they do occur they may need medical attention.

Check with your doctor as soon as possible if any of the following side effects occur:

Less common

Trembling or shaking

Rare

Blisters on skin; cough or shortness of breath; fever or chills; irregular heartbeats; peeling or scaling of skin; skin rash (severe); sores in mouth; unusual bleeding or bruising

Other side effects may occur that usually do not need

medical attention. These side effects may go away during
treatment as your body adjusts to the medicine. However,
check with your doctor if any of the following side effects
continue or are bothersome:

More common

Dizziness or lightheadedness; loss of appetite; nausea

Less common

Blurred vision; confusion; headache; nervousness; numbness or tingling of fingers and toes; skin rash; sweating; vomiting

Other side effects not listed above may also occur in some
patients. If you notice any other effects, check with your
doctor.

TORSEMIDE   Systemic†

A commonly used brand name in the U.S. is Demadex.

---

†Not commercially available in Canada.

Description

Torsemide (TORE-se-mide) belongs to the group of medicines called loop diuretics. Torsemide is given to help
reduce the amount of water in the body in certain conditions, such as congestive heart failure, severe liver disease
(cirrhosis), or kidney disease. It works by acting on the
kidneys to increase the flow of urine.

Torsemide is also used to treat high blood pressure (hypertension). High blood pressure adds to the workload of the
heart and arteries. If it continues for a long time, the heart
and arteries may not function properly. This can damage
the blood vessels of the brain, heart, and kidneys, resulting
in a stroke, heart failure, or kidney failure. High blood
pressure may also increase the risk of heart attacks. These
problems may be less likely to occur if blood pressure
is controlled.

Torsemide is available only with your doctor's prescription, in the following dosage forms:

Oral
- Tablets (U.S.)

Parenteral
- Injection (U.S.)

Before Using This Medicine

In deciding to use a medicine, the risks of taking the medicine must be weighed against the good it will do. This is a decision you and your doctor will make. For torsemide, the following should be considered:

Allergies—Tell your doctor if you have ever had any unusual or allergic reaction to bumetanide, ethacrynic acid, furosemide, sulfonamides (sulfa drugs), or thiazide diuretics (water pills). Also, tell your health care professional if you are allergic to any other substances, such as foods, preservatives, or dyes.

Pregnancy—Studies have not been done in pregnant women. In general, diuretics are not useful for normal swelling of feet and hands that occurs during pregnancy. Diuretics should not be taken during pregnancy unless recommended by your doctor.

Breast-feeding—It is not known whether torsemide passes into breast milk. Although most medicines pass into breast milk in small amounts, many of them may be used safely while breast-feeding. Mothers who are taking this medicine and who wish to breast-feed should discuss this with their doctor.

Children—Studies on this medicine have been done only in adult patients, and there is no specific information comparing use of torsemide in children with use in other age groups.

Older adults—Many medicines have not been studied specifically in older people. Therefore, it may not be known whether they work exactly the same way they do in younger adults. Although there is no specific information comparing use of torsemide in the elderly with use in other age groups, this medicine is not expected to cause different side effects or problems in older people than it does in younger adults.

Other medicines—Although certain medicines should not be used together at all, in other cases two different medicines may be used together even if an interaction might occur. In these cases, your doctor may want to change the dose, or other precautions may be necessary. When you are taking torsemide, it is especially important that your health care professional know if you are taking any of the following:

- Acetazolamide (e.g., Diamox) or
- Alcohol or
- Amphotericin B by injection (e.g., Fungizone) or
- Azlocillin (e.g., Azlin) or
- Capreomycin (e.g., Capastat) or
- Carbenicillin by injection (e.g., Geopen) or
- Corticosteroids (cortisone-like medicine) or
- Corticotropin (ACTH) or
- Dichlorphenamide (e.g., Daranide) or
- Diuretics (water pills) or
- Insulin or
- Laxatives (with overdose or chronic misuse) or
- Methazolamide (e.g., Neptazane) or
- Mezlocillin (e.g., Mezlin) or
- Piperacillin (e.g., Pipracil) or
- Salicylates or
- Sodium bicarbonate (e.g., baking soda) or
- Ticarcillin (e.g., Ticar) or
- Ticarcillin and clavulanate (e.g., Timentin) or
- Vitamin B_{12} (e.g., AlphaRedisol, Rubramin-PC) (when used in megaloblastic anemia) or
- Vitamin D—Use of these medicines with torsemide may increase the chance of potassium loss
- Aldesleukin (e.g., Proleukin) or
- Anti-infectives by mouth or by injection (medicine for infection) or

- Carmustine (e.g., BiCNU) or
- Cisplatin (e.g., Platinol) or
- Combination pain medicine containing acetaminophen and aspirin (e.g., Excedrin) or other salicylates (with large amounts taken regularly) or
- Cyclosporine (e.g., Sandimmune) or
- Deferoxamine (e.g., Desferal) (with long-term use) or
- Gold salts (medicine for arthritis) or
- Inflammation or pain medicine, except narcotics, or
- Methotrexate (e.g., Mexate) or
- Penicillamine (e.g., Cuprimine) or
- Pentamidine (e.g., Pentam 300) or
- Plicamycin (e.g., Mithracin) or
- Streptozocin (e.g., Zanosar) or
- Tiopronin (e.g., Thiola)—Use of these medicines with torsemide may increase the chance of kidney damage
- Anticoagulants (blood thinners)—Torsemide may decrease the effects of these medicines
- Lithium (e.g., Lithane)—Use of lithium with torsemide may increase the chance of kidney damage; also, the chance of side effects of lithium may be increased

Other medical problems—The presence of other medical problems may affect the use of torsemide. Make sure you tell your doctor if you have any other medical problems, especially:

- Diabetes mellitus (sugar diabetes)—Torsemide may increase the amount of sugar in the blood
- Gout or
- Hearing problems—Torsemide may make these conditions worse
- Heart attack (recent)—Use of torsemide after a recent heart attack may make this condition worse
- Kidney disease (severe) or
- Liver disease—Higher blood levels of torsemide may occur, which may increase the chance of side effects

---

Proper Use of This Medicine

This medicine may cause you to have an unusual feeling of tiredness when you begin to take it. You may also notice an increase in the amount of urine or in your frequency of urination. After you have taken the medicine for a while, these effects should lessen.

It is best to plan your dose or doses according to a schedule that will least affect your personal activities and sleep. Ask your health care professional to help you plan the best time to take this medicine.

To help you remember to take your medicine, try to get into the habit of taking it at the same time each day.

For patients taking this medicine for *high blood pressure:*

- In addition to the use of the medicine your doctor has prescribed, treatment for your high blood pressure may include weight control and care in the types of foods you eat, especially foods high in sodium. Your doctor will tell you which of these are most important for you. You should check with your doctor before changing your diet.

- Many patients who have high blood pressure will not notice any signs of the problem. In fact, many may feel normal. It is very important that you *take your medicine exactly as directed* and that you keep your appointments with your doctor even if you feel well.

- Remember that this medicine will not cure your high blood pressure but it does help control it. Therefore, you must continue to take it as directed if you expect to lower your blood pressure and keep it down. *You may have to take high blood pressure medicine for the rest of your life.* If high blood pressure is not treated, it can cause serious problems, such as heart failure, blood vessel disease, stroke, or kidney disease.

Dosing—The dose of torsemide will be different for different patients. *Follow your doctor's orders or the directions on the label.* The following information includes only the average doses of torsemide. *If your dose is different, do not change it* unless your doctor tells you to do so.

The number of tablets that you take depends on the strength of the medicine. Also, *the length of time you take the medicine depends on the medical problem for which you are taking torsemide.*

- For *oral* dosage form (tablets):
    —For lowering the amount of water in the body:
    - Adults—Dose is usually 5 to 20 milligrams (mg) once a day. However, your doctor may increase your dose as needed.
    - Children—Use and dose must be determined by your doctor.
    —For high blood pressure:
    - Adults—5 to 10 mg once a day.
    - Children—Use and dose must be determined by your doctor.
- For *injection* dosage form:
    —For lowering the amount of water in the body:
    - Adults—Dose is usually 5 to 20 mg injected into a vein once a day. However, your doctor may increase your dose as needed.
    - Children—Use and dose must be determined by your doctor.

Missed dose—If you miss a dose of this medicine, take it as soon as possible. However, if it is almost time for your next dose, skip the missed dose and go back to your regular dosing schedule. Do not double doses.

Storage—To store this medicine:

- Keep out of the reach of children.
- Store away from heat and direct light.
- Do not store in the bathroom, near the kitchen sink, or in other damp places. Heat or moisture may cause the medicine to break down.
- Keep the medicine from freezing. Do not refrigerate.
- Do not keep outdated medicine or medicine no longer

needed. Be sure that any discarded medicine is out
of the reach of children.

Precautions While Using This Medicine

It is important that your doctor check your progress at
regular visits to make sure that this medicine is working
properly.

*This medicine may cause a loss of potassium from your
body:*

- To help prevent this, your doctor may want you to:
   —eat or drink foods that have a high potassium content (for example, orange or other citrus fruit
   juices), or
   —take a potassium supplement, or
   —take another medicine to help prevent the loss of
   the potassium in the first place.
- It is very important to follow these directions. Also,
   it is important not to change your diet on your own.
   This is more important if you are already on a special
   diet (as for diabetes) or if you are taking a potassium
   supplement or a medicine to reduce potassium loss.
   Extra potassium may not be necessary and, in some
   cases, too much potassium could be harmful.

To prevent the loss of too much water and potassium, tell
your doctor if you become sick, especially with severe or
continuing nausea and vomiting or diarrhea.

Before having any kind of surgery (including dental surgery) or emergency treatment, make sure the medical doctor or dentist in charge knows that you are taking this
medicine.

*Dizziness, lightheadedness, or fainting may occur, espe-
cially when you get up from a lying or sitting position.
This is more likely to occur in the morning. Getting up*

slowly may help. When you get up from lying down, sit on the edge of the bed with your feet dangling for 1 or 2 minutes. Then stand up slowly. If the problem continues or gets worse, check with your doctor.

The dizziness, lightheadedness, or fainting is also more likely to occur if you drink alcohol, stand for long periods of time, or exercise, or if the weather is hot. *While you are taking this medicine, be careful to limit the amount of alcohol you drink. Also, use extra care during exercise or hot weather or if you must stand for long periods of time.*

For *diabetic patients:*
- This medicine may affect blood sugar levels. While you are using this medicine, be especially careful in testing for sugar in your blood or urine.

For patients taking this medicine for *high blood pressure:*
- *Do not take other medicines unless they have been discussed with your doctor.* This especially includes over-the-counter (nonprescription) medicines for appetite control, asthma, colds, cough, hay fever, or sinus problems, since they may tend to increase your blood pressure.

Side Effects of This Medicine

Along with its needed effects, a medicine may cause some unwanted effects. Although not all of these side effects may occur, if they do occur they may need medical attention.

Check with your doctor as soon as possible if any of the following side effects occur:

Less common

    Dryness of mouth; fast or irregular heartbeat; increased thirst; mood or mental changes; muscle pain or cramps; nausea or vomiting; unusual tiredness or weakness

Rare

> Black, tarry stools; dizziness when getting up from a sitting or lying position; ringing or buzzing in the ears or any hearing loss; skin rash

Other side effects may occur that usually do not need medical attention. These side effects may go away during treatment as your body adjusts to the medicine. However, check with your doctor if any of the following side effects continue or are bothersome:

More common

> Constipation; dizziness; headache; stomach upset

GLOSSARY

Abdomen—The body area between the chest and pelvis.

Abortifacient—Medicine that causes abortion.

Abrade—Scrape or rub away the outer cover or layer of a part.

Absorption—Passing into the body; incorporation of substances into or across tissues of the body, for example, digested food into the blood from the small intestine, or poisons through the skin.

Achlorhydria—Absence of acid that normally would be found in the stomach.

Acidifier, urinary—Medicine that makes the urine more acidic.

Acidosis—Too much acidity or loss of alkalinity in the body fluids and tissues.

Acromegaly—Enlargement of the face, hands, and feet because of too much growth hormone.

Acute—Sharp or intense; describes a condition that begins suddenly, has severe symptoms, and usually lasts a short time.

Addison's disease—Disease caused by not enough secretion of corticosteroid hormones by the adrenal glands; causes weakness, salt loss, and low blood pressure.

Adhesion—The union by connective tissue of two parts that are normally separate (such as parts of a joint).

Adjunct—An additional or secondary treatment that is helpful but is not necessary to treatment of a particular condition; not effective for that condition if used alone.

Adjuvant—1. A substance added to or used with another substance to assist its action. 2. Something that assists or enhances the effectiveness of medical treatment.

Adrenal cortex—Outer layer of tissue of the adrenal gland, which produces corticosteroid hormones.

Adrenal glands—Two organs located next to the kidneys.

They produce the hormones epinephrine and norepinephrine and corticosteroid hormones, such as cortisol.

Adrenaline—See Epinephrine.

Adrenal medulla—Inner part of the adrenal gland, which produces epinephrine and norepinephrine.

Adrenocorticoids—See Corticosteroids.

Aerosol—Suspension of very small liquid or solid particles in compressed gas; drugs in aerosol form are dispensed in the form of a mist by releasing the gas.

African sleeping sickness—See Trypanosomiasis, African.

Agent—A force or substance capable of causing a change.

Agoraphobia—Fear of public places or open spaces.

Agranulocytosis—Disorder in which there is a severe decrease in the number of granulocytes normally present in the blood.

AIDS (acquired immunodeficiency syndrome)—Disease caused by human immunodeficiency virus (HIV). The disease results in a breakdown of the body's immune system, which makes a person more likely to get some other infections and some forms of cancer.

Alcohol-abuse deterrent—Medicine used to help alcoholics avoid the use of alcohol.

Alkaline—Having a pH of more than 7. Opposite of acidic.

Alkalizer, urinary—Medicine that makes the urine more alkaline.

Alkalosis—Too much alkalinity or loss of acidity in the body fluids and tissues.

Alopecia—Loss or absence of hair from areas where it normally is present; baldness.

Altitude sickness agent—Medicine used to prevent or lessen some of the effects of high altitude on the body.

Alzheimer's disease—Progressive disorder of thinking and other mental processes, usually beginning in late middle age.

Aminoglycosides—A class of chemically related antibiotics used to treat some serious types of bacterial infections.

Anabolic steroids—Synthetic forms of male hormones.

Analgesic—Medicine that relieves pain without causing unconsciousness.

Anaphylaxis—Sudden, severe allergic reaction.

Androgen—Substance, such as testosterone, that stimulates development of male characteristics.

Anemia—Reduction, to below normal, of hemoglobin in the blood.

Anesthesiologist—A physician who is qualified to give an anesthetic and other medicines to a patient before and during surgery.

Anesthetic—Medicine that causes a loss of feeling or sensation, especially of pain, sometimes through loss of consciousness.

Aneurysm—Abnormal dilatation or saclike swelling of an artery, vein, or the heart.

Angina—Pain, tightness, or feeling of heaviness in the chest, due mostly to lack of oxygen for the heart muscle. The pain may be felt in the left shoulder, jaw, or arm instead of or in addition to the chest. Symptoms often occur during exercise.

Angioedema—Allergic condition marked by continuing swelling and severe itching of areas of the skin.

Anorexia—Loss of appetite for food.

Anoxia—Absence of oxygen. The term is sometimes incorrectly used for hypoxia, which means an abnormally low amount of oxygen in the body.

Antacid—Medicine used to neutralize excess acid in the stomach.

Antagonist—Drug or other substance that blocks or works against the action of another.

Anthelmintic—Medicine used to destroy or expel intestinal worms.

Antiacne agent—Medicine used to treat acne.

Antianemic—Agent that prevents or corrects anemia.

Antianginal—Medicine used to prevent or treat angina attacks.

Antianxiety agent—Medicine used to treat excessive nervousness, tension, or anxiety.

Antiarrhythmic—Medicine used to treat irregular heartbeats.

Antiasthmatic—Medicine used to treat asthma.

Antibacterial—Medicine that kills or stops the growth of bacteria.

Antibiotic—Chemical substance used to treat infections.

Antibody—Special kind of blood protein that helps the body fight infection.

Antibulimic—Medicine used to treat bulimia.

Anticholelithic—Medicine used to dissolve gallstones.

Anticoagulant—Medicine used to prevent formation of blood clots in the blood vessels.

Anticonvulsant—Medicine used to prevent or treat convulsions (seizures).

Antidepressant—Medicine used to treat mental depression.

Antidiabetic agent—Medicine used to control blood sugar levels in patients with diabetes mellitus (sugar diabetes).

Antidiarrheal—Medicine used to treat diarrhea.

Antidiuretic—Medicine used to decrease formation of urine (for example, in patients with diabetes insipidus).

Antidote—Medicine used to prevent or treat harmful effects of another medicine or a poison.

Antidyskinetic—Medicine used to help treat the loss of muscle control caused by certain diseases or by some other medicines.

Antidysmenorrheal—Medicine used to treat menstrual cramps.

Antiemetic—Medicine used to prevent or treat nausea and vomiting.

Antiendometriotic—Medicine used to treat endometriosis.

Antienuretic—Medicine used to help prevent bedwetting.

Antifibrotic—Medicine used to treat fibrosis.

Antiflatulent—Medicine used to help relieve excess gas in the stomach or intestines.

Antifungal—Medicine used to treat infections caused by a fungus.

Antiglaucoma agent—Medicine used to treat glaucoma.

Antigout agent—Medicine used to prevent or relieve gout attacks.

Antihemorrhagic—Medicine used to prevent or help stop serious bleeding.

Antihistamine—Medicine used to prevent or relieve the symptoms of allergies (such as hay fever).

Antihypercalcemic—Medicine used to help lower the amount of calcium in the blood.

Antihyperlipidemic—Medicine used to help lower high levels of lipids in the blood.

Antihyperphosphatemic—Medicine used to help lower the amount of phosphate in the blood.

Antihypertensive—Medicine used to treat high blood pressure.

Antihyperuricemic—Medicine used to prevent or treat gout or other medical problems caused by too much uric acid in the blood.

Antihypocalcemic—Medicine used to increase calcium blood levels in patients with too little calcium.

Antihypoglycemic—Medicine used to increase blood sugar levels in patients with low blood sugar.

Antihypokalemic—Medicine used to increase potassium blood levels in patients with too little potassium.

Anti-infective—Medicine used to treat infection.

Anti-inflammatory—Medicine used to relieve pain, swelling, and other symptoms of inflammation.

Anti-inflammatory, nonsteroidal—An anti-inflammatory medicine that is not a cortisone-like medicine.

Anti-inflammatory, steroidal—A cortisone-like anti-inflammatory medicine.

Antimetabolite—Medicine that interferes with the normal processes within cells, preventing their growth.

Antimuscarinic—Medicine used to block the effects of a certain chemical in the body; often used to reduce smooth muscle spasms, especially abdominal or stomach cramps or spasms.

Antimyasthenic—Medicine used to treat myasthenia gravis.

Antimyotonic—Medicine used to prevent or relieve nighttime leg cramps or muscle spasms.

Antineoplastic—Medicine used to treat cancer.

Antineuralgic—Medicine used to treat neuralgia.

Antiprotozoal—Medicine used to treat infections caused by protozoa.

Antipsoriatic—Medicine used to treat psoriasis.

Antipsychotic—Medicine used to treat certain nervous, mental, and emotional conditions.

Antipyretic—Medicine used to reduce fever.

Antirheumatic—Medicine used to treat arthritis (rheumatism).

Antirosacea—Medicine used to treat rosacea.

Antiseborrheic—Medicine used to treat dandruff and seborrhea.

Antiseptic—Medicine that stops the growth of germs. Used on the surface of the skin to prevent infections in cuts, scrapes, and wounds.

Antispasmodic—Medicine used to reduce smooth muscle spasms (for example, stomach, intestinal, or urinary tract spasms).

Antispastic—Medicine used to treat muscle spasms.

Antithyroid agent—Medicine used to treat an overactive thyroid gland.

Antitremor agent—Medicine used to treat tremors (trembling or shaking).

Antitubercular—Medicine used to treat tuberculosis (TB).

Antitussive—Medicine used to relieve cough.

Antiulcer agent—Medicine used to treat stomach and duodenal ulcers.

Antivertigo agent—Medicine used to prevent dizziness.

Antiviral—Medicine used to treat infections caused by a virus.

Anus—The opening at the end of the digestive tract through which bowel contents are passed.

Anxiety—An emotional state with apprehension, worry, or tension in reaction to real or imagined danger or dread of a situation; accompanied by sweating, increased pulse, trembling, weakness, and fatigue.

Apnea—Temporary absence of breathing.

Apoplexy—See Stroke.

Appendicitis—Inflammation of the appendix.

Appetite stimulant—Medicine used to help increase the desire for food.

Appetite suppressant—Medicine used in weight control programs to help decrease the desire for food.

Arrhythmia—Abnormal heart rhythm.

Arteritis, temporal—Inflammatory disease of arteries, usually of the head; occurs in older people.

Arthralgia—Pain in a joint.

Arthritis, rheumatoid—Chronic disease, especially of the joints, marked by pain and swelling.

Ascites—Accumulation of fluid in the abdominal cavity.

Asthma—Disease marked by inflammation of the bronchial tubes (air passages). During an attack, air passages become constricted, causing wheezing and difficult breathing. Attacks may be brought on by allergens, virus infection, cold air, or exercise.

Atherosclerosis—Common disease of the arteries in which artery walls thicken and harden.

Avoid—To keep away from deliberately.

Bacteremia—Presence of bacteria in the blood.

Bacterium—Tiny, one-celled organism. Different types of bacteria are responsible for a number of diseases and infections.

Bancroft's filariasis—Disease transmitted by mosquitos in which an infection with the filarial worm occurs. Affects the lymph system, producing inflammation.

Beriberi—Disorder caused by too little vitamin B_1 (thiamine), marked by an accumulation of fluid in the body, extreme weight loss, inflammation of nerves, or paralysis.

Bile—Thick fluid produced by the liver and stored in the gallbladder. Bile helps in the digestion of fats.

Bile duct—Tubular passage which carries bile from the liver to the gallbladder, or from the gallbladder to the intestine.

Bilharziasis—See Schistosomiasis.

Biliary—Relating to bile, the bile duct, or the gallbladder.

Bilirubin—The bile pigment that is orange-colored or yellow; an excess in the blood may cause jaundice.

Bipolar disorder—Severe mental illness marked by repeated episodes of depression and mania. Also called *manic-depressive illness.*

Bisexual—One who is sexually attracted to both sexes.

Black fever—See Leishmaniasis, visceral.

Blackwater fever—Condition, marked by dark urine, rarely seen as a complication of malaria.

Bone marrow—Soft material filling the cavities of bones.

Bone marrow depression—Condition in which the production of red blood cells, leukocytes, or platelets by the red bone marrow is decreased.

Bone resorption inhibitor—Medicine used to prevent or treat certain types of bone disorders, such as Paget's disease of the bone; helps prevent bone loss.

Bowel disease, inflammatory, suppressant—Medicine used to treat certain intestinal disorders, such as colitis.

Bradycardia—Slow heart rate, usually less than 60 beats per minute.

Bronchitis—Inflammation of the bronchial tubes (air passages) of the lungs.

Bronchodilator—Medicine used to open up the bronchial tubes (air passages) of the lungs to increase the flow of air through them.

Buccal—Relating to the cheek. A buccal medicine is taken by placing it in the pocket between the cheek and the gum and letting it slowly dissolve.

Bulimia—Disturbance in eating behavior marked by bouts of excessive eating followed by self-induced vomiting and diarrhea, hard exercise, or fasting.

Bursa—Small fluid-filled sac present where body parts move over one another (such as in a joint) to help reduce friction.

Bursitis—Inflammation of a bursa.

Candidiasis of the mouth—Overgrowth of the yeast *Candida* in the mouth marked by white patches on the tongue or inside the mouth. Also called *thrush* or *white mouth*.

Candidiasis of the vagina—Yeast infection of the vagina caused by the yeast *Candida;* associated with itching, burning, and a cheesy or curd-like white discharge.

Cardiac—Relating to the heart.

Cardiac arrhythmia—Irregularity or loss of the normal rhythm of the heartbeat.

Cardiac load–reducing agent—Medicine used to ease the

workload of the heart by allowing the blood to flow through the blood vessels more easily.

Cardiotonic—Medicine used to improve the strength and efficiency of the heart.

Caries, dental—Tooth decay, sometimes causing pain, leading to the crumbling of the tooth. Also called *cavities*.

Cataract—An opacity (cloudiness) in the eye lens that impairs vision or causes blindness.

Catheter—Tube inserted into a small opening in the body so that fluids can be put in or taken out.

Caustic—Burning or corrosive agent; irritating and destructive to living tissue.

Cavity—1. Hollow space within the body. 2. Hole in a tooth, caused by dental caries.

Central nervous system—Part of the nervous system that is composed of the brain and spinal cord.

Cerebral palsy—Permanent disorder of motor weakness and loss of coordination due to damage to the brain.

Cervix—Lower end or necklike opening of the uterus to the vagina.

Chemotherapy—Treatment of illness or disease by chemical agents. The term most commonly refers to the use of drugs to treat cancer.

Chickenpox—See Varicella.

Chlamydia—A family of microorganisms that cause a variety of diseases in humans. One form is transmitted by sexual contact.

Cholesterol—Fatlike substance made by the liver but also absorbed from the diet; found only in animal tissues. Too much blood cholesterol is associated with several potential health risks, especially atherosclerosis (hardening of the arteries).

Chromosome—The structure in the cell nucleus that contains the DNA; in humans, there are normally 46.

Chronic—Describes a condition of long duration, which

is often of gradual onset and may involve very slow changes. Note that the term ''chronic'' has nothing to do with how serious the condition is.

Cirrhosis—Chronic liver disease marked by destruction of its cells and abnormal tissue growth.

Clitoris—Small, erectile body, being a part of the female external sex organs.

CNS—See Central nervous system.

Cold sores—See Herpes simplex.

Colic—Waves of sudden severe abdominal pain, which are usually separated by relatively pain-free intervals.

Colitis—Inflammation of the colon (bowel).

Colony stimulating factor—Protein that stimulates the production of one or more kinds of cells made in the bone marrow.

Colostomy—Operation in which part of the colon (bowel) is brought through the abdominal wall to create an artificial opening. The contents of the intestine are discharged through the opening, bypassing the rest of the intestines.

Coma—State of unconsciousness from which the patient cannot be aroused.

Coma, hepatic—Disturbances in mental function and the nervous system caused by severe liver disease.

Condom—Thin sheath or cover worn over the penis during sexual intercourse to prevent pregnancy or infection; made of latex (rubber) or animal intestine.

Congestive heart failure—Condition resulting from inability of the heart to pump strongly enough to maintain adequate blood flow; characterized by breathlessness and edema.

Conjunctiva—Delicate mucous membrane covering the front of the eye and the inside of the eyelid.

Conjunctivitis—Inflammation of the conjunctiva.

Constriction—Squeezing together and becoming narrower

or smaller, such as constriction of blood vessels or eye pupils.

Contagious disease—Disease that can be transmitted from one person to another.

Contamination—The introduction of germs or unclean material into or on normally sterile substances or objects.

Contraceptive—Medicine or device used to prevent pregnancy.

Contraction—A shortening or tightening, as in the normal function of muscles.

Convulsion—Sudden involuntary contraction or series of jerkings of muscles.

Corticosteroids—Group of cortisone-like hormones that are secreted by the adrenal cortex and are critical to the body. The two major groups of corticosteroids are glucocorticoids, which affect fat and body metabolism, and mineralocorticoids, which regulate salt/water balance. Also called *adrenocorticoids*.

Cortisol—Natural hormone produced by the adrenal cortex, important for carbohydrate, protein, and fat metabolism and for the normal response to stress; synthetic cortisol (hydrocortisone) is used to treat inflammations, allergies, collagen diseases, rheumatic disorders, and adrenal failure.

Cot death—See Sudden infant death syndrome (SIDS).

Cowpox—See Vaccinia.

Creutzfeldt-Jakob disease—Rare disease, probably caused by a slow-acting virus that affects the brain and nervous system.

Crib death—See Sudden infant death syndrome (SIDS).

Crohn's disease—Chronic, inflammatory disease of the digestive tract, usually the lower small intestine.

Croup—Inflammation and blockage of the larynx (voice box) in young children.

Crystalluria—Crystals in the urine.

Cushing's syndrome—Condition in which the adrenal gland produces too much cortisone-like hormone, leading to weight gain, round face, and high blood pressure.

Cycloplegia—Paralysis of certain eye muscles; can be induced by medication for certain eye examinations.

Cycloplegic—Medicine used to induce cycloplegia.

Cyst—Abnormal sac or closed cavity filled with liquid or semisolid matter.

Cystic—Marked by cysts.

Cystic fibrosis—Hereditary disease of children and young adults which predominantly affects the lungs. Exocrine glands do not function normally, and excess mucus is produced.

Cystine—An amino acid found in most proteins; it is produced by the digestion of the protein.

Cystitis, interstitial—Inflammation of the bladder, predominantly in women, with frequent urge to urinate and painful urination.

Cytomegalovirus—One of a group of viruses. One form may be sexually transmitted and can be fatal in patients with weakened immune systems.

Cytoplasm—The contents of a cell outside the nucleus.

Cytotoxic agent—Chemical that kills cells or stops cell division; used to treat cancer.

Decongestant, nasal—Medicine used to help relieve nasal congestion (stuffy nose).

Decongestant, ophthalmic—Medicine used in the eye to relieve redness, burning, itching, or other irritation.

Decubitus—The position taken in lying down.

Decubitus ulcer—Bedsore; damage to the skin and underlying tissues caused by constant pressure.

Dental—Related to the teeth and gums.

Depression, mental—Condition marked by deep sadness; associated with lack of any pleasurable interest in life. Other symptoms include disturbances in sleep, appetite, and concentration, and difficulty in performing day-to-day tasks.

Dermatitis herpetiformis—Skin disease marked by sores and itching.

Dermatitis, seborrheic—Type of eczema found on the scalp and face.

Dermatomyositis—Inflammatory disorder of the skin and underlying tissues, including breakdown of muscle fibers.

Diabetes insipidus—Disorder in which the patient produces large amounts of dilute urine and is constantly thirsty. Also called *water diabetes.*

Diabetes mellitus—Disorder in which the body cannot process sugars to release energy; either the body does not produce enough insulin or the body tissues are unable to use the insulin present. This leads to too much sugar in the blood (hyperglycemia). Also called *sugar diabetes.*

Diagnose—Find out the cause or nature of a disorder by examination and laboratory tests.

Diagnostic procedure—A process carried out to determine the cause or nature of a condition, disease, or disorder.

Dialysis, renal—Artificial technique for removing waste materials or poisons from the blood when the kidneys are not working properly.

Digestant—Agent that will help in digestion.

Diplopia—Awareness of two images of a single object at one time; double vision.

Diuretic—Medicine used to increase the amount of urine produced by helping the kidneys get rid of water and salt. Also called *water pill.*

Diverticulitis—Inflammation of a diverticulum in the intestinal tract.

Diverticulum—Sac or pouch opening from a canal or cavity.

DNA—Deoxyribonucleic acid; the genetic material that controls heredity. DNA is located in the cell nucleus.

Down syndrome—Mental retardation associated with the presence of an extra chromosome 21. Patients with Down syndrome are marked physically by a round head, flat nose, slightly slanted eyes, and short stature. Also called *mongolism*.

Duct—Tube or channel, especially one that serves to carry secretions from a gland.

Dumdum fever—See Leishmaniasis, visceral.

Duodenal ulcer—Open sore in that part of the small intestine closest to the stomach.

Duodenum—First of the three parts of the small intestine.

Dyskinesia—Refers to abnormal, involuntary movement or a defect in voluntary movement.

Dyspnea—Shortness of breath; difficult breathing.

Eczema—Inflammation of the skin, marked by itching and rash.

Edema—Swelling of body tissue due to accumulation of fluids, usually first noticed in the feet or lower legs.

Eighth-cranial-nerve disease—Disease of the eighth cranial nerve, serving the inner ear; results in dizziness, loss of balance, loss of hearing, nausea, or vomiting.

Electrolyte—In medical use, chemicals (ions) in body fluids that are needed for normal functioning of the body. Body electrolytes include bicarbonate, chloride, sodium, potassium, etc.

Embolism—Sudden blocking of a blood vessel by a blood clot or foreign substances carried to the place of obstruction by the blood.

Embryo—In humans, a developing fertilized egg within the uterus (womb) from about two to eight weeks after fertilization.

Emergency—Extremely serious unexpected or sudden happening or situation that calls for immediate action.

Emollient—Substance that soothes and softens an irritated surface, such as the skin.

Emphysema—Lung condition in which destructive changes occur in the air spaces; air is not exchanged normally during the process of breathing in and out.

Encephalitis—Inflammation of the brain.

Encephalopathy—Any degenerative disease of the brain; caused by many different medical conditions.

Endocarditis—Inflammation of the lining of the heart, leading to fever, heart murmurs, and heart failure.

Endocrine gland—A gland that has no duct; releases its secretion directly into the blood.

Endometriosis—Condition in which material similar to the lining of the uterus (womb) appears at other sites within the pelvic cavity, causing pain and bleeding.

Enteric coating—Coating on tablets which allows them to pass through the stomach unchanged before being broken up in the intestine and being absorbed. Used to protect the stomach from the medicine and/or the medicine from the stomach's acid.

Enteritis—Inflammation of the small intestine, usually causing diarrhea.

Enuresis—Urinating while asleep (bedwetting).

Enzyme—Type of protein produced by cells that may bring about or speed up a normal chemical reaction in the body.

Eosinophil—One type of white blood cells readily stained by the dye eosin; important in allergic reactions and parasitic infections.

Eosinophilia—Condition in which the number of eosinophils in the blood is abnormally high.

Epidural space—Area in the spinal column into which medicines (usually for pain) can be administered.

Epilepsy—Any of a group of brain disorders featuring sudden attacks of seizures and other symptoms.

Epinephrine—Hormone secreted by the adrenal medulla.

It stimulates the heart, constricts blood vessels, and relaxes some smooth muscles. Also called *adrenaline*.

EPO—See Erythropoietin.

Ergot alkaloids—A class of medicines that cause narrowing of blood vessels; used to treat migraine headaches, and to reduce bleeding in childbirth.

Erythropoietin—Hormone secreted by the kidney. It controls the production of red blood cells by the bone marrow; also available as a synthetic drug (EPO).

Esophagus—The part of the digestive tract connecting the pharynx to the stomach.

Estrogen—Principal female sex hormone necessary for the normal sexual development of the female; during the menstrual cycle, its actions help prepare for possible pregnancy. Estrogen is often used to treat discomforts of menopause.

Exocrine gland—Any gland that discharges its secretion through a duct that opens on a surface (not into the blood).

Exophthalmos—Thrusting forward of the eyeballs in their sockets giving the appearance of the eyes sticking out too far; commonly associated with hyperthyroidism.

Expectorant—Medicine used to help remove mucus or phlegm in the lungs by coughing or spitting it up.

Extrapyramidal symptoms—Movement disorders occurring with certain diseases or with use of certain drugs, including trembling and shaking of hands and fingers, twisting movements of the body, shuffling walk, and stiffness of arms or legs.

Familial Mediterranean fever—Inherited condition involving inflammation of the lining of the chest, abdomen, and joints. Also called *recurrent polyserositis*.

Fasciculation—Small, spontaneous contraction of a few muscle fibers, which is visible through the skin; muscular twitching.

Favism—Inherited condition resulting from sensitivity to broad (fava) beans; marked by fever, vomiting, diarrhea, and acute destruction of red blood cells.

Fertility—Capacity to bring about the start of pregnancy.

Fertilization—Union of an ovum with a sperm.

Fetus—In humans, a developing baby within the uterus (womb) from about the beginning of the third month of pregnancy.

Fibrocystic—Having benign (noncancerous) tumors of connective tissue.

Fibroid tumor—A noncancerous tumor of the uterus formed of fibrous or fully developed connective tissue.

Fibrosis—Condition in which the skin and underlying tissues tighten and become less flexible.

Fistula—Abnormal tubelike passage connecting two internal organs or one that leads from an abscess or internal organ to the body surface.

Flatulence—Excessive amount of air or gas in the stomach or intestine.

Flu—See Influenza.

Flushing—Temporary redness of the face and/or neck.

Fungus—Any of a group of simple organisms, including molds and yeasts.

Fungus infection—Infection caused by a fungus. Some common fungus infections are tinea pedis (athlete's foot), tinea capitis (ringworm of the scalp), tinea cruris (ringworm of the groin or jock itch), and mouth or vaginal candidiasis (yeast infections).

Gait—Manner of walk.

Gamma globulin—The portion of the blood that contains most of the antibodies associated with the body's immunity to infection.

Gastric—Relating to the stomach.

Gastric acid secretion inhibitor—Medicine used to decrease the amount of acid produced by the stomach.

Gastroenteritis—Inflammation of the stomach and intestine.

Gastroesophageal reflux—Backward flow into the esophagus of the contents of the stomach and duodenum. The condition is often characterized by "heartburn."

Generic—General in nature; relating to an entire group or class. In relation to medicines, the general name of a drug substance; not owned by one specific group as would be true for a trademark or brand name.

Genital—1. Relating to the organs concerned with reproduction; the sexual organs. 2. Relating to reproduction.

Genital warts—Small growths found on the genitals or around the anus; caused by a virus. The disease may be transmitted by sexual contact.

Gilles de la Tourette syndrome—See Tourette's disorder.

Gingiva—Gums.

Gingival hyperplasia—Overgrowth of the gums.

Gingivitis—Inflammation of the gums.

Glandular fever—See Mononucleosis.

Glaucoma—Condition of abnormally high pressure in the eye; may lead to loss of vision if not treated.

Glomeruli—Clusters of capillaries in the nephrons of the kidney that act as filters of the blood.

Glomerulonephritis—Inflammation of the glomeruli of the kidney not directly caused by infection.

Glucose-6-phosphate dehydrogenase (G6PD) deficiency—Lack of or reduced amounts of an enzyme (glucose-6-phosphate dehydrogenase) that helps the breakdown of certain sugar compounds in the body.

Gluten—Type of protein found primarily in wheat and rye.

Goiter—Enlargement of the thyroid gland that causes the neck to swell. Condition usually results from a lack of iodine or overactivity of the thyroid gland.

Gonadotropin—Any hormone that stimulates the activities of the ovaries or testes.

Gonorrhea—An infectious disease, usually transmitted by sexual contact. It causes infection in the genital organs in both men and women, and may also result in systemic disease.

Gout—Disease in which too much uric acid builds up in the blood and joints, leading to inflammation of the joints.

Granulation—Small, fleshy outgrowths on the healing surface of a wound or ulcer; a normal stage in healing.

Granulocyte—A class of white blood cell.

Granulocytopenia—Abnormal reduction of the number of granulocytes in the blood; agranulocytosis.

Granuloma—A growth or mass of granulation tissue produced in response to chronic infection, inflammation, a foreign body, or to unknown causes.

Graves' disease—Disorder that causes thyrotoxicosis, goiter, and exophthalmos. Also called *exophthalmic goiter.*

Groin—The area between the abdomen and thigh.

Guillain-Barré syndrome—Nerve disease marked by sudden numbness and weakness in the limbs that may progress to complete paralysis.

Gynecomastia—Excessive development of the breasts in the male.

Hair follicle—Sheath of tissue surrounding a hair root.

Hansen's disease—See Leprosy.

Hartnup disease—Hereditary disease in which the body has trouble processing certain chemicals, leading to mental retardation, rough skin, and problems with muscle coordination.

Heart attack—See Myocardial infarction.

Hematuria—Presence of blood or red blood cells in the urine.

Hemoglobin—Iron-containing substance found in red blood cells that transports oxygen from the lungs to the tissues of the body.

Hemolytic anemia—Type of anemia resulting from breakdown of red blood cells.

Hemophilia—Hereditary disease in males in which blood clotting is delayed, leading to excessive and uncontrolled bleeding even after minor injuries.

Hemorrhoids—Enlarged veins in the walls of the anus. Also called *piles*.

Hepatic—Relating to the liver.

Hepatitis—Inflammation of the liver.

Hernia, hiatal—Condition in which the stomach passes partly into the chest through the opening for the esophagus in the diaphragm.

Herpes simplex—The virus that causes "cold sores." These are an inflammation of the skin resulting in small, painful blisters. Infection may occur either in or around the mouth or, in the case of genital herpes, on the genitals (sex organs).

Herpes zoster—An infectious disease usually marked by pain and blisters along one nerve, often on the face, chest, stomach, or back. The infection is caused by the virus that also causes chickenpox. Also called *shingles*.

Heterosexual—One who is sexually attracted to persons of the opposite sex.

High blood pressure—See Hypertension.

Hirsutism—Adult male pattern of hair growth in women.

HIV (human immunodeficiency virus)—Virus that causes AIDS.

Hodgkin's disease—Malignant condition marked by swelling of the lymph nodes, with weight loss and fever.

Homosexual—One who is sexually attracted to persons of the same sex.

Hormone—Substance produced in one part of the body (such as a gland), which then passes into the bloodstream and travels to other organs or tissues, where it carries out its effect.

Hot flashes—Sensations of heat of the face, neck, and

upper body, often accompanied by sweating and flushing; commonly associated with menopause.

Hydrocortisone—See Cortisol.

Hyperactivity—Abnormally increased activity.

Hypercalcemia—Too much calcium in the blood.

Hypercalciuria—Too much calcium in the urine.

Hypercholesterolemia—Excessive amount of cholesterol in the blood.

Hyperglycemia—Abnormally high blood sugar.

Hyperkalemia—Abnormally high amount of potassium in the blood.

Hyperkeratosis—Overgrowth or thickening of the outer horny layer of the skin.

Hyperlipidemia—General term for an abnormally high level of any or all of the lipids in the blood.

Hyperphosphatemia—Too much phosphate in the blood.

Hypersensitivity—Condition in which the body has an abnormally increased reaction to a foreign substance.

Hypertension—Blood pressure in the arteries (blood vessels) that is higher than normal for the patient's age group. Hypertension may lead to a number of serious health problems. Also called *high blood pressure*.

Hyperthermia—Abnormally high body temperature.

Hyperthyroidism—Excessive secretion of thyroid hormones by the thyroid gland, causing thyrotoxicosis.

Hypocalcemia—Too little calcium in the blood.

Hypoglycemia—Abnormally low blood sugar.

Hypokalemia—Abnormally low amount of potassium in the blood.

Hypotension, orthostatic—Excessive fall in blood pressure that occurs when standing or upon standing up.

Hypothalamus—Area of the brain that controls many body functions, including body temperature, certain metabolic and endocrine processes, and some activities of the nervous system.

Hypothermia—Abnormally low body temperature.

Hypothyroidism—Condition caused by thyroid hormone deficiency, which results in a decrease in metabolism.

Hypoxia—Broad term meaning intake of oxygen or its use by the body is inadequate.

Ileostomy—Operation in which the ileum is brought through the abdominal wall to create an artificial opening. The contents of the intestine are discharged through the opening, bypassing the colon (bowel).

Ileum—Last of the three portions of the small intestine.

Immune deficiency condition—Lack of immune response to protect against infectious disease.

Immune system—Complex network of the body that defends against foreign substances or organisms that may harm the body.

Immunizing agent, active—Agent that causes the body to produce its own antibodies for protection against certain infections.

Immunocompromised—Decreased natural immunity caused by irradiation, certain medicine or diseases, or other conditions.

Immunosuppressant—Medicine that reduces the body's natural immunity.

Impair—To cause to decrease, weaken, or damage, usually because of injury or disease.

Impetigo—Contagious bacterial skin infection common in babies and children in which skin redness develops into blisters that break and form a thick crust.

Implant—1. Special form of medicine, often a small pellet or rod, that is inserted into the body or beneath the skin so that the medicine will be released continuously over a period of time. 2. To insert or graft material or an object into a body site. 3. Material or an object inserted into a body site, such as a lens implant or a breast implant. 4. Action of a fertilized ovum becoming attached or embedded in the uterus.

Impotence—Difficulty or inability of a male to have or maintain an erection of the penis.

Incontinence—Inability to control natural passage of urine or of bowel movements.

Induce—To cause or bring about.

Infertility—Medical condition which results in the difficulty or inability of a woman to become pregnant or of a man to cause pregnancy.

Inflammation—Pain, redness, swelling, and heat in a part of the body, usually in response to injury or illness.

Influenza—Highly contagious respiratory virus infection, marked by coughing, headache, chills, fever, muscle pain, and general weakness. Also called *flu*.

Ingredient—One of the parts or substances that make up a mixture or compound.

Inhalation—1. Act of drawing in the breath or drawing air into the lungs. 2. Medicine that is used when breathed (inhaled) into the lungs. Some inhalations work locally in the lungs, while others produce their effects elsewhere in the body.

Inhibitor—Substance that prevents a process or reaction.

Inner ear—Inner portion of the ear; a liquid filled system of cavities and ducts that make up the organs of hearing and balance.

Insomnia—Inability to sleep or remain asleep.

Insulin—Hormone that increases the efficiency with which the body uses sugar. Injections of insulin are used in the treatment and control of diabetes mellitus (sugar diabetes).

Intra-amniotic—Within the sac that contains the fetus and amniotic fluid.

Intra-arterial—Within an artery.

Intracavernosal—Into the corpus cavernosa (cavities in the penis that, when filled with blood, produce an erection).

Intracavitary—Into a body cavity (for example, the chest cavity or bladder).

Intramuscular—Into a muscle.

Intrauterine device (IUD)—Small plastic or metal device placed in the uterus (womb) to prevent pregnancy.

Intravenous—Into a vein.

Ion—Atom or group of atoms carrying an electric charge.

Irrigation—Washing of a body cavity or wound with a stream of sterile water or a solution of a medicine.

Ischemia—Condition caused by inadequate blood flow to a part of the body; usually caused by constriction or blocking of blood vessels that supply the part of the body affected.

Jaundice—Yellowing of the eyes and skin due to excess bilirubin in the blood.

Jock itch—Ringworm of the groin.

Kala-azar—See Leishmaniasis, visceral.

Kaposi's sarcoma—Malignant tumor of blood vessels; often appears in the skin. One form occurs in immuno-compromised patients, for example, transplant recipients and AIDS patients.

Keratolytic—Medicine used to soften hardened areas of the skin, such as warts.

Ketoacidosis—Type of acidosis associated with diabetes.

Lactation—Secretion of breast milk.

Larva—The immature form of life of some insects and other animal groups that hatch from eggs.

Larynx—Organ that serves as a passage for air from the pharynx to the lungs; it contains the vocal cords.

Laxative—Medicine used to encourage bowel movements.

Laxative, bulk-forming—Laxative that acts by absorbing liquid and swelling to form a soft, bulky stool. The bowel is then stimulated normally by the presence of the bulky mass.

Laxative, hyperosmotic—Laxative that acts by drawing

water into the bowel from surrounding body tissues. This provides a soft stool mass and increased bowel action.

Laxative, lubricant—Laxative that acts by coating the bowel and the stool mass with a waterproof film. This keeps moisture in the stool. The stool remains soft and its passage is made easier.

Laxative, stimulant—Laxative that acts directly on the intestinal wall. The direct stimulation increases the muscle contractions that move the stool mass along. Also called *contact laxative.*

Laxative, stool softener—Laxative that acts by helping liquids mix into the stool and prevent dry, hard stool masses. The stool remains soft and its passage is made easier. Also called *emollient laxative.*

Legionnaires' disease—Lung infection caused by a certain bacterium.

Leishmaniasis, visceral—Tropical disease, transmitted by sandfly bites, which causes liver and spleen enlargement, anemia, weight loss, and fever. Also called *black fever, Dumdum fever,* or *kala-azar.*

Lennox-Gastaut syndrome—Type of childhood epilepsy.

Leprosy—Chronic infectious disease characterized by lesions, especially in the skin and nerves, leading to loss of feeling, paralysis in the hands and feet, and deformity. Also called *Hansen's disease.*

Leukemia—Disease of the blood and bone marrow in which too many white blood cells are produced, resulting in anemia, bleeding, and low resistance to infections.

Leukocyte—White blood cell.

Leukoderma—See Vitiligo.

Leukopenia—Abnormal reduction in the total number of leukocytes in the blood.

Lipid—Term applied generally to dietary fat or fatlike substances not soluble in water.

Local effect—Affecting only the area to which something is being applied.

Lugol's solution—Transparent, deep brown liquid containing iodine and potassium iodide.

Lupus—See Lupus erythematosus, systemic.

Lupus erythematosus, systemic—Chronic inflammatory disease most often affecting the skin, joints, and various internal organs. Also called *lupus* or *SLE* (systemic lupus erythematosus).

Lymph—Fluid that bathes the tissues. It is formed in tissue spaces in all parts of the body and circulated by the lymphatic system.

Lymphatic system—Network of vessels that conveys lymph from the spaces between the cells of the body back to the bloodstream.

Lymph node—A small rounded body found at intervals along the lymphatic system. The nodes act as filters for the lymph by keeping bacteria and other foreign particles from entering the bloodstream. They also produce lymphocytes.

Lymphocyte—Any of a number of white blood cells found in the blood, lymph, and lymphatic tissues. They are involved in immunity.

Lymphoma—Malignant tumor of lymph nodes or tissue.

Lyse—To cause breakdown. In cells, damage or rupture of the membrane results in destruction of the cell.

Macrobiotic—Vegetarian diet consisting mostly of whole grains.

Malaria—Tropical blood infection caused by a protozoa; symptoms include chills, fever, sweats, headaches, and anemia. Malaria is spread to humans by the bite of an infected mosquito.

Malignant—Describing a condition that becomes continually worse if untreated; also used to mean cancerous.

Malnutrition—Condition caused by unbalanced or insufficient diet.

Mammogram—X-ray picture of the breast.

Mania—Mental state in which fast talking and excited feelings or actions are out of control.

Mast cells—Cells in the connective tissue that store histamine; they release substances that bring about inflammation and produce signs of allergic reactions.

Mastocytosis—Accumulation of too many mast cells in tissues.

Mediate—To bring about or accomplish indirectly.

Megavitamin therapy—Taking very large doses of vitamins to prevent or treat certain medical problems.

Melanoma—Highly malignant cancer tumor, usually occurring on the skin.

Ménière's disease—Disease affecting the inner ear that is characterized by ringing in the ears, hearing loss, and dizziness.

Meningitis—Inflammation of the tissues that surround the brain and spinal cord.

Menopause—The time in a woman's life when the ovaries no longer produce an egg cell at regular times and menstruation stops.

Methemoglobin—Substance formed when hemoglobin has been oxidized; in this form, hemoglobin cannot act as an oxygen carrier.

Methemoglobinemia—Presence of methemoglobin in the blood.

Middle ear—Chamber of the ear lying behind the eardrum and containing the structures that conduct sound.

Migraine—Throbbing headache, usually affecting one side of the head; often accompanied by nausea, vomiting, and sensitivity to light.

Miotic—Medicine used in the eye that causes the pupil to constrict (become smaller).

Mongolism—See Down syndrome.

Mono—See Mononucleosis.

Monoclonal—Derived from a single cell; related to production of drugs by genetic engineering, such as monoclonal antibodies.

Mononucleosis—Infectious viral disease occurring mostly in adolescents and young adults, marked by fever, sore throat, swelling of the lymph nodes in the neck and armpits, and severe fatigue. Also called *mono* or *glandular fever.*

Motility—Ability to move without outside aid, force, or cause.

Motor—Relating to structures that bring about movement, such as nerves and muscles.

Mucolytic—Medicine that breaks down or dissolves mucus.

Mucosal—Relating to the mucous membrane.

Mucous membrane—Moist layer of tissue surrounding or lining many body structures and cavities, including the mouth, lips, inside of nose, anus, and vagina.

Mucus—Thick fluid produced by the mucous membranes and glands.

Multiple sclerosis (MS)—Chronic, inflammatory nerve disease marked by weakness, unsteadiness, shakiness, and speech and vision problems.

Myasthenia gravis—Chronic disease marked by abnormal weakness, and sometimes paralysis, of certain muscles.

Mydriatic—Medicine used in the eye that causes the pupil to dilate (become larger).

Myelogram—X-ray picture of the spinal cord.

Myeloma, multiple—Cancerous bone marrow disease.

Myocardial infarction—Interruption of blood supply to the heart, leading to sudden, severe chest pain, and damage to the heart muscle. Also called *heart attack.*

Myocardial reinfarction prophylactic—Medicine used to help prevent additional heart attacks in patients who have already had one attack.

Myotonia congenita—Hereditary muscle disorder marked

by difficulty in relaxing a muscle or releasing a grip after any strong effort.

Narcolepsy—Extreme tendency to fall asleep suddenly.

Nasal—Relating to the nose.

Nasogastric (NG) tube—Tube that is inserted through the nose, down the throat, and into the stomach. It may be used to remove fluid or gas from the stomach or to administer medicine, food, fluid, or nutrients to the patient.

Nebulizer—Instrument that administers liquid in the form of a fine spray.

Necrosis—Death of tissue, cells, or a part of a structure or organ, surrounded by healthy parts.

Neoplasm—New and abnormal growth of tissue in or on a part of the body, in which the multiplication of cells is uncontrolled and progressive. Also called *tumor*.

Nephron—Unit of the kidney that acts as a filter of the blood in forming urine.

Neuralgia—Severe stabbing or throbbing pain along the course of one or more nerves.

Neuralgia, trigeminal—Severe burning or stabbing pain along certain nerves in the face. Also called *tic douloureux*.

Neuritis, optic—Disease of the nerves in the eye.

Neuritis, peripheral—Inflammation of terminal nerves or the nerve endings, usually associated with pain, muscle wasting, and loss of reflexes.

Neutropenia—Abnormally small number of neutrophils in the blood.

Neutrophil—The most common type of granulocyte; important in the body's protection against infection.

Nodule—Small, rounded mass, lump, or swelling.

Nonsuppurative—Not discharging pus.

NSAID (nonsteroidal anti-inflammatory drug)—See Anti-inflammatory, nonsteroidal.

Nucleus—The part of the cell that contains the chromosomes.

Nystagmus—Rapid, rhythmic, involuntary movements of the eyeball; may be from side to side, up and down, or around.

Obesity—Excess accumulation of fat in the body along with an increase in body weight that exceeds the healthy range for the body's frame.

Obstetrics—Field of medicine concerned with the care of women during pregnancy and childbirth.

Obstruction—Something that blocks or closes up a passage or structure.

Occlusive dressing—Dressing (such as plastic kitchen wrap) that completely cuts off air to the skin.

Occult—Concealed, hidden, or of unknown cause; cannot be seen by the human eye; detectable only by microscope or chemical testing, as for occult blood in the stools or feces.

Ophthalmic—Relating to the eye.

Opioid—1. Any synthetic narcotic with opium-like actions; not derived from opium. 2. Natural chemicals that produce opium-like effects by acting at the same cell sites where opium exerts action.

Oral—Relating to the mouth.

Orchitis—Inflammation of the testis.

Osteitis deformans—See Paget's disease.

Osteomalacia—Softening of the bones due to lack of vitamin D.

Osteoporosis—Loss of calcium from bone tissue, resulting in bones that are brittle and easily fractured.

OTC (over the counter)—Refers to medicine or devices available without a prescription.

Otic—Relating to the ear.

Otitis media—Inflammation of the middle ear.

Ototoxicity—Having a harmful effect on the organs or nerves of the ear concerned with hearing and balance.

Ovary—Female sex organ that produces egg cells and sex hormones. The two ovaries are in the lower abdomen, one on each side.

Overactive thyroid—See Hyperthyroidism.

Ovulation—Process by which an ovum is released from the ovary. In human menstruating females, this usually occurs once a month.

Ovum—Mature female sex or reproductive cell, or egg cell. It is capable of developing into a new organism if fertilized.

Paget's disease—Chronic bone disease, marked by thickening of the bones and severe pain. Also called *osteitis deformans.*

Pancreatitis—Inflammation of the pancreas.

Pancytopenia—Reduction in the number of red cells, all types of white cells, and platelets in the blood.

Paralysis agitans—See Parkinson's disease.

Parathyroid glands—Four small bodies situated beside the thyroid gland; secrete parathyroid hormone that regulates calcium and phosphorus metabolism.

Parenteral—Any method of administering medicine when the medicine cannot be given by mouth; most often refers to injecting a medicine into the body using a needle and syringe.

Parkinsonism—See Parkinson's disease.

Parkinson's disease—Brain disease marked by tremor (shaking), stiffness, and difficulty in moving. Also called *Parkinsonism, paralysis agitans,* or *shaking palsy.*

Patent ductus arteriosus (PDA)—Condition in babies in which an important blood vessel adjacent to the heart fails to close as it should, resulting in faulty circulation and serious health problems.

Pediculicide—Medicine that kills lice.

Pediculosis—Infestation of the body, pubis, or scalp with lice.

Pellagra—Disease caused by too little niacin, which results in scaly skin, diarrhea, and mental depression.

Pemphigus—Skin disease marked by successive outbreaks of blisters.

Peptic ulcer—Open sore in esophagus, stomach, or duodenum.

Peritoneum—Membrane sac lining the abdominal wall and covering the liver, stomach, spleen, gallbladder, and intestines.

Peritonitis—Inflammation of the peritoneum.

Peyronie's disease—Dense, fiber-like growth in the penis, which can be felt as an irregular hard lump, and which usually causes bending and pain when the penis is erect.

Pharynx—Space just behind the mouth that serves as a passageway for food from the mouth to the esophagus and for air from the nose and mouth to the larynx.

Phenol—Substance used as a preservative for some injectable medicines.

Pheochromocytoma—Tumor of the adrenal medulla.

Phlebitis—Inflammation of a vein.

Phlegm—Thick mucus produced in the respiratory passages.

Piles—See Hemorrhoids.

Pituitary gland—Pea-sized body located at the base of the skull. It produces a number of hormones that are essential to normal body growth and functioning.

Placebo—Medicine that, unknown to the patient, has no active medicinal substance; its use may relieve or improve a condition because the patient believes it will. Also called *sugar pill.*

Plaque, dental—Mixture of saliva, bacteria, and carbohydrates that forms on the teeth, leading to caries (cavities) and gum disease.

Platelet—Small, disk-shaped body found in the blood that plays an important role in blood clotting.

Platelet aggregation inhibitor—Medicine used to help

prevent the platelets in the blood from clumping together. This effect reduces the chance of heart attack or stroke in certain patients.

Pleura—Membrane covering the lungs and lining the chest cavity.

Pneumococcal—Relating to certain bacteria that cause pneumonia.

Pneumocystis carinii—Organism that causes pneumocystis carinii pneumonia.

Pneumocystis carinii pneumonia—A pulmonary disease of infants and weakened persons, including those with AIDS or those receiving drugs that weaken the immune system.

Polymorphous light eruption—A skin problem in certain people, which results from exposure to sunlight.

Polymyalgia rheumatica—A rheumatic disease, most common in elderly patients, which causes aching and stiffness in the shoulders and hips.

Polyp—Tumor or mass of tissue attached with a stalk or broad base; found in cavities such as the nose, uterus, or rectum.

Porphyria—A group of uncommon, usually inherited diseases of defective porphyrin metabolism.

Porphyrin—One of a number of pigments occurring in living organisms throughout nature; porphyrins are constituents of bile pigment, hemoglobin, and certain enzymes.

Prevent—To stop or to keep from happening.

Priapism—Prolonged abnormal, painful erection of the penis.

Proctitis—Inflammation of the rectum.

Progesterone—Natural steroid hormone responsible for preparing the uterus for pregnancy. If fertilization occurs, progesterone's actions carry on or maintain the pregnancy.

Progestin—A natural or synthetic hormone that has progesterone-like actions.

Prolactin—Hormone secreted by the pituitary gland that stimulates and maintains milk flow in women following childbirth.

Prolactinoma—A pituitary tumor; results in secretion of excess prolactin.

Prophylactic—1. Agent or medicine used to prevent the occurrence of a specific condition. 2. Condom.

Prostate—Gland surrounding the neck of the male urethra just below the base of the bladder. It secretes a fluid that constitutes a major portion of the semen.

Prosthesis—Any artificial substitute for a missing body part.

Protozoa—Tiny, one-celled animals; some cause diseases in humans.

Psoralen—Chemical found in plants and used in certain perfumes and medicines. Exposure to a psoralen and then to sunlight may increase the risk of severe burning.

Psoriasis—Chronic skin disease marked by itchy, scaly, red patches.

Psychosis—Severe mental illness marked by loss of contact with reality, often involving delusions, hallucinations, and disordered thinking.

Purpura—Condition marked by bleeding into the skin; skin rash or spots are first red, darken to purple, then fade to brownish-yellow.

PUVA—Treatment for psoriasis by use of a psoralen, such as methoxsalen or trioxsalen, and long-wave ultraviolet light.

Rachischisis—See Spina bifida.

Radiopaque agent—Substance that makes it easier to see an area of the body with x-rays. Radiopaque agents are used to help diagnose a variety of medical problems.

Radiopharmaceutical—Radioactive agent used to diagnose certain medical problems or treat certain diseases.

Raynaud's syndrome—Condition marked by paleness, numbness, and discomfort in the fingers when they are exposed to cold.

Rectal—Relating to the rectum.

Renal—Relating to the kidneys.

Reye's syndrome—Serious disease affecting the liver and brain that sometimes occurs after a virus infection, such as influenza or chickenpox. It occurs most often in young children and teenagers. The first sign of Reye's syndrome is usually severe, prolonged vomiting.

Rheumatic heart disease—Heart disease marked by scarring and chronic inflammation of the heart and its valves, occurring after rheumatic fever.

Rhinitis—Inflammation of the mucous membrane inside the nose.

Rickets—Bone disease usually caused by too little vitamin D, resulting in soft and malformed bones.

Ringworm—See Tinea.

Risk—The possibility of injury or of suffering harm.

River blindness—Tropical disease produced by infection with worms of the Onchocerca type. The condition usually causes severe itching and may cause blindness. Also called *Roble's disease, blinding filarial disease,* and *craw-craw.*

Rosacea—Skin disease of the face, usually in middle-aged and older persons. Also called *adult acne.*

Sarcoidosis—Chronic disorder in which the lymph nodes in many parts of the body are enlarged, and small fleshy swellings develop in the lungs, liver, and spleen.

Scabicide—Medicine used to treat scabies (itch mite) infection.

Scabies—Contagious dermatitis caused by a mite burrowing into the skin; characterized by tiny skin eruptions and severe itching.

Schistosomiasis—Tropical infection in which worms enter the skin from infested water and settle in the bladder or intestines, causing inflammation and scarring. Also called *bilharziasis*.

Schizophrenia—Severe mental disorder in which thinking, mood, and behavior are disturbed.

Scintigram—Image obtained by detecting radiation emitted from a radiopharmaceutical introduced into the body.

Scleroderma—Chronic disease first characterized by hardening, thickening, and shrinking of the skin; later, certain organs also are affected.

Scotoma—Area of decreased vision or total loss of vision in a part of the visual field; blind spot.

Scrotum—Sac that holds the testes (male sex glands).

Scurvy—Disease caused by a deficiency of vitamin C (ascorbic acid), marked by bleeding gums, bleeding beneath the skin, and body weakness.

Sebaceous gland—Skin gland that secretes sebum.

Seborrhea—Skin condition caused by the excess release of sebum from the sebaceous glands, accompanied by dandruff and oily skin.

Sebum—Fatty secretion produced by sebaceous (oil) glands of the skin.

Secretion—1. Process in which a gland in the body or on the surface of the body releases a substance for use. 2. The substance released by the gland.

Sedative-hypnotic—Medicine used to treat excessive nervousness, restlessness, or insomnia.

Sedation—A profoundly relaxed or calmed state.

Seizure—A sudden attack or convulsion, as in epilepsy or other disorders.

Semen—Fluid released from the penis at sexual climax. It is made up of sperm suspended in secretions from the reproductive tract.

Severe—Of a great degree, such as very serious pain or distress.

Shaking palsy—See Parkinson's disease.

Shingles—See Herpes zoster.

Shock—Severe disruption of cellular metabolism associated with reduced blood volume and blood pressure too low to supply adequate blood to the tissues.

Shunt—Surgical tube used to transfer blood or other fluid from one part of the body to another.

SIADH (secretion of inappropriate antidiuretic hormone) syndrome—Disease in which the body retains (keeps) more fluid than normal.

Sickle cell anemia—Hereditary disorder that predominantly affects blacks; caused by abnormal hemoglobin. The name comes from the sickle-shaped red blood cells found in the blood of patients.

Sinusitis—Inflammation of a sinus.

Sjögren's syndrome—Condition usually occurring in older women, marked by dry eyes, dry mouth, and rheumatoid arthritis.

Skeletal muscle relaxant—Medicine used to relax certain muscles and help relieve the pain and discomfort caused by strains, sprains, or other injury to the muscles.

SLE—See Lupus erythematosus, systemic.

Soluble—Able to be dissolved in a fluid.

Spasticity—Increase in normal muscular tone, causing stiff, awkward movements.

Spastic paralysis—Paralysis marked by muscle rigidity or spasticity in the part of the body that is paralyzed.

Sperm—Mature male reproductive or sex cell.

Spermicide—Substance that kills sperm.

Spina bifida—Birth defect in which the infant's spinal cord is partially exposed through a hole in the backbone. Also called *rachischisis*.

Stenosis—Abnormal narrowing of a passage or duct of the body.

Sterility—1. Inability to produce offspring. 2. The state of being free of living microorganisms.

Stimulant, respiratory—Medicine used to stimulate breathing.

Stomatitis—Inflammation of the mucous membrane of the mouth.

Streptokinase—Enzyme that dissolves blood clots.

Stroke—Very serious event which occurs when an artery to the brain becomes clogged by a blood clot or bursts and causes hemorrhage. Stroke can affect speech, memory, behavior, and other life patterns, and may result in paralysis. Also called *apoplexy.*

Stye—Infection of one or more sebaceous glands of the eyelid, marked by swelling.

Subcutaneous—Under the skin.

Sublingual—Under the tongue. A sublingual medicine is taken by placing it under the tongue and letting it slowly dissolve.

Sudden infant death syndrome (SIDS)—Death of an infant, usually while asleep, from an unknown cause. Also called *crib death* or *cot death.*

Sugar diabetes—See Diabetes mellitus.

Sugar pill—See Placebo.

Sulfite—Type of preservative; causes allergic reactions, such as asthma, in sensitive patients.

Sunscreen—Substance, usually a cream or lotion, that blocks ultraviolet light and helps prevent sunburn when applied to the skin.

Suppository—Mass of medicated material shaped for insertion into the rectum, vagina, or urethra. Suppository is solid at room temperature but melts at body temperature.

Suppressant—Medicine that stops an action or condition.

Suspension—A form of medicine in which the drug is mixed with a liquid but is not dissolved in it. When the liquid is left standing, particles settle at the bottom and the top portion turns clear. When shaken it is ready for use.

Syncope—Sudden loss of consciousness due to inadequate blood flow to the brain; fainting.

Syphilis—An infectious disease, usually transmitted by sexual contact. The three stages of the disease may be separated by months or years.

Syringe—Device used to inject liquids into the body, remove material from a part of the body, or wash out a body cavity.

Systemic—For general effects throughout the body; applies to most medicines when taken by mouth or given by injection.

Tachycardia—Abnormal rapid beating of the heart, usually at a rate over 100 beats per minute in adults.

Temporomandibular joint (TMJ)—Hinge that connects the lower jaw to the skull.

Tendinitis—Inflammation of a tendon.

Teratogenic—Causing abnormal development in an embryo or fetus resulting in birth defects.

Testosterone—Principal male sex hormone.

Tetany—Condition marked by spasm and twitching of the muscles, particularly those of the hands, feet, and face; caused by a decrease in the calcium ion concentration in the blood.

Therapeutic—Relating to the treatment of a specific condition.

Thimerosal—Chemical used as a preservative in some medicines, and as an antiseptic and disinfectant.

Thrombolytic agent—Substance that dissolves blood clots.

Thrombophlebitis—Inflammation of a vein accompanied by the formation of a blood clot.

Thrombus—Blood clot that obstructs a blood vessel or a cavity of the heart.

Thrush—See Candidiasis of the mouth.

Thyroid gland—Gland in the lower front of the neck. It

releases thyroid hormones, which control body metabolism.

Thyrotoxicosis—Condition resulting from excessive amounts of thyroid hormones in the blood, causing increased metabolism, fast heartbeat, tremors, nervousness, and increased sweating.

Tic—Repeated involuntary movement or spasm of a muscle.

Tic douloureux—See Neuralgia, trigeminal.

Tinea—Fungus infection of the surface of the skin, particularly the scalp, feet, and nails. Also called *ringworm.*

Tone—The slight, continuous tension present in resting muscles.

Topical—For local effects when applied directly to the skin.

Tourette's disorder—Condition usually marked with motor tics (jerking movements) and vocal tics (grunts, sniffs). Also called *Gilles de la Tourette syndrome.*

Toxemia—Blood poisoning caused by bacterial production of toxins.

Toxemia of pregnancy—Condition occurring in pregnant women marked by hypertension, edema, excess protein in the urine, convulsions, and possibly coma.

Toxic—Poisonous; related to or caused by a toxin or poison.

Toxin—A substance produced by an animal or plant that is poisonous to another organism.

Toxoplasmosis—Disease caused by a blood protozoan, usually transmitted to humans from cats or by eating raw meat; generally the symptoms are mild and self-limited.

Tracheostomy—A surgical opening through the throat into the trachea (windpipe) to bypass an obstruction to breathing.

Tranquilizer—Medicine that produces a calming effect. It is used to relieve mental anxiety and tension.

Transdermal—A means of administering medicine into the body by use of skin patches or disks, or ointment; medicine contained in the patch or disk or the ointment is absorbed through the skin.

Trichomoniasis—Infection of the vagina resulting in inflammation of genital tissues and discharge. It can be passed on to males.

Triglyceride—A molecular form in which fats are present in food and the body; triglycerides are stored in the body as fat.

Trypanosome fever—See Trypanosomiasis, African.

Trypanosomiasis, African—Tropical disease, transmitted by tsetse fly bites, which causes fever, headache, and chills, followed by enlarged lymph nodes and anemia. Months or even years later, the disease affects the central nervous system, causing drowsiness and lethargy, coma, and death. Also called *African sleeping sickness*.

Tuberculosis (TB)—Infectious disease which may affect any organ but most commonly the lungs; symptoms include fever, night sweats, weight loss, and spitting up blood.

Tumor—Abnormal growth or enlargement in or on a part of the body.

Tyramine—Chemical present in many foods and beverages. Its structure and action in the body are similar to epinephrine.

Ulcer—Open sore or break in the skin or mucous membrane; often fails to heal and is accompanied by inflammation.

Ulcerative colitis—Chronic, recurrent inflammation and ulceration of the colon.

Ulceration—1. Formation or development of an ulcer. 2. Condition of an area marked with ulcers loosely associated with one another.

Underactive thyroid—See Hypothyroidism.

Ureter—Tube through which urine passes from the kidney to the bladder.

Urethra—Tube through which urine passes from the bladder to the outside of the body.

Urticaria—Hives; an eruption of itching wheals on the skin.

Vaccine—Medicine given by mouth or by injection to produce immunity to a certain infection.

Vaccinia—The skin and sometimes body reactions associated with smallpox vaccine. Also called *cowpox*.

Vaginal—Relating to the vagina.

Varicella—Very infectious virus disease marked by fever and itchy rash that develops into blisters and then scabs. Also called *chickenpox*.

Vascular—Relating to the blood vessels.

Vasodilator—Medicine that dilates the blood vessels, permitting increased blood flow.

Ventricular fibrillation—Life-threatening condition of fine, quivering, irregular movements of many individual muscle fibers of the ventricular muscle; replaces the normal heartbeat and interrupts pumping function.

Ventricle—A small cavity, such as one of the two lower chambers of the heart or one of the several cavities of the brain.

Vertigo—Sensation of whirling motion or dizziness, either of oneself or of one's surroundings.

Veterinary—Relating to animals and their diseases and treatment.

Virus—Any of a group of simple microbes too small to be seen by a light microscope. They can grow and reproduce only in living cells. Many cause diseases in humans, including the common cold.

Vitiligo—Condition in which some areas of skin lose pigment and turn white. Also called *leukoderma*.

von Willebrand's disease—Hereditary blood disease in which blood clotting is delayed, leading to excessive and uncontrolled bleeding even after minor injuries.

Water diabetes—See Diabetes insipidus.

Water pill—See Diuretic.

Wheal—Temporary, small, raised area of the skin, usually accompanied by itching or burning; welt.

Wheezing—A whistling sound made when there is difficulty in breathing.

White mouth—See Candidiasis of the mouth.

Wilson's disease—Inborn defect in the body's ability to process copper. Too much copper may lead to jaundice, cirrhosis, mental retardation, or symptoms like those of Parkinson's disease.

Zollinger-Ellison syndrome—Disorder in which the stomach produces too much acid, leading to ulcers.

CONTRIBUTORS

USP People 1990–1995

OFFICERS

Mark Novitch, M.D., *President*, Washington, DC
Donald R. Bennett, M.D., Ph.D., *Vice-President*, Chicago, IL
John T. Fay, Jr., Ph.D., *Treasurer*, San Clemente, CA
Arthur Hull Hayes, Jr., M.D., *Past President*, New
    Rochelle, NY
Jerome A. Halperin, *Secretary*, Rockville, MD

BOARD OF TRUSTEES

James T. Doluisio, Ph.D.[1], *Chair*, Austin, TX
Donald R. Bennett, M.D., Ph.D., *ex officio*, Chicago, IL
John V. Bergen, Ph.D.[2], *Vice Chair*, Villanova, PA
Edwin D. Bransome, Jr., M.D.[3], Augusta, GA
Jordan L. Cohen, Ph.D.[1], Lexington, KY
J. Richard Crout, M.D.[3], Rockville, MD
John T. Fay, Jr., Ph.D., *ex officio*, San Clemente, CA
Arthur Hull Hayes, Jr., M.D., *ex officio*, New Rochelle, NY
Joseph A. Mollica, Ph.D.[2], Wilmington, DE
Grace Powers Monaco, J.D.[4], Washington, DC
Mark Novitch, M.D., *ex officio*, Washington, DC

GENERAL COMMITTEE OF REVISION

Jerome A. Halperin[5], *Executive Director, USPC, Chairman*
Lee T. Grady, Ph.D.[5], *Director, Drug Standards Division*
Keith W. Johnson[5], *Director, Drug Information Division*
Loyd V. Allen, Jr., Ph.D., Oklahoma City, OK
Jerry R. Allison, Ph.D., New Brunswick, NJ
Thomas J. Ambrosio, Ph.D., Somerville, NJ
Gregory E. Amidon, Ph.D., Kalamazoo, MI
Norman W. Atwater, Ph.D., Hopewell, NJ

---

[1]Representing pharmacy.
[2]At large.
[3]Representing medicine.
[4]Public member.
[5]12601 Twinbrook Parkway, Rockville, MD 20852.

Henry L. Avallone, B.Sc., North Brunswick, NJ
Leonard C. Bailey, Ph.D., Piscataway, NJ
John A. Belis, M.D., Hershey, PA
Leslie Z. Benet, Ph.D., San Francisco, CA
Judy P. Boehlert, Ph.D., Nutley, NJ
James C. Boylan, Ph.D., Abbott Park, IL
Lynn R. Brady, Ph.D.[6], (1990–1992), Seattle, WA
R. Edward Branson, Ph.D., Beltsville, MD
William H. Briner, Capt., B.S., Durham, NC
Stephen R. Byrn, Ph.D., West Lafayette, IN
Peter R. Byron, Ph.D., Richmond, VA
Herbert S. Carlin, D.Sc., Florham Park, NJ
Dennis L. Casey, Ph.D., Raritan, NJ
Lester Chafetz, Ph.D., Kansas City, MO
Virginia C. Chamberlain, Ph.D., Rockville, MD
Wei-Wei, Chang, Ph.D., (1992–), Morris Plains, NJ
Mary Beth Chenault, B.S., Harrisonburg, VA
Zak T. Chowhan, Ph.D., Palo Alto, CA
Sebastian G. Ciancio, D.D.S., Buffalo, NY
Murray S. Cooper, Ph.D., Islamorada, FL
Lloyd E. Davis, Ph.D., D.V.M., Urbana, IL
Leon Ellenbogen, Ph.D., Clifton, NJ
R. Michael Enzinger, Ph.D., (1990–1992), Kalamazoo, MI
Clyde R. Erskine, B.S., M.B.A., Newtown Square, PA
Edward A. Fitzgerald, Ph.D., Bethesda, MD
Everett Flanigan, Ph.D., Kankakee, IL
Klaus G. Florey, Ph.D., Princeton, NJ
Thomas S. Foster, Pharm.D., Lexington, KY
Joseph F. Gallelli, Ph.D., Bethesda, MD
Robert L. Garnick, Ph.D., So. San Francisco, CA
Douglas D. Glover, M.D., R.Ph., Morgantown, WV
Alan M. Goldberg, Ph.D., Baltimore, MD
Burton J. Goldstein, M.D., Williams Island, FL
Dennis K. J. Gorecki, Ph.D., Saskatoon, Saskatchewan,
  Canada
Michael J. Groves, Ph.D., Lake Forest, IL
Robert M. Guthrie, M.D., Columbus, OH
Samir A. Hanna, Ph.D., Lawrenceville, NJ
Stanley L. Hem, Ph.D., West Lafayette, IN
Joy Hochstadt, Ph.D., New York, NY

---

[6]Deceased.

David W. Hughes, Ph.D., (1990–1993), Nepean, Ontario, Canada

Norman C. Jamieson, Ph.D., St. Louis, MO

Richard D. Johnson, Pharm.D., Ph.D., Kansas City, MO

Judith K. Jones, M.D., Ph.D., Arlington, VA

Stanley A. Kaplan, Ph.D., Baltimore, MD

Herbert E. Kaufman, M.D., New Orleans, LA

Donald Kaye, M.D., Philadelphia, PA

Paul E. Kennedy, Ph.D., West Conshohocken, PA

Jay S. Keystone, M.D., Toronto, Ontario, Canada

Rosalyn C. King, Pharm.D., M.P.H., Silver Spring, MD

Gordon L. Klein, M.D., Galveston, TX

Joseph E. Knapp, Ph.D., Pittsburgh, PA

John B. Landis, Ph.D. (1990–1992), Kalamazoo, MI

Thomas P. Layloff, Ph.D., St. Louis, MO

Lewis J. Leeson, Ph.D., Summit, NJ

John W. Levchuk, Ph.D., Rockville, MD

Robert D. Lindeman, M.D., Albuquerque, NM

Charles H. Lochmüller, Ph.D., Durham, NC

Edward G. Lovering, Ph.D., Nepean, Ontario, Canada

Catherine M. MacLeod, M.D., Chicago, IL

Carol S. Marcus, Ph.D., M.D., Torrance, CA

Tibor I. Matula, Ph.D., (1993–), Ottawa, Ontario, Canada

Thomas Medwick, Ph.D., Piscataway, NJ

Robert F. Morrissey, Ph.D., New Brunswick, NJ

Terry E. Munson, B.S., Fairfax, VA

Harold S. Nelson, M.D., Denver, CO

Wendel L. Nelson, Ph.D., Seattle, WA

Maria I. New, M.D., New York, NY

Sharon C. Northup, Ph.D., Round Lake, IL

Jeffery L. Otto, Ph.D., (1992–), Broomfield, CO

Garnet E. Peck, Ph.D., West Lafayette, IN

Robert V. Petersen, Ph.D., Salt Lake City, UT

Rosemary C. Polomano, R.N., M.S.N., Philadelphia, PA

Thomas P. Reinders, Pharm.D., Richmond, VA

Christopher T. Rhodes, Ph.D., West Kingston, RI

Joseph R. Robinson, Ph.D., Madison, WI

Lary A. Robinson, M.D., Tampa, FL

David B. Roll, Ph.D., Salt Lake City, UT

Theodore J. Roseman, Ph.D., Round Lake, IL

Sanford H. Roth, M.D., Phoenix, AZ

Leonard P. Rybak, M.D., Springfield, IL

Robert V. Petersen, Ph.D.
Robert S. Stern, M.D.
Paul F. White, Ph.D., M.D.

DRUG INFORMATION DIVISION EXECUTIVE COMMITTEE (1994–1995)

Herbert S. Carlin, D.Sc., *Chair*

James C. Boylan, Ph.D.
Sebastian G. Ciancio, D.D.S.
Lloyd E. Davis, D.V.M., Ph.D.
Jay S. Keystone, M.D.
Robert D. Lindeman, M.D.
Maria I. New, M.D.
Rosemary C. Polomano, R.N., M.S.N.
Thomas P. Reinders, Pharm.D.
Gordon D. Schiff, M.D.
Albert L. Sheffer, M.D.
Theodore G. Tong, Pharm.D.
Robert E. Vestal, M.D.
John W. Yarbro, M.D., Ph.D.

DRUG STANDARDS DIVISION EXECUTIVE COMMITTEE (1994–1995)

James T. Stewart, Ph.D. *Chair*

Jerry R. Allison, Ph.D.
Judy P. Boehlert, Ph.D.
Capt. William H. Briner, B.S.
Herbert S. Carlin, D.Sc.
Lester Chafetz, Ph.D.
Zak T. Chowhan, Ph.D.
Murray S. Cooper, Ph.D.
Klaus G. Florey, Ph.D.
Joseph F. Gallelli, Ph.D.
Robert L. Garnick, Ph.D.
Thomas P. Layloff, Ph.D.
Lewis J. Leeson, Ph.D.
Thomas Medwick, Ph.D.
Robert F. Morrissey, Ph.D.
Sharon C. Northup, Ph.D.
Ralph F. Shangraw, Ph.D.

DRUG NOMENCLATURE COMMITTEE
(1994–1995)

Herbert S. Carlin, D.Sc., *Chair*

William M. Heller, Ph.D., *Consultant/Advisor*

Lester Chafetz, Ph.D.

Lloyd E. Davis, D.V.M., Ph.D.

Everett Flanigan, Ph.D.

Douglas D. Glover, M.D.

Richard D. Johnson, Pharm.D., Ph.D.

Edward G. Lovering, Ph.D.

Rosemary C. Polomano, R.N., M.S.N.

Thomas P. Reinders, Pharm.D.

Eric B. Sheinin, Ph.D.

Philip D. Walson, M.D.

Drug Information Division Advisory Panels

Members who serve as Chairs are listed first.

The information presented in this text represents an ongoing review of the drugs contained herein and represents a consensus of various viewpoints expressed. The individuals listed below have served on the USP Advisory Panels for the 1993–1994 revision period and have contributed to the development of the 1995 USP DI database. Such listing does not imply that these individuals have reviewed all of the material in this text or that they individually agree with all statements contained herein.

Anesthesiology

Paul F. White, Ph.D., M.D., *Chair*, Dallas, TX; Eugene Y. Cheng, M.D., Milwaukee, WI; Charles J. Coté, M.D., Chicago, IL; Robert Feinstein, M.D., St. Louis, MO; Peter S.A. Glass, M.D., Durham, NC; Michael B. Howie, M.D., Columbus, OH; Beverly A. Krause, C.R.N.A., M.S., St. Louis, MO; Carl Lynch, III, M.D., Ph.D., Charlottesville, VA; Carl Rosow, M.D., Ph.D., Boston, MA; Peter S. Sebel, M.B., Ph.D., Atlanta, GA; Walter L. Way, M.D., Greenbrae, CA; Matthew B. Weinger, M.D., San Diego, CA; Richard Weiskopf, M.D., San Francisco, CA; David H. Wong, Pharm.D., M.D., Long Beach, CA

Cardiovascular and Renal Drugs
Burton E. Sobel, M.D., *Chair*, St. Louis, MO; William P. Baker, M.D., Ph.D., Bethesda, MD; Nils U. Bang, M.D., Indianapolis, IN; Emmanuel L. Bravo, M.D., Cleveland, OH; Mary Jo Burgess, M.D., Salt Lake City, UT; James H. Chesebro, M.D., Boston, MA; Peter Corr, Ph.D., St. Louis, MO; Dwain L. Eckberg, M.D., Richmond, VA; Ruth Eshleman, Ph.D., W. Kingston, RI; William H. Frishman, M.D., Bronx, NY; Edward D. Frohlich, M.D., New Orleans, LA; Martha Hill, Ph.D., R.N., Baltimore, MD; Norman M. Kaplan, M.D., Dallas, TX; Michael Lesch, M.D., Detroit, MI; Manuel Martinez-Maldonado, M.D., Decatur, GA; Patrick A. McKee, M.D., Oklahoma City, OK; Dan M. Roden, M.D., Nashville, TN; Michael R. Rosen, M.D., New York, NY; Jane Schultz, R.N., B.S.N., Rochester, MN; Robert L. Talbert, Pharm.D., San Antonio, TX; Raymond L. Woosley, M.D., Ph.D., Washington, DC

Clinical Immunology/Allergy/Rheumatology
Albert L. Sheffer, M.D., *Chair*, Boston, MA; John A. Anderson, M.D., Detroit, MI; Emil Bardana, Jr., M.D., Portland, OR; John Baum, M.D., Rochester, NY; Debra Danoff, M.D., Montreal, Quebec; Daniel G. de Jesus, M.D., Ph.D., Vanier, Ontario; Elliott F. Ellis, M.D., Jacksonville, FL; Patricia A. Fraser, M.D., Boston, MA; Frederick E. Hargreave, M.D., Hamilton, Ontario; Evelyn V. Hess, M.D., Cincinnati, OH; Jean M. Jackson, M.D., Boston, MA; Stephen R. Kaplan, M.D., Buffalo, NY; Sandra M. Koehler, Milwaukee, WI; Richard A. Moscicki, M.D., Newton, MA; Shirley Murphy, M.D., Albuquerque, NM; Gary S. Rachelefsky, M.D., Los Angeles, CA; Robert E. Reisman, M.D., Buffalo, NY; Robert L. Rubin, Ph.D., La Jolla, CA; Daniel J. Stechschulte, M.D., Kansas City, KS; Virginia S. Taggert, Bethesda, MD; Joseph A. Tami, Pharm.D., San Antonio, TX; John H. Toogood, M.D., London, Ontario; Martin D. Valentine, M.D., Baltimore, MD; Michael Weinblatt, M.D., Boston, MA; Dennis Michael Williams, Pharm.D., Chapel Hill, NC; Stewart Wong, Ph.D., Annandale, VA

Clinical Toxicology/Substance Abuse
Theodore G. Tong, Pharm.D., *Chair*, Tucson, AZ; John Ambre, M.D., Ph.D., Chicago, IL; Usoa E. Busto, Pharm.D., Toronto, Ontario; Darryl Inaba, Pharm.D., San Francisco, CA; Edward P. Krenzelok, Pharm.D., Pittsburgh, PA; Michael Montagne,

Ph.D., Boston, MA; Sven A. Normann, Pharm.D., Tampa, FL; Gary M. Oderda, Pharm.D., Salt Lake City, UT; Paul Pentel, M.D., Minneapolis, MN; Rose Ann Soloway, R.N., Washington, DC; Daniel A. Spyker, M.D., Ph.D., Rockville, MD; Anthony R. Temple, M.D., Ft. Washington, PA; Anthony Tommasello, Pharm.D., Baltimore, MD; Joseph C. Veltri, Pharm.D., Salt Lake City, UT; William A. Watson, Pharm.D., Kansas City, MO

Consumer Interest/Health Education

Gordon D. Schiff, M.D., *Chair*, Chicago, IL; Michael J. Ackerman, Ph.D., Bethesda, MD; Barbara Aranda-Naranjo, R.N., San Antonio, TX; Frank J. Ascione, Pharm.D., Ph.D., Ann Arbor, MI; Judith I. Brown, Silver Spring, MD; Jose Camacho, Austin, TX; Margaret A. Charters, Ph.D., Syracuse, NY; Jennifer Cross, San Francisco, CA; William G. Harless, Ph.D., Bethesda, MD; Louis H. Kompare, Lake Buena Vista, FL; Margo Kroshus, R.N., B.S.N., Rochester, MN; Marilyn Lister, Wakefield, Quebec; Margaret Lueders, Seattle, WA; Frederick S. Mayer, R.Ph., M.P.H., Sausalito, CA; Nancy Milio, Ph.D., Chapel Hill, NC; Irving Rubin, Port Washington, NY; T. Donald Rucker, Ph.D., River Forest, IL; Stephen B. Soumerai, Sc.D., Boston, MA; Carol A. Vetter, Rockville, MD

Critical Care Medicine

Catherine M. MacLeod, M.D., *Chair*, Chicago, IL; William Banner, Jr., M.D., Salt Lake City, UT; Philip S. Barie, M.D., New York, NY; Thomas P. Bleck, M.D., Charlottesville, VA; Roger C. Bone, M.D., Toledo, OH; Susan S. Fish, Pharm.D., Boston, MA; Edgar R. Gonzalez, Pharm.D., Richmond, VA; Robert Gottesman, Rockville, MD; John W. Hoyt, M.D., Pittsburgh, PA; Sheldon A. Magder, M.D., Montreal, Quebec; Joseph E. Parrillo, M.D., Chicago, IL; Sharon Peters, M.D., St. John's, Newfoundland; Domenic A. Sica, M.D., Richmond, VA; Martin G. Tweeddale, M.B., Ph.D., Vancouver, British Columbia

Dentistry

Sebastian G. Ciancio, D.D.S., *Chair*, Buffalo, NY; Donald F. Adams, D.D.S., Portland, OR; Karen A. Baker, M.S. Pharm., Iowa City, IA; Stephen A. Cooper, D.M.D., Ph.D., Philadelphia, PA; Frederick A. Curro, D.M.D., Ph.D., Jersey City, NJ; Paul J. Desjardins, D.M.D., Ph.D., Newark, NJ; Tommy W. Gage, D.D.S., Ph.D., Dallas, TX; Stephen F. Goodman,

D.D.S., New York, NY; Daniel A. Haas, D.D.S., Ph.D., Toronto, Ontario; Richard E. Hall, D.D.S., Ph.D., Buffalo, NY; Lireka P. Joseph, Dr.P.H., Rockville, MD; Janice Lieberman, Fort Lee, NJ; Laurie Lisowski, Lewiston, NY; Clarence L. Trummel, D.D.S., Ph.D., Farmington, CT; Joel M. Weaver, II, D.D.S., Ph.D., Columbus, OH; Clifford W. Whall, Jr., Ph.D., Chicago, IL; Raymond P. White, Jr., D.D.S., Ph.D., Chapel Hill, NC; Ray C. Williams, D.M.D., Boston, MA

Dermatology

Robert S. Stern, M.D., *Chair*, Boston, MA; Beatrice B. Abrams, Ph.D., Somerville, NJ; Richard D. Baughman, M.D., Hanover, NH; Michael Bigby, M.D., Boston, MA; Janice T. Chussil, R.N., M.S.N., Portland, OR; Stuart Maddin, M.D., Vancouver, British Columbia; Milton Orkin, M.D., Robbinsdale, MN; Neil H. Shear, M.D., Toronto, Ontario; Edgar Benton Smith, M.D., Galveston, TX; Dennis P. West, M.S. Pharm., Lincolnshire, IL; Gail M. Zimmerman, Portland, OR

Diagnostic Agents—Nonradioactive

Robert L. Siegle, M.D., *Chair*, San Antonio, TX; Kaizer Aziz, Ph.D., Rockville, MD; Robert C. Brasch, M.D., San Francisco, CA; Nicholas Harry Malakis, M.D., Bethesda, MD; Robert F. Mattrey, M.D., San Diego, CA; James A. Nelson, M.D., Seattle, WA; Jovitas Skucas, M.D., Rochester, NY; Gerald L. Wolf, Ph.D., M.D., Charlestown, MA

Drug Information Science

James A. Visconti, Ph.D., *Chair*, Columbus, OH; Marie A. Abate, Pharm.D., Morgantown, WV; Ann B. Amerson, Pharm.D., Lexington, KY; Philip O. Anderson, Pharm.D., San Diego, CA; Danial E. Baker, Pharm.D., Spokane, WA; C. David Butler, Pharm.D., M.B.A., Naperville, IL; Linda L. Hart, Pharm.D., Saddle River, NJ; Edward J. Huth, M.D., Philadelphia, PA; John M. Kessler, Pharm.D., Chapel Hill, NC; R. David Lauper, Pharm.D., Emeryville, CA; Domingo R. Martinez, Pharm.D., Birmingham, AL; William F. McGhan, Pharm.D., Ph.D., Philadelphia, PA; John K. Murdoch, B.Sc.Phm., Toronto, Ontario; Kurt A. Proctor, Ph.D., Alexandria, VA; Arnauld F. Scafidi, M.D., M.P.H., Rockville, MD; John A. Scarlett, M.D., Austin, TX; Gary H. Smith, Pharm.D., Tucson, AZ; Dennis F. Thompson, Pharm.D., Oklahoma City, OK; William G. Troutman, Pharm.D., Albuquerque, NM; Lee A. Wanke, M.S., Houston, TX

Drug Utilization Review

Judith K. Jones, M.D., Ph.D., *Chair*, Arlington, VA; John F.
Beary, III, M.D., Washington, DC; James L. Blackburn,
Pharm.D., Saskatoon, Saskatchewan; Richard S. Blum, M.D.,
East Hills, NY; Amy Cooper-Outlaw, Pharm.D., Stone Moun-
tain, GA; Joseph W. Cranston, Jr., Ph.D., Chicago, IL;
W. Gary Erwin, Pharm.D., Philadelphia, PA; Jere E. Goyan,
Ph.D., Saddle River, NJ; Duane M. Kirking, Ph.D., Ann
Arbor, MI; Karen E. Koch, Pharm.D., Tupelo, MS; Aida A.
LeRoy, Pharm.D., Arlington, VA; Jerome Levine, M.D., Bal-
timore, MD; Richard W. Lindsay, M.D., Charlottesville, VA;
M. Laurie Mashford, M.D., Melbourne, Victoria, Australia;
Deborah M. Nadzam, R.N., Ph.D., Oakbrook Terrace, IL;
William Z. Potter, M.D., Ph.D., Bethesda, MD; Louise R.
Rodriquez, M.S., Washington, DC; Stephen P. Spielberg,
M.D., Ph.D., West Point, PA; Suzan M. Streichenwein, M.D.,
Houston, TX; Brian L. Strom, M.D., Philadelphia, PA; Mi-
chael Weintraub, M.D., Rockville, MD; Antonio Carlos Za-
nãini, M.D., Ph.D., Sao Paulo, Brazil

Endocrinology

Maria I. New, M.D., *Chair*, New York, NY; Ronald D. Brown,
M.D., Oklahoma City, OK; R. Keith Campbell, Pharm.D.,
Pullman, WA; David S. Cooper, M.D., Baltimore, MD; Betty
J. Dong, Pharm.D., San Francisco, CA; Andrea Dunaif, M.D.,
New York, NY; Anke A. Ehrhardt, Ph.D., New York, NY;
Nadir R. Farid, M.D., Durham, N.C.; John G. Haddad, Jr.,
M.D., Philadelphia, PA; Michael M. Kaplan, M.D., Southfield,
MI; Harold E. Lebovitz, M.D., Brooklyn, NY; Marvin E. Levin,
M.D., Chesterfield, MO; Marvin M. Lipman, M.D., Scarsdale,
NY; Barbara J. Maschak-Carey, R.N., M.S.N., Philadelphia,
PA; James C. Melby, M.D., Boston, MA; Walter J. Meyer, III,
M.D., Galveston, TX; Rita Nemchik, R.N., M.S., C.D.E., Flor-
ence, NJ; Daniel A. Notterman, M.D., New York, NY; Ron
Gershon Rosenfeld, M.D., Stanford, CA; Paul Saenger, M.D.,
Bronx, NY; Leonard Wartofsky, M.D., Washington, DC

Family Practice

Robert M. Guthrie, M.D., *Chair*, Columbus, OH; Jack A. Brose,
D.O., Athens, OH; Jannet M. Carmichael, Pharm.D., Reno,
NV; Jacqueline A. Chadwick, M.D., Scottsdale, AZ; Mark E.
Clasen, M.D., Ph.D., Dayton, OH; Lloyd P. Haskell, M.D.,
West Borough, MA; Luis A. Izquierdo-Mora, M.D., Rio Pie-
dras, PR; Edward L. Langston, M.D., Houston, TX; Stephen

T. O'Brien, M.D., Enfield, CT; Charles D. Ponte, Pharm.D.,
Morgantown, WV; Jack M. Rosenberg, Pharm.D., Ph.D.,
Brooklyn, NY; John F. Sangster, M.D., London, Ontario;
Theodore L. Yarboro, Sr., M.D., M.P.H., Sharon, PA

Gastroenterology
Gordon L. Klein, M.D., *Chair*, Galveston, TX; Karl E. Anderson,
M.D., Galveston, TX; William Balistreri, M.D., Cincinnati,
OH; Paul Bass, Ph.D., Madison, WI; Rosemary R. Berardi,
Pharm.D., Ann Arbor, MI; Raymond F. Burk, M.D., Nash-
ville, TN; Thomas Q. Garvey, III, M.D., Potomac, MD; Don-
ald J. Glotzer, M.D., Boston, MA; Flavio Habal, M.D.,
Toronto, Ontario; Paul E. Hyman, M.D., Torrance, CA; Ber-
nard Mehl, D.P.S., New York, NY; William J. Snape, Jr.,
M.D., Torrance, CA; Ronald D. Soltis, M.D., Minneapolis,
MN; C. Noel Williams, M.D., Halifax, Nova Scotia; Hyman
J. Zimmerman, M.D., Bethesda, MD

Geriatrics
Robert E. Vestal, M.D., *Chair*, Boise, ID; Darrell R. Abernethy,
M.D., Washington, DC; William B. Abrams, M.D., West
Point, PA; Jerry Avorn, M.D., Boston, MA; Robert A. Blouin,
Pharm.D., Lexington, KY; S. George Carruthers, M.D., Hali-
fax, Nova Scotia; Lynn E. Chaitovitz, Rockville, MD; Terry
Fulmer, R.N., Ph.D., New York, NY; Philip P. Gerbino,
Pharm.D., Philadelphia, PA; Pearl S. German, Sc.D., Balti-
more, MD; David J. Greenblatt, M.D., Boston, MA; Martin
D. Higbee, Pharm.D., Tucson, AZ; Brian B. Hoffman, M.D.,
Palo Alto, CA; J. Edward Jackson, M.D., San Diego, CA;
Joseph V. Levy, Ph.D., San Francisco, CA; Paul A. Mitenko,
M.D., FRCPC, Nanaimo, British Columbia; John E. Morley,
M.B., B.Ch., St. Louis, MO; Jay Roberts, Ph.D., Philadelphia,
PA; Louis J. Rubenstein, R.Ph., Alexandria, VA; Janice B.
Schwartz, M.D., San Francisco, CA; Alexander M.M. Shep-
herd, M.D., San Antonio, TX; William Simonson, Pharm.D.,
Portland, OR; Daniel S. Sitar, Ph.D., Winnipeg, Manitoba;
Mary K. Walker, R.N., Ph.D., Lexington, KY; Alastair J. J.
Wood, M.D., Nashville, TN

Hematologic and Neoplastic Disease
John W. Yarbro, M.D., Ph.D., *Chair*, Springfield, IL; Joseph S.
Bailes, M.D., McAllen, TX; Laurence H. Baker, D.O., Ann
Arbor, MI; Barbara D. Blumberg-Carnes, Albuquerque, NM;
Helene G. Brown, B.S., Los Angeles, CA; Nora L. Burnham,

Pharm.D., Princeton, NJ; William J. Dana, Pharm.D., Houston, TX; Connie Henke-Yarbro, R.N., B.S.N., Springfield, IL; William H. Hryniuk, M.D., San Diego, CA; B. J. Kennedy, M.D., Minneapolis, MN; Barnett Kramer, M.D., Rockville, MD; Michael J. Mastrangelo, M.D., Philadelphia, PA; David S. Rosenthal, M.D., Cambridge, MA; Richard L. Schilsky, M.D., Chicago, IL; Rowena N. Schwartz, Pharm.D., Pittsburgh, PA; Roy L. Silverstein, M.D., New York, NY; Samuel G. Taylor, IV, M.D., Chicago, IL; Raymond B. Weiss, M.D., Washington, DC

Infectious Disease Therapy

Donald Kaye, M.D., *Chair*, Philadelphia, PA; Robert Austrian, M.D., Philadelphia, PA; C. Glenn Cobbs, M.D., Birmingham, AL; Joseph W. Cranston, Jr., Ph.D., Chicago, IL; John J. Dennehy, M.D., Danville, PA; Courtney V. Fletcher, Pharm. D., Minneapolis, MN; Earl H. Freimer, M.D., Toledo, OH; Marc LeBel, Pharm.D., Quebec, Quebec; John D. Nelson, M.D., Dallas, TX; Lindsay E. Nicolle, M.D., Winnipeg, Manitoba; Alvin Novick, M.D., New Haven, CT; Charles G. Prober, M.D., Stanford, CA; Douglas D. Richman, M.D., San Diego, CA; Spotswood L. Spruance, M.D., Salt Lake City, UT; Roy T. Steigbigel, M.D., Stony Brook, NY; Paul F. Wehrle, M.D., San Clemente, CA

International Health

Rosalyn C. King, Pharm.D., M.P.H., *Chair*, Silver Spring, MD; Walter M. Batts, Rockville, MD; Eugenie Brown, Pharm.D., Kingston, Jamaica; Alan Cheung, Pharm.D., M.P.H., Washington, DC; Mary Couper, M.D., Geneva, Switzerland; Gabriel Daniel, Washington, DC; S. Albert Edwards, Pharm.D., Lincolnshire, IL; Enrique Fefer, Ph.D., Washington, DC; Peter H. M. Fontilus, Curaçao, Netherlands Antilles; Gan Ee Kiang, Penang, Malaysia; Marcellus Grace, Ph.D., New Orleans, LA; George B. Griffenhagen, Washington, DC; Margareta Helling-Borda, Geneva, Switzerland; Thomas Langston, Silver Spring, MD; Thomas Lapnet-Moustapha, Yaounde, Cameroon; David Lee, B.A., M.D., Arlington, VA; Aissatov Lo, Ka-Olack, Senegal; Stuart M. MacLeod, M.D., Hamilton, Ontario; Russell E. Morgan, Jr., Dr.P.H., Chevy Chase, MD; David Ofori-Adjei, M.D., Accra, Ghana; S. Ofosu-Amaah, M.D., New York, NY; James Rankin, Arlington, VA; Olikoye Ransome-Kuti, M.D., Lagos, Nigeria; Budiono Santoso, M.D., Ph.D., Yogyakarta, Indonesia; Carmen Selva, Ph.D., Madrid, Spain;

Valentin Vinogradov, Moscow, Russia; Fela Viso-Gurovich, Mexico City, Mexico; William B. Walsh, M.D., Chevy Chase, MD; Lawrence C. Weaver, Ph.D., Minneapolis, MN; Albert I. Wertheimer, Ph.D., Glen Allen, VA

Neurology

Stanley van den Noort, M.D., *Chair*, Irvine, CA; William T. Beaver, M.D., Washington, DC; Elizabeth U. Blalock, M.D., Anaheim, CA; James C. Cloyd, Pharm.D., Minneapolis, MN; David M. Dawson, M.D., West Roxbury, MA; Kevin Farrell, M.D., Vancouver, British Columbia; Kathleen M. Foley, M.D., New York, NY; Anthony E. Lang, M.D., Toronto, Ontario; Ira T. Lott, M.D., Orange, CA; James R. Nelson, M.D., La Jolla, CA; J. Kiffin Penry, M.D., Winston-Salem, NC; Neil H. Raskin, M.D., San Francisco, CA; Alfred J. Spiro, M.D., Bronx, NY; M. DiAnn Turek, R.N., Holt, MI

Nursing Practice

Rosemary C. Polomano, R.N., M.S.N., *Chair*, Philadelpia, PA; Mecca S. Cranley, R.N., Ph.D., Buffalo, NY; Jan M. Ellerhorst-Ryan, R.N., M.S.N., Cincinnati, OH; Linda Felver, Ph.D., R.N., Portland, OR; Hector Hugo Gonzalez, R.N., Ph.D., San Antonio, TX; Mary Harper, R.N., Ph.D., Rockville, MD; Ada K. Jacox, R.N., Ph.D., Baltimore, MD; Patricia Kummeth, R.N., M.S., Rochester, MN; Ida M. Martinson, R.N., Ph.D., San Francisco, CA; Carol P. Patton, R.N., Ph.D., J.D., Detroit, MI; Ginette A. Pepper, R.N., Ph.D., Englewood, CO; Geraldine A. Peterson, R.N., M.A., Potomac, MD; Linda C. Pugh, R.N., Ph.D., York, PA; Sharon S. Rising, R.N., C.N.M., Cheshire, CT; Marjorie Ann Spiro, R.N., B.S., C.S.N., Scarsdale, NY

Nutrition and Electrolytes

Robert D. Lindeman, M.D., *Chair*, Albuquerque, NM; Hans Fisher, Ph.D., New Brunswick, NJ; Walter H. Glinsmann, M.D., Washington, DC; Helen Andrews Guthrie, M.S., Ph.D., State College, PA; Steven B. Heymsfield, M.D., New York, NY; K. N. Jeejeebhoy, M.D., Toronto, Ontario; Leslie M. Klevay, M.D., Grand Forks, ND; Linda S. Knox, M.S.N., Philadelphia, PA; Bonnie Liebman, M.S., Washington, DC; Sudesh K. Mahajan, M.D., Grosse Point Woods, MI; Craig J. McClain, M.D., Lexington, KY; Jay M. Mirtallo, M.S., Columbus, OH; Sohrab Mobarhan, M.D., Maywood, IL; Robert M. Russell, M.D., Boston, MA; Harold H. Sandstead,

M.D., Galveston, TX; William J. Stone, M.D., Nashville, TN; Carlos A. Vaamonde, M.D., Miami, FL; Stanley Wallach, M.D., New York, NY

Obstetrics and Gynecology

Douglas D. Glover, M.D., *Chair*, Morgantown, WV; Rudi Ansbacher, M.D., Ann Arbor, MI; Florence Comite, M.D., New Haven, CT; James W. Daly, M.D., Columbia, MO; Marilynn C. Frederiksen, M.D., Chicago, IL; Charles B. Hammond, M.D., Durham, NC; Barbara A. Hayes, M.A., New Rochelle, NY; Art Jacknowitz, Pharm.D., Morgantown, WV; William J. Ledger, M.D., New York, NY; Andre-Marie Leroux, M.D., Ottawa, Ontario; William A. Nahhas, M.D., Dayton, OH; Warren N. Otterson, M.D., Shreveport, LA; Samuel A. Pasquale, M.D., New Brunswick, NJ; Johanna Perlmutter, M.D., Boston, MA; Robert W. Rebar, M.D., Cincinnati, OH; Richard H. Reindollar, M.D., Boston, MA; G. Millard Simmons, M.D., Morgantown, WV; J. Benjamin Younger, M.D., Birmingham, AL

Ophthalmology

Herbert E. Kaufman, M.D., *Chair*, New Orleans, LA; Steven R. Abel, Pharm.D., Indianapolis, IN; Jules Baum, M.D., Boston, MA; Lee R. Duffner, M.D., Miami, FL; David L. Epstein, M.D., Durham, NC; Allan J. Flach, Pharm.D., M.D., Corte Madera, CA; Vincent H. L. Lee, Ph.D., Los Angeles, CA; Steven M. Podos, M.D., New York, NY; Kirk R. Wilhelmus, M.D., Houston, TX; Thom J. Zimmerman, M.D., Ph.D., Louisville, KY

Otorhinolaryngology

Leonard P. Rybak, M.D., Ph.D., *Chair*, Springfield, IL; Robert E. Brummett, Ph.D., Portland, OR; Robert A. Dobie, M.D., San Antonio, TX; Linda J. Gardiner, M.D., Fort Myers, FL; David Hilding, M.D., Price, UT; David B. Hom, M.D., Minneapolis, MN; Helen F. Krause, M.D., Pittsburgh, PA; Richard L. Mabry, M.D., Dallas, TX; Lawrence J. Marentette, M.D., Ann Arbor, MI; Robert A. Mickel, M.D., Ph.D., San Francisco, CA; Randal A. Otto, M.D., San Antonio, TX; Richard W. Waguespack, M.D., Birmingham, AL; William R. Wilson, M.D., Washington, DC

Parasitic Disease

Jay S. Keystone, M.D., *Chair*, Toronto, Ontario; Michele Barry, M.D., New Haven, CT; Frank J. Bia, M.D., M.P.H., Guilford,

CT; David Botero, M.D., Medellín, Colombia; David O. Freedman, M.D., Birmingham, AL; Elaine C. Jong, M.D., Seattle, WA; Dennis D. Juranek, M.D., Atlanta, GA; Donald J. Krogstad, M.D., New Orleans, LA; Douglas W. MacPherson, M.D., Hamilton, Ontario; Edward K. Markell, M.D., Berkeley, CA; Theodore Nash, M.D., Bethesda, MD; Murray Wittner, M.D., Bronx, NY

Patient Counseling (Ad Hoc)
Frank J. Ascione, Pharm.D., Ph.D., *Chair*, Ann Arbor, MI; John E. Arradondo, M.D., Houston, TX; Candace Barnett, Atlanta, GA; Karin Bolte, Washington, DC; Allan H. Bruckheim, M.D., Harrison, NY; Mark Clasen, M.D., Ph.D., Dayton, OH; Amy Cooper-Outlaw, Pharm.D., Stone Mountain, GA; Frederick A. Curro, D.M.D., Ph.D., Jersey City, NJ; Robin DiMatteo, Ph.D., Riverside, CA; Diane B. Ginsburg, Austin, TX; Denise Grimes, R.N., Jackson, MI; Richard Herrier, Tucson, AZ; Barry Kass, R.Ph., Boston, MA; Thomas Kellenberger, Pharm.D., Montvale, NJ; Alice Kimball, Darnestown, MD; Pat Kramer, Bismarck, ND; Patti Kummeth, R.N., Rochester, MN; Ken Leibowitz, Philadelphia, PA; Colleen Lum Lung, R.N., Denver, CO; Louise Matte, Quebec, Canada; Scotti Milley, Richmond, VA; Constance Pavlides, R.N., D.N.Sc., Rockville, MD; Lisa Tedesco, Ph.D., Ann Arbor, MI

Pediatric Anesthesiology (Ad Hoc)
Charles J. Coté, M.D., *Chair*, Chicago, IL; J. Michael Badgwell, M.D., Lubbock, TX; Barbara Brandom, M.D., Pittsburgh, PA; Ryan Cook, M.D., Pittsburgh, PA; John J. Downes, M.D., Philadelphia, PA; Dennis Fisher, M.D., San Francisco, CA; John E. Forestner, M.D., Fort Worth, TX; Helen W. Karl, M.D., Seattle, WA; Harry G. G. Kingston, M.B., Portland, OR; Anne Marie Lynn, M.D., Seattle, WA; Mark Shriner, M.D. Philadelphia, PA; Victoria Simpson, M.D., Ph.D., Denver, CO; Meb Watcha, M.D., St. Louis, MO

Pediatrics
Philip D. Walson, M.D., *Chair*, Columbus, OH; Susan Alpert, Ph.D., M.D., Rockville, MD; Jacob V. Aranda, M.D., Ph.D., Montreal, Quebec; Cheston M. Berlin, Jr., M.D., Hershey, PA; Nancy Jo Braden, M.D., Phoenix, AZ; Patricia J. Bush, Ph.D., Washington, DC; Marion J. Finkel, M.D., Morris Township, NJ; George S. Goldstein, M.D., Briarcliff Manor, NY; Ralph E. Kauffman, M.D., Detroit, MI; Gideon Koren,

M.D., Toronto, Ontario; Joan M. Korth-Bradley, Pharm.D., Ph.D., Philadelphia, PA; Richard Leff, Pharm.D., Kansas City, KS; Carolyn Lund, R.N., M.S., San Francisco, CA; Wayne Snodgrass, M.D., Galveston, TX; Celia A. Viets, M.D., Ottawa, Canada; John T. Wilson, M.D., Shreveport, LA; Sumner J. Yaffe, M.D., Bethesda, MD; Karin E. Zenk, Pharm.D., Irvine, CA

Pharmacy Practice

Thomas P. Reinders, Pharm.D., *Chair*, Richmond, VA; Olya Duzey, M.S., Big Rapids, MI; Yves Gariepy, B.Sc.Pharm., Quebec, Quebec; Ned Heltzer, M.S., New Castle, DE; Lester S. Hosto, B.S., Little Rock, AR; Martin J. Jinks, Pharm.D., Pullman, WA; Frederick Klein, B.S., Montvale, NJ; Calvin H. Knowlton, Ph.D., Lumberton, NJ; Patricia A. Kramer, B.S., Bismarck, ND; Dennis McCallum, Pharm.D., Minneapolis, MN; Shirley P. McKee, B.S., Houston, TX; William A. McLean, Pharm.D., Ottawa, Ontario; Gladys Montañez, B.S., Santurce, PR; Donald L. Moore, B.S., Kokomo, IN; John E. Ogden, M.S., Washington, DC; Henry A. Palmer, Ph.D., Storrs, CT; Lorie G. Rice, B.A., M.P.H., San Francisco, CA; Mike R. Sather, M.S., Albuquerque, NM; Albert Sebok, B.S., Hudson, OH; William E. Smith, Pharm.D., Ph.D., Boston, MA; Susan East Torrico, B.S., Orlando, FL; J. Richard Wuest, Pharm.D., Cincinnati, OH; Glenn Y. Yokoyama, Pharm.D., Pasadena, CA

Psychiatric Disease

Burton J. Goldstein, M.D., *Chair*, Williams Island, FL; Magda Campbell, M.D., New York, NY; Alex A. Cardoni, M.S. Pharm., Hartford, CT; James L. Claghorn, M.D., Houston, TX; N. Michael Davis, M.S., Miami, FL; Larry Ereshefsky, Pharm.D., San Antonio, TX; W. Edwin Fann, M.D., Houston, TX; Alan J. Gelenberg, M.D., Tucson, AZ; Tracy R. Gordy, M.D., Austin, TX; Paul Grof, M.D., Ottawa, Ontario; Russell T. Joffe, M.D., Toronto, Ontario; Nathan Rawls, Pharm.D., Memphis, TN; Ruth Robinson, Saskatoon, Saskatchewan; Matthew V. Rudorfer, M.D., Rockville, MD; Karen A. Theesen, Pharm.D., Omaha, NE

Pulmonary Disease

Harold S. Nelson, M.D., *Chair*, Denver, CO; Richard C. Ahrens, M.D., Iowa City, IA; Eugene R. Bleecker, M.D., Baltimore, MD; William W. Busse, M.D., Madison, WI; Christopher

Fanta, M.D., Boston, MA; Mary K. Garcia, R.N., Sugarland, TX; Nicholas Gross, M.D., Hines, IL; Leslie Hendeles, Pharm.D., Gainesville, FL; Elliot Israel, M.D., Boston, MA; Susan Janson-Bjerklie, R.N., Ph.D., San Francisco, CA; John W. Jenne, M.D., Hines, IL; H. William Kelly, Pharm.D., Albuquerque, NM; James P. Kemp, M.D., San Diego, CA; Henry Levison, M.D., Toronto, Ontario; Gail Shapiro, M.D., Seattle, WA; Stanley J. Szefler, M.D., Denver, CO

Radiopharmaceuticals
Carol S. Marcus, Ph.D., M.D., *Chair*, Torrance, CA; Capt. William H. Briner, B.S., Durham, NC; Ronald J. Callahan, Ph.D., Boston, MA; Janet F. Eary, M.D., Seattle, WA; Joanna S. Fowler, Ph.D., Upton, NY; David L. Gilday, M.D., Toronto, Ontario; David A. Goodwin, M.D., Palo Alto, CA; David L. Laven, N.Ph., C.R.Ph., FASCP, Bay Pines, FL; Andrea H. McGuire, M.D., Des Moines, IA; Peter Paras, Ph.D., Rockville, MD; Barry A. Siegel, M.D., St. Louis, MO; Edward B. Silberstein, M.D., Cincinnati, OH; Dennis P. Swanson, M.S., Pittsburgh, PA; Mathew L. Thakur, Ph.D., Philadelphia, PA; Henry N. Wellman, M.D., Indianapolis, IN

Surgical Drugs and Devices
Lary A. Robinson, M.D., *Chair*, Tampa, FL; Gregory Alexander, M.D., Rockville, MD; Norman D. Anderson, M.D., Baltimore, MD; Alan R. Dimick, M.D., Birmingham, AL; Jack Hirsh, M.D., Hamilton, Ontario; Manucher J. Javid, M.D., Madison, WI; Henry J. Mann, Pharm.D., Bloomington, MN; Kurt M. W. Niemann, M.D., Birmingham, AL; Robert P. Rapp, Pharm.D., Lexington, KY; Ronald Rubin, M.D., West Newton, MA

Urology
John A. Belis, M.D., *Chair*, Hershey, PA; Culley C. Carson, M.D., Chapel Hill, NC; Richard A. Cohen, M.D., Red Bank, NJ; B. J. Reid Czarapata, R.N., North Potomac, MD; Jean B. de Kernion, M.D., Los Angeles, CA; Warren Heston, Ph.D., New York, NY; Mark V. Jarowenko, M.D., Hershey, PA; Mary Lee, Pharm.D., Chicago, IL; Marguerite C. Lippert, M.D., Charlottesville, VA; Penelope A. Longhurst, Ph.D., Philadelphia, PA; Tom F. Lue, M.D., San Francisco, CA; Michael G. Mawhinney, Ph.D., Morgantown, WV; Martin G. McLoughlin, M.D., Vancouver, British Columbia; Randall G. Rowland, M.D., Ph.D., Indianapolis, IN; J. Patrick Spirnak,

M.D., Cleveland, OH; William F. Tarry, M.D., Morgantown, WV; Keith N. Van Arsdalen, M.D., Philadelphia, PA

Veterinary Medicine
Lloyd E. Davis, D.V.M., Ph.D., *Chair*, Urbana, IL; Arthur L. Aronson, D.V.M., Ph.D., Raleigh, NC; Gordon W. Brumbaugh, D.V.M., Ph.D., College Station, TX; Peter Conlon, D.V.M., Ph.D., Guelph, Ontario; Gordon L. Coppoc, D.V.M., Ph.D., West Lafayette, IN; Sidney A. Ewing, D.V.M., Ph.D., Stillwater, OK; Stuart D. Forney, M.S., Fort Collins, CO; William G. Huber, D.V.M., Ph.D., Sun City West, AZ; Vernon Corey Langston, D.V.M., Ph.D., Mississippi State, MS; Mark G. Papich, D.V.M., Raleigh, NC; John W. Paul, D.V.M., Somerville, NJ; Thomas E. Powers, D.V.M., Ph.D., Columbus, OH; Charles R. Short, D.V.M., Ph.D., Baton Rouge, LA; Richard H. Teske, D.V.M., Ph.D., Rockville, MD; Jeffrey R. Wilcke, D.V.M., M.S., Blacksburg, VA

Drug Information Division
Additional Contributors

The information presented in this text represents an ongoing review of the drugs contained herein and represents a consensus of various viewpoints expressed. In addition to the individuals listed below, many schools, associations, pharmaceutical companies, and governmental agencies have provided comment or otherwise contributed to the development of the 1995 USP DI data base. Such listing does not imply that these individuals have reviewed all of the material in this text or that they individually agree with all statements contained herein.

Donald I. Abrams, M.D., San Francisco, CA
Jonathan Abrams, M.D., Albuquerque, NM
Bruce H. Ackerman, Pharm.D., Philadelphia, PA
N. Franklin Adkinson, M.D., Baltimore, MD
Allen C. Alfrey, M.D., Denver, CO
Joanne Allard, M.D., Toronto, Ontario, Canada
Carmen Allegra, M.D., Bethesda, MD
Mike Apley, D.V.M., Greeley, CO
Martin Bacon, M.D., Bethesda, MD
José M. Ballester, M.D., La Habana, Cuba
Rick Barbarash, Pharm.D., St. Louis, MO
Patsy Barnett, Pharm.D., Birmingham, AL

LuAnne Barron, Birmingham, AL
Robert W. Beightol, Pharm.D., Roanoke, VA
William Bell, M.D., Baltimore, MD
Gladys Bendahan Barchilón, Barcelona, Spain
Patricia Bennett, B.S.Pharm., Cincinnati, OH
David L. Benowitz, M.D., San Francisco, CA
Byron S. Berlin, M.D., Lansing, MI
Frederick A. Berry, M.D., Charlottesville, VA
Ernest Beutler, M.D., La Jolla, CA
Christine A. Bezouska, M.D., Morgantown, WV
S. Bruce Binder, M.D., Ph.D., Dayton, OH
Martin Black, M.D., Philadelphia, PA
Laura Boehnke, Pharm.D., Houston, TX
Halcy Bohen, Ph.D., Washington, DC
Wayne E. Bradley, Duluth, GA
Michael Brady, M.D., Columbus, OH
Edward L. Braud, M.D., Springfield, IL
Robert E. Braun, D.D.S., Buffalo, NY
Kenneth Bridges, M.D., Boston, MA
Paul J. Brown, M.D., Bedford, NH
Louis Buttino, Jr., M.D., Dayton, OH
Wesley G. Byerly, Pharm.D., Winston-Salem, NC
Karim A. Calis, Pharm.D., Bethesda, MD
Mary E. Carman, Ottawa, Ontario
Charles C.J. Carpenter, M.D., Providence, RI
Peggy Carver, M.D., Ann Arbor, MI
Marcel Casavant, M.D., Columbus, OH
Bruce A. Chabner, M.D., Bethesda, MD
Erin S. Champagne, D.V.M., Blacksburg, VA
Chih Wen Chang, Pharm.D., Maywood, IL
Te-Wen Chang, M.D., Boston, MA
Kenneth R. Chapman, M.D., Toronto, Ontario
Bruce D. Cheson, M.D., Bethesda, MD
Henry Chilton, Pharm.D., Winston-Salem, NC
Frank Chytil, Ph.D., Nashville, TN
Scott B. Citino, D.V.M., Yulee, FL
Cyril R. Clarke, Ph.D., Stillwater, OK
Jackson Como, M.D., Birmingham, AL
Betsy Jane Cooper, M.D., Washington, DC
James W. Cooper, Ph.D., Athens, GA
Deborah Cotton, M.D., Boston, MA
Fred F. Cowan, Ph.D., Portland, OR

Donald W. Cox, M.D., Morgantown, WV
Mark V. Crisman, D.V.M., Blacksburg, VA
Craig Darby, R.Ph., Twinsburg, OH
Michael Davidson, D.V.M., Raleigh, NC
Ann J. Davis, M.D., Boston, MA
Janet Davis, M.D., Miami, FL
Ken Davis, M.D., New York, NY
Thomas D. DeCillis, North Port, FL
Carel P. de Haseth, Ph.D., Netherland Antilles
Daniel Deykin, M.D., Boston, MA
Nick Diamant, M.D., Toronto, Ontario, Canada
Annette Dickinson, Ph.D., Washington, DC
Barry D. Dickinson, Ph.D., Chicago, IL
Christine Z. Dickinson, M.D., Royal Oak, MI
John B. DiMarco, M.D., Ph.D., Charlottesville, VA
James E. Doherty, M.D., Little Rock, AR
Donald C. Doll, M.D., Columbia, MO
Jerry Dolovich, M.D., Hamilton, Ontario
R. Gordon Douglas, M.D., Rahway, NJ
Ed Drea, Pharm.D., Phoenix, AZ
Bonnie Driggers, R.N., Portland, OR
Marion Dugdale, M.D., Memphis, TN
Carol Duncan, R.N., Portland, OR
Suzanne Eastman, M.S., R.Ph., Columbus, OH
John E. Edwards, Jr., M.D., Torrance, CA
Robert Edwards, Pharm.D., Columbus, OH
Lawrence H. Einhorn, M.D., Indianapolis, IN
Augustin Escalante, M.D., Downey, CA
Gary Euler, Dr.P.H., Atlanta, GA
William Fant, Pharm.D., Cincinnati, OH
Martin N. Farlow, M.D., Indianapolis, IN
R. Edward Faught, M.D., Birmingham, AL
David S. Fedson, M.D., Charlottesville, VA
John P. Feighner, La Mesa, CA
James M. Ferguson, M.D., Salt Lake City, UT
Paul Ferrell, M.D., Bethesda, MD
Anne Gilbert Feuer, R.Ph., Cincinnati, OH
Suzanne Fields, Pharm.D., San Antonio, TX
J.R. Fontilus, M.D., Netherland Antilles
Tammy Fox, R.Ph., Fairfield, OH
Charles W. Francis, M.D., Rochester, NY
Ruth Francis-Floyd, D.V.M., Gainesville, FL

Rudolph M. Franklin, M.D., New Orleans, LA
H. H. Frey, Berlin, Germany
Dorothy Friedberg, M.D., New York, NY
Alan Friedman, M.D., New York, NY
José P.B. Gallardo, R.Ph., Iowa City, IA
Gloria Garber, R.Ph., Cincinnati, OH
Arthur Garson, M.D., Durham, NC
S. Gauthier, M.D., Montreal, PQ, Canada
Edward Genton, M.D., New Orleans, LA
Anne A. Gershon, M.D., New York, NY
Larry N. Gever, Pharm.D., Cranbury, NJ
Michael J. Glade, Ph.D., Chicago, IL
Charles J. Glueck, M.D., Cincinnati, OH
Maryanne Godlewski-Vagnini, R.Ph., Brooklyn, NY
Lewis Goldfrank, M.D., New York, NY
J. Max Goodson, D.D.S., Ph.D., Boston, MA
Fred Gordin, M.D., Washington, DC
John D. Grabenstein, M.S., Fort Sam Houston, TX
Roni Grad, M.D., Albuquerque, NM
Nina M. Graves, Pharm.D., Minneapolis, MN
Terri Graves Davidson, Pharm.D., Atlanta, GA
David Green, M.D., Chicago, IL
Harry Green, M.D., Evansville, IN
Martin D. Green, M.D., Rockville, MD
Philip C. Greig, M.D., Durham, NC
Vincent Habiyambere, M.D., Geneva, Switzerland
Angela M. Hadbavny, Pharm.D., Pittsburgh, PA
Benjamin F. Hammond, D.D.S., Ph.D., Philadelphia, PA
Kenneth R. Hande, M.D., Nashville, TN
Edward A. Hartshorn, Ph.D., League City, TX
Robert C. Hastings, M.D., Carville, LA
William E. Hathaway, Denver, CO
Frederick G. Hayden, M.D., Charlottesville, VA
Cleopatra L. Hazel, Pharm.D., Netherland Antilles
Murk-Hein Heinemann, M.D., New York, NY
Peter Hellyer, D.V.M., Raleigh, NC
Bryan N. Henderson, II, D.D.S., Dallas, TX
William Herbert, M.D., Durham, NC
Barbara Herwaldt, M.D., Atlanta, GA
Monto Ho, M.D., Pittsburgh, PA
Vincent C. Ho, M.D., British Columbia, Canada
M.E. Hoar, Springfield, MA

Robert Hodgeman, M.S., R.Ph., Cincinnati, OH
Gary N. Holland, M.D., Los Angeles, CA
Richard A. Holmes, M.D., Columbia, MO
William Hopkins, Pharm.D., Atlanta, GA
Richard B. Hornick, M.D., Orlando, FL
Raymond W. Houde, M.D., New York, NY
Colin W. Howden, M.D., Columbia, SC
Walter T. Hughes, M.D., Memphis, TN
B. Thomas Hutchinson, M.D., Boston, MA
John Iazzetta, Pharm.D., Toronto, Ontario, Canada
Rodney D. Ice, Ph.D., Atlanta, GA
Frederick Jacobsen, M.D., Washington, DC
Mark Jacobson, M.D., San Francisco, CA
Robert Jacobson, M.D., Carville, LA
Ann L. Janer, M.S., Auburn, AL
Janet P. Jaramilla, Pharm.D., Chicago, IL
James W. Jefferson, M.D., Madison, WI
Alan Jenkins, M.D., Charlottesville, VA
Leslye Johnson, Ph.D., Bethesda, MD
Joseph L. Jorizzo, M.D., Winston-Salem, NC
Gunnar Juliusson, M.D., Ph.D., Huddinge, Sweden
Hugh F. Kabat, Ph.D., Albuquerque, NM
James Kahn, M.D., San Francisco, CA
Alan Kanada, Pharm.D., Denver, CO
John J. Kavanagh, M.D., Houston, TX
Michael J. Keating, M.D., Houston, TX
Michael Kelley, M.D., Columbus, OH
David C. Kem, M.D., Oklahoma City, OK
N. David Kennedy, R.Ph., Washington, DC
Joseph M. Khoury, M.D., Bethesda, MD
Agnes V. Klein, M.D., Vanier, Ontario
Anne Klibanski, M.D., Boston, MA
Sandra Knowles, B.Pharm., Toronto, Ontario, Canada
John Koepke, Pharm.D., Columbus, OH
Joseph A. Kovacs, M.D., Bethesda, MD
Paul A. Krusinski, M.D., Burlington, VT
Paul B. Kuehn, Ph.D., Woodinville, WA
R.W. Kuncl, M.D., Baltimore, MD
Thomas L. Kurt, M.D., Dallas, TX
Lyle Laird, Pharm.D., San Antonio, TX
John S. Lambert, M.D., Rochester, NY
John R. LaMontagne, Bethesda, MD

Michael Lange, M.D., New York, NY
Victor J. Lanzotti, M.D., Springfield, IL
P. Reed Larsen, M.D., Boston, MA
Eugene Laska, M.D., Orangeburg, NY
Oscar L. Laskin, M.D., East Hanover, NJ
John Laszlo, M.D., Atlanta, GA
Belle Lee, Pharm.D., San Francisco, CA
Ilo E. Leppik, M.D., Minneapolis, MN
Raymond Levy, London, England
Richard A. Lewis, M.D., Houston, TX
William Lieber, M.D., Waterbury, CT
Charles Liebow, II, D.D.S., Ph.D., Buffalo, NY
Christopher D. Lind, M.D., Nashville, TN
Charles H. Livengood, III, M.D., Durham, NC
Don M. Long, M.D., Ph.D., Baltimore, MD
Julio R. Lopez, M.D., Martinez, CA
Colleen Lum Lung, R.N., Denver, CO
Howard I. Maibach, M.D., San Francisco, CA
Marilyn Manco-Johnson, Denver, CO
Victor J. Marder, M.D., Rochester, NY
Joseph E. Margarone, II, D.D.S., Buffalo, NY
Maurie Markman, M.D., Cleveland, OH
Jon Markovitz, M.D., Phoenix, AZ
William C. Matthews, M.D., San Diego, CA
Harry R. Maxon, III, M.D., Cincinnati, OH
Alice Lorraine McAfee, Pharm.D., San Pedro, CA
Lisa Y. McDonald, Pharm.D., Emeryville, CA
Norman L. McElroy, San Jose, CA
Charles McGrath, D.V.M., Blacksburg, VA
Ross E. McKinney, M.D., Durham, NC
Anne McNulty, M.D., Waterbury, CT
Wallace B. Mendelson, M.D., Cleveland, OH
Dean D. Metcalfe, M.D., Bethesda, MD
Donald Miller, Pharm.D., Fargo, ND
John Mills, M.D., Fairfield, Victoria, Australia
Joel S. Mindel, M.D., Ph.D., New York, NY
Bernard L. Mirkin, M.D., Chicago, IL
Janet L. Mitchell, M.D., New York, NY
John R. Modlin, M.D., Hanover, NH
C. Craig Moldenhauer, M.D., San Diego, CA
Garreth A. Moore, Blacksburg, VA
Mary E. Mortensen, M.D., Columbus, OH

Robyn Mueller, R.Ph., Cincinnati, OH
R.I. Ogilvie, M.D., Toronto, Ontario
Linda K. Ohri, Pharm.D., Omaha, NE
James M. Oleske, M.D., Newark, NJ
Robert O'Mara, M.D., Rochester, NY
Michael J. O'Neill, R.Ph., Twinsburg, OH
Walter A. Orenstein, M.D., Atlanta, GA
James R. Oster, M.D., Miami, FL
Judith M. Ozbun, R.Ph., M.S., Fargo, ND
David C. Pang, Ph.D., Chicago, IL
Michael F. Para, M.D., Columbus, OH
Satyapal R. Pareddy, B.Pharm., Brooklyn, NY
Robert C. Park, M.D., Washington, DC
William W. Parmly, M.D., San Francisco, CA
Albert Patterson, Hines, IL
James A. Pederson, M.D., Oklahoma City, OK
Ronald Peterson, M.D., Ph.D., Rochester, MN
Melenie Petropoulos, R.Ph., Twinsburg, OH
Lawrence D. Piro, M.D., La Jolla, CA
Philip A. Pizzo, M.D., Bethesda, MD
Christopher V. Plowe, M.D., Bethesda, MD
Therese Poirier, Pharm.D., Pittsburgh, PA
Michael A. Polis, M.D., Bethesda, MD
James A. Ponto, R.Ph., Iowa City, IA
Carol M. Proudfit, Ph.D., Chicago, IL
Nixa Ramos, Arecibo, Puerto Rico
Norbert P. Rapoza, Ph.D., Chicago, IL
Gary Raskob, M.Sc., Oklahoma City, OK
Terry D. Rees, D.D.S., Dallas, TX
Alfred J. Remillard, Pharm.D., Saskatoon, Saskatchewan, Canada
Robert Roberts, M.D., Houston, TX
David Robertson, M.D., Nashville, TN
Daniel C. Robinson, Pharm.D., Los Angeles, CA
John E. Roney, R.Ph., Cincinnati, OH
Jeff Rosner, R.Ph., Twinsburg, OH
Douglas S. Ross, M.D., Boston, MA
Phillip J. Rubin, M.D., Phoenix, AZ
Michael S. Saag, M.D., Birmingham, AL
Henry S. Sacks, Ph.D., M.D., New York, NY
Sharon Safrin, M.D., San Francisco, CA
Evelyn Salerno, Pharm.D., Hialeah, FL
Hugh A. Sampson, Jr., M.D., Baltimore, MD

Subbiah Sangiah, D.V.M., Ph.D., Stillwater, OK
Victor M. Santana, Memphis, TN
Belinda Sartor, M.D., Shreveport, LA
Donald C. Sawyer, East Lansing, MI
Elliot Schecter, M.D., Oklahoma City, OK
Udo P. Schmiedl, M.D., Ph.D., Seattle, WA
Gabriel Schmunis, M.D., Washington, DC
Steven M. Schnittman, M.D., Rockville, MD
George Schuster, M.D., Augusta, GA
Stephen Schuster, M.D., Philadelphia, PA
Dorothy Schwartz-Porsche, Berlin, Germany
Douglas A. Sears, Tenafly, NJ
Jerome Seidenfeld, Ph.D., Chicago, IL
Charles F. Seifert, Pharm.D., Oklahoma City, OK
Allen Shaughnessy, Pharm.D., Harrisburg, PA
Donald J. Sherrard, M.D., Seattle, WA
Yvonne M. Shevchuk, Pharm.D., Saskatoon, Saskatchewan, Canada
Harold M. Silverman, Pharm.D., Silver Spring, MD
Irv Siven, M.D., New York, NY
Barry H. Smith, M.D., Ph.D., New York, NY
Dance Smith, Pharm.D., Ft. Steilacoom, WA
Geralynn B. Smith, M.S., Detroit, MI
John R. Smith, M.S., Ph.D., Portland, OR
Steven J. Smith, Ph.D., Chicago, IL
Elliott M. Sogol, Ph.D., Research Triangle Park, NC
Nicholas Soter, M.D., New York, NY
William Speliacy, M.D., Tampa, FL
Joan Stachnik, Chicago, IL
William Steers, M.D., Charlottesville, VA
John J. Stern, M.D., Philadelphia, PA
Irwin Strathman, M.D., Lutz, FL
Kris Strohbehn, M.D., Boston, MA
David Stuhr, Denver, CO
Alan Sugar, M.D., Boston, MA
Linda Gore Sutherland, Pharm.D., Laramie, WY
Sandra Tailor, Pharm.D., Toronto, Ontario, Canada
David A. Taylor, M.D., Morgantown, WV
Mary E. Teresi, Iowa City, IA
Cheryl Nunn Thompson, Chicago, IL
John C. Thurman, D.V.M., Urbana, IL
Roger C. Toffle, M.D., Morgantown, WV
Douglas M. Tollefsen, M.D., St. Louis, MO

Eric J. Topol, M.D., Ann Arbor, MI
Jayme Trott, Pharm.D., San Antonio, TX
Donald G. Vidt, M.D., Cleveland, OH
Richard Vogel, D.D.S., Newark, NJ
Georgia Vogelsang, M.D., Baltimore, MD
Paul A. Volberding, M.D., San Francisco, CA
Andrea Wall, R.Ph., Cincinnati, OH
William Warner, Ph.D., New York, NY
Michael Weber, M.D., Irvine, CA
Krisantha Weerasuriya, M.D., Geneva, Switzerland
G. John Weir, M.D., Marshfield, WI
Timothy E. Welty, Pharm.D., Cincinnati, OH
Stanford Wessler, M.D., Rye, NY
Carolyn Westhoff, New York, NY
John White, Pharm.D., Spokane, WA
Richard J. Whitley, M.D., Birmingham, AL
Catherine Wilfert, M.D., Durham, NC
Robert G. Wolfangel, Ph.D., St. Louis, MO
M. Michael Wolfe, M.D., Boston, MA
William Wonderlin, Ph.D., Morgantown, WV
Richard J. Wood, M.D., Boston, MA
Curtis Wright, M.D., Rockville, MD
Catharine Wuest, R.Ph., Cincinnati, OH
Robert Yarchoan, M.D., Bethesda, MD
John M. Zajecka, M.D., Chicago, IL
Stephanie Zarus, Pharm.D., Philadelphia, PA
Frederic J. Zucchero, M.A., R.Ph., Chesterfield, MO
Jane R. Zucker, Atlanta, GA

Headquarters Staff

DRUG INFORMATION DIVISION

Director: Keith W. Johnson

Assistant Director: Georgie M. Cathey

Administrative Staff: Jaime A. Ramirez *(Administrative Assistant),* Albert Crucillo, Mayra L. Rios

Senior Drug Information Specialists: Sandra Lee Boyer, Nancy Lee Dashiell, Debra A. Edwards, Esther H. Klein *(Supervisor),* Angela Méndez Mayo *(Spanish Publications Coordinator)*

Drug Information Specialists: Katherine M. Bennett, Joyce

Carpenter, Ann Corken, Jymeann King, Doris Lee *(Supervisor)*, Robin Schermerhorn, Denise Seldon, Daniel W. Seyoum

Veterinary Drug Information Specialist: Amy Neal

Coordinator, Patient Counseling and Education Programs: Stacy M. Hartranft

Computer Applications: Richard Allen *(Programmer)*, Bernard G. Silverstein *(Computer Applications Specialist)*

Publications Development Staff: Diana M. Blais *(Manager)*, Anne M. Lawrence *(Associate)*, Dorothy Raymond *(Assistant)*, Darcy Schwartz *(Assistant)*

Library Services: Florence A. Hogan *(Manager)*, Terri Rikhy *(Assistant)*, Madeleine Welsch

Research Associate, International Programs: David D. Housley

Research Assistant: Annamarie J. Sibik

Consultants: Janet Elgert, Lourdes de Gonzalez, David W. Hughes, S. Ramakrishnan Iyer, Wanda Janicki, Kate Phelan, Marcelo Vernengo

Scholar in Residence: Patricia J. Bush, Georgetown University

Student Interns/Externs: Robyn Dubinsky, University of Missouri at Kansas City; Rachel Ellis, Nottingham University, England; Kevin Garey, Dalhousie University, Nova Scotia; Bereket Melaku, Howard University; Kavita Nair, University of Toledo; Ken Rogers, University of Arizona; Yván Sánchez-Huamaní, National University of Trujillo, Peru

Visiting Scholars: Giulia Cingolani, Rome, Italy; Elena Oshkalova, Moscow, Russian Federation; Svetlana Udotova, Moscow, Russian Federation

USP ADMINISTRATIVE STAFF

Executive Director: Jerome A. Halperin
Associate Executive Director: Joseph G. Valentino
Assistant Executive Director for Professional and Public Affairs: Jacqueline L. Eng
Director, Finance: Abe Brauner
Director, Operations: J. Robert Strang

Director, Personnel: Arlene Bloom

Director, Fulfillment/Facilities: Drew J. Lutz

Legal: Kim Keller (Staff Attorney), John Lindow (Associate Legal Counsel for Business Affairs), Colleen Ottoson (Staff Attorney)

DRUG STANDARDS DIVISION

Director: Lee T. Grady

Assistant Directors: Charles H. Barnstein *(Revision)*, Barbara B. Hubert *(Scientific Administration)*, Robert H. King *(Technical Services)*

Senior Scientists: Roger Dabbah, V. Srinivasan, William W. Wright

Scientists: Frank P. Barletta, Vivian A. Gray, W. Larry Paul

Senior Scientific Associate: Todd L. Cecil

Technical Editors: Ann K. Ferguson, Melissa M. Smith

Supervisor of Administration: Anju K. Malhotra

Support Staff: Patricia Barnhill, Glenna Etherton, Theresa H. Lee, Cecilia Luna, Maureen Rawson, Ernestene Williams

Drug Research and Testing Laboratory: Richard F. Lindauer *(Director)*

Hazard Communications: Linda Shear

Consultants: J. Joseph Belson, Zorach R. Glaser, Martin Golden, Aubrey S. Outschoorn

MARKETING

Director: Joan Blitman

Senior Product Manager: Mark A. Sohasky *(Electronic Information)*

Product Manager: Kathleen Bagas *(Publications)*

Marketing Associates: Jennifer C. Glenn, Dana L. McCullah, Steven Saars

Marketing Representative: Susan M. Williams *(Electronic Applications)*

Marketing Communications Manager: Derek Rice

Marketing Research Analyst: Deborah King

PUBLICATION SERVICES

Acting Director: Gail M. Oring

Managing Editors: A. V. Precup *(USP DI)*, Sandra Boynton *(USP-NF)*

Editorial Associates: *USP DI*—Ellen R. Loeb *(Senior Editorial Associate)*, Carol M. Griffin, Carol N. Hankin, Marie Kotomori, Harriet S. Nathanson, Ellen D. Smith, Barbara A. Visco; *USP-NF*—Jesusa D. Cordova *(Senior Editorial Associate)*, Ellen Elovitz, John Pahle, Margaret Kay Walshaw

USAN Staff: Carolyn A. Fleeger *(Editor)*, Gerilynne Seigneur

Typesetting Systems Coordinator: Jean E. Dale

Typesetting Staff: Susan L. Entwistle *(Supervisor)*, Donna Alie, Deborah R. Connelly, Lauren Taylor Davis, Deborah James, M. T. Samahon, Micheline Tranquille

Graphics: Cristy Gonzalez, Todd Hodges, Tia C. Morfessis, Greg Varhola

Word Processing: Barbara A. Bowman *(Supervisor)*, Frances Rampp, Susan Schartman, Jane Shulman

Also Contributing: Barbara Arnold, Proofreading; Brian Dillon and Paul Widem of Editech Services, Inc., Proofreading; Terri A. DeIuliis, Graphics; Michelle Thomas, Clerical Assistance.

PRACTITIONER REPORTING PROGRAMS

Assistant Executive Director for Practitioner Reporting Programs: Diane D. Cousins

Staff: Robin A. Baldwin, Shawn C. Becker, Jean Canada, Alice C. Curtis, Ilze Mohseni, Joanne Pease, Susmita Samanta, Anne Paula Thompson, Mary Susan Zmuda

---

Members of the USPC and the Institutions and Organizations Represented
(as of March 15, 1994)

Officers and Board of Trustees

President: Mark Novitch, M.D.
Vice President: Donald R. Bennett, M.D., Ph.D.
Treasurer: John T. Fay, Jr., Ph.D.
Trustees Representing Medical Sciences: Edwin D. Bransome, Jr., M.D.; J. Richard Crout, M.D.

Association of Food and Drug Officials: David R. Work, J.D.

Association of Official Analytical Chemists: Thomas Layloff, Jr.

Chemical Manufacturers Association: Andrew J. Schmitz, Jr. *(deceased)*

Cosmetic, Toiletry & Fragrance Association, Inc.: G.N. McEwen, Jr., Ph.D., J.D.

Council for Responsible Nutrition: Annette Dickinson, Ph.D.

Drug Information Association: Elizabeth B. D'Angelo, Ph.D.

Generic Pharmaceutical Industry Association: William F. Haddad

Health Industry Manufacturers Association: Dee Simons

National Association of Boards of Pharmacy: Carmen Catizone

National Association of Chain Drug Stores, Inc.: Saul Schneider

National Pharmaceutical Alliance: Christina F. Sizemore

National Wholesale Druggists' Association: Bruce R. Siecker, R.Ph., Ph.D.

Nonprescription Drug Manufacturers Association: R. William Soller, Ph.D.

Parenteral Drug Association, Inc.: Peter E. Manni, Ph.D.

Pharmaceutical Manufacturers Association: Maurice Q. Bectel

Other Organizations and Institutions

Alabama

Auburn University, School of Pharmacy: Kenneth N. Barker, Ph.D.

Samford University School of Pharmacy: H. Anthony McBride, Ph.D.

University of Alabama School of Medicine: Robert B. Diasio, M.D.

University of South Alabama, College of Medicine: Samuel J. Strada, Ph.D.

Medical Association of the State of Alabama: Paul A. Palmisano, M.D.

Alabama Pharmaceutical Association: Mitchel C. Rothholz

Alaska

Alaska Pharmaceutical Association: Jackie Warren, R.Ph.

Arizona

University of Arizona, College of Medicine: John D. Palmer, Ph.D., M.D.

University of Arizona, College of Pharmacy: Michael Mayersohn, Ph.D.

Arizona Pharmacy Association: Edward Armstrong

Arkansas

University of Arkansas for Medical Sciences, College of Pharmacy: Kenneth G. Nelson, Ph.D.

Arkansas Pharmacists Association: Norman Canterbury, P.D.

California

Loma Linda University Medical Center: Ralph Cutler, M.D.

Stanford University School of Medicine: Brian B. Hoffman, M.D.

University of California, Davis, School of Medicine: Larry Stark, Ph.D.

University of California, San Diego, School of Medicine: Harold J. Simon, M.D., Ph.D.

University of California, San Francisco, School of Medicine: Walter L. Way, M.D.

University of Southern California, School of Medicine: Wayne R. Bidlack, Ph.D.

University of California, San Francisco, School of Pharmacy: Richard H. Guy, Ph.D.

University of Southern California, School of Pharmacy: Robert T. Koda, Pharm.D., Ph.D.

University of the Pacific, School of Pharmacy: Alice Jean Matuszak, Ph.D.

California Pharmacists Association: Robert P. Marshall, Pharm.D.

Colorado

University of Colorado School of Pharmacy: Merrick Lee Shively, Ph.D.

Colorado Pharmacists Association: Thomas G. Arthur, R.Ph.

Connecticut

University of Connecticut, School of Medicine: Paul F. Davern

University of Connecticut, School of Pharmacy: Karl A. Nieforth, Ph.D.

Connecticut Pharmaceutical Association: Henry A. Palmer, Ph.D.

Delaware

Delaware Pharmaceutical Society: Charles J. O'Connor

Medical Society of Delaware: John M. Levinson, M.D.

District of Columbia

George Washington University: Janet Elgert-Madison, Pharm.D.

Georgetown University, School of Medicine: Arthur Raines, Ph.D.

Howard University, College of Medicine: Sonya K. Sobrian, Ph.D.

Howard University, College of Pharmacy & Pharmacal Sciences: Wendell T. Hill, Jr., Pharm.D.

Florida

Southeastern College of Pharmacy: William D. Hardigan, Ph.D.

University of Florida, College of Medicine: Thomas F. Muther, Ph.D.

University of Florida, College of Pharmacy: Michael A. Schwartz, Ph.D.

University of South Florida, College of Medicine: Joseph J. Krzanowski, Jr., Ph.D.

Florida Pharmacy Association: "Red" Camp

Georgia

Medical College of Georgia, School of Medicine: David W. Hawkins, Pharm.D.

Mercer University School of Medicine: W. Douglas Skelton, M.D.

Mercer University, Southern School of Pharmacy: Hewitt W. Matthews, Ph.D.

Morehouse School of Medicine: Ralph W. Trottier, Jr., Ph.D., J.D.

University of Georgia, College of Pharmacy: Stuart Feldman, Ph.D.

Medical Association of Georgia: E. D. Bransome, Jr., M.D.

Georgia Pharmaceutical Association, Inc.: Larry R. Braden

Idaho

Idaho State University, College of Pharmacy: Eugene I. Isaacson, Ph.D.

Idaho State Pharmaceutical Association: Doris Denney

Illinois

Chicago Medical School/University of Health Sciences: Velayudhan Nair, Ph.D., D.Sc.

Loyola University of Chicago, Stritch School of Medicine: Erwin Coyne, Ph.D.

Northwestern University Medical School: Marilynn C. Frederiksen, M.D.

Rush Medical College of Rush University: Paul G. Pierpaoli, M.S.

Southern Illinois University, School of Medicine: Leonard Rybak, M.D., Ph.D.

University of Chicago, Pritzker School of Medicine: Patrick T. Horn, M.D., Ph.D.

University of Illinois, College of Medicine: Marten M. Kernis, Ph.D.

University of Illinois, College of Pharmacy: Henri R. Manasse, Jr., Ph.D.

Chicago College of Pharmacy: David J. Slatkin, Ph.D.

Illinois Pharmacists Association: Ronald W. Gottrich

Illinois State Medical Society: Vincent A. Costanzo, Jr., M.D.

Indiana

Butler University, College of Pharmacy: Wagar H. Bhatti, Ph.D.

Purdue University, School of Pharmacy and Pharmacal Sciences: Garnet E. Peck, Ph.D.

Indiana State Medical Association: Edward Langston, R.Ph., M.D.

Iowa

Drake University, College of Pharmacy: Sidney L. Finn, Ph.D.

University of Iowa, College of Medicine: John E. Kasik, M.D., Ph.D.

University of Iowa, College of Pharmacy: Robert A. Wiley, Ph.D.

Iowa Pharmacists Association: Steve C. Firman, R.Ph.

Kansas

University of Kansas, School of Pharmacy: Prof. Christopher Riley

Kansas Pharmacists Association: Robert R. Williams

Kentucky

University of Kentucky, College of Medicine: John M. Carney, Ph.D.

University of Kentucky, College of Pharmacy: Patrick P. De-Luca, Ph.D.

University of Louisville, School of Medicine: Peter P. Rowell, Ph.D.

Kentucky Medical Association: Ellsworth C. Seeley, M.D.

Kentucky Pharmacists Association: Chester L. Parker, Pharm.D.

Louisiana

Louisiana State University School of Medicine in New Orleans: Paul L. Kirkendol, Ph.D.

Northeast Louisiana University, School of Pharmacy: William M. Bourn, Ph.D.

Tulane University, School of Medicine: Floyd R. Domer, Ph.D.

Xavier University of Louisiana: Barry A. Bleidt, Ph.D., R.Ph.
Louisiana State Medical Society: Henry W. Jolly, Jr., M.D.
Louisiana Pharmacists Association: Mona J. Davis

Maryland

Johns Hopkins University, School of Medicine: E. Robert Feroli, Jr., Pharm.D.
University of Maryland, School of Medicine: Edson X. Albuquerque, M.D., Ph.D.
Uniformed Services University of the Health Sciences, F. Edward Hebert School of Medicine: Louis R. Cantilena, Jr., M.D., Ph.D.
University of Maryland, Baltimore, School of Pharmacy: Larry L. Augsburger, Ph.D.
Medical and Chirurgical Faculty of the State of Maryland: Frederick Wilhelm, M.D.
Maryland Pharmacists Association: Nicholas C. Lykos, P.D.

Massachusetts

Boston University, School of Medicine: J. Worth Estes, M.D.
Harvard Medical School: Peter Goldman, M.D.
Massachusetts College of Pharmacy and Allied Health Sciences: David A. Williams, Ph.D.
Northeastern University, College of Pharmacy and Allied Health Professions: John L. Neumeyer, Ph.D.
Tufts University, School of Medicine: John Mazzullo, M.D.
University of Massachusetts Medical School: Brian Johnson, M.D.
Massachusetts Medical Society: Errol Green, M.D.

Michigan

Ferris State University, School of Pharmacy: Gerald W.A. Slywka, Ph.D.
Michigan State University, College of Human Medicine: John Penner, M.D.
University of Michigan, College of Pharmacy: Ara G. Paul, Ph.D.
University of Michigan Medical Center: Jeoffrey K. Stross, M.D.
Wayne State University, School of Medicine: Ralph E. Kauffman, M.D.
Wayne State University, College of Pharmacy and Allied Health Professions: Janardan B. Nagwekar, Ph.D.
Michigan Pharmacists Association: Patrick L. McKercher, Ph.D.

Minnesota

Mayo Medical School: James J. Lipsky, M.D.

University of Minnesota, College of Pharmacy: E. John Staba, Ph.D.

University of Minnesota Medical School, Minneapolis: Jack W. Miller, Ph.D.

Minnesota Medical Association: Harold Seim, M.D.

Minnesota Pharmacists Association: Arnold D. Delger

Mississippi

University of Mississippi, School of Medicine: James L. Achord, M.D.

University of Mississippi, School of Pharmacy: Robert W. Cleary, Ph.D.

Mississippi State Medical Association: Charles L. Mathews

Mississippi Pharmacists Association: Mike Kelly

Missouri

St. Louis College of Pharmacy: John W. Zuzack, Ph.D.

St. Louis University, School of Medicine: Alvin H. Gold, Ph.D.

University of Missouri, Columbia, School of Medicine: John W. Yarbro, M.D.

University of Missouri, Kansas City, School of Medicine: Paul Cuddy, Pharm.D.

University of Missouri, Kansas City, School of Pharmacy: Lester Chafetz, Ph.D.

Washington University, School of Medicine: H. Mitchell Perry, Jr., M.D.

Missouri Pharmaceutical Association: George L. Oestreich

Montana

The University of Montana, School of Pharmacy & Allied Health Sciences: David S. Forbes, Ph.D.

Nebraska

Creighton University, School of Medicine: Michael C. Makoid, Ph.D.

Creighton University School of Pharmacy and Allied Health Professions: Kenneth R. Keefner, Ph.D.

University of Nebraska, College of Medicine: Manuchair Ebadi, Ph.D.

University of Nebraska, College of Pharmacy: Clarence T. Ueda, Pharm.D., Ph.D.

Nebraska Pharmacists Association: Rex C. Higley, R.P.

Nevada

Nevada Pharmacists Association: Steven P. Bradford

New Hampshire

Dartmouth Medical School: James J. Kresel, Ph.D.

New Hampshire Pharmaceutical Association: William J. Lancaster, P.D.

New Jersey

University of Medicine and Dentistry of New Jersey, New Jersey Medical School: Sheldon B. Gertner, Ph.D.

Rutgers, The State University of New Jersey, College of Pharmacy: John L. Colaizzi, Ph.D.

Medical Society of New Jersey: Joseph N. Micale, M.D.

New Jersey Pharmaceutical Association: Stephen J. Csubak, Ph.D.

New Mexico

University of New Mexico, College of Pharmacy: William M. Hadley, Ph.D.

New Mexico Pharmaceutical Association: Hugh Kabat, Ph.D.

New York

Albert Einstein College of Medicine of Yeshiva University: Walter G. Levine, Ph.D.

City University of New York, Mt. Sinai School of Medicine: Joel S. Mindel, M.D., Ph.D.

Columbia University College of Physicians and Surgeons: Michael R. Rosen, M.D.

Cornell University Medical College: Lorraine J. Gudas, Ph.D.

Long Island University, Arnold and Marie Schwartz College of Pharmacy and Health Sciences: Jack M. Rosenberg, Ph.D.

New York Medical College: Mario A. Inchiosa, Jr., Ph.D.

New York University School of Medicine: Norman Altzuler, Ph.D.

State University of New York, Buffalo, School of Medicine: Robert J. McIsaac, Ph.D.

State University of New York, Buffalo, School of Pharmacy: Robert M. Cooper

State University of New York, Health Science Center, Syracuse: Oliver M. Brown, Ph.D.

St. John's University, College of Pharmacy and Allied Health Professions: Albert A. Belmonte, Ph.D.

Union University, Albany College of Pharmacy: David W. Newton, Ph.D.

University of Rochester, School of Medicine and Dentistry: Michael Weintraub, M.D., Ph.D.

Medical Society of the State of New York: Richard S. Blum, M.D.
Pharmaceutical Society of the State of New York: Bruce Moden

North Carolina

Bowman Gray School of Medicine, Wake Forest University: Jack W. Strandhoy, Ph.D.

Campbell University, School of Pharmacy: Antoine Al-Achi, Ph.D.

Duke University Medical Center: William J. Murray, M.D., Ph.D.

East Carolina University, School of Medicine: A-R.A. Abdel-Rahman, Ph.D.

University of North Carolina, Chapel Hill, School of Medicine: George Hatfield, Ph.D.

University of North Carolina, Chapel Hill, School of Pharmacy: Richard J. Kowalsky, Pharm.D.

North Carolina Pharmaceutical Association: George H. Cocolas, Ph.D.

North Carolina Medical Society: T. Reginald Harris, M.D.

North Dakota

University of North Dakota, School of Medicine: David W. Hein, Ph.D.

North Dakota State University, College of Pharmacy: William M. Henderson, Ph.D.

North Dakota Medical Association: Vernon E. Wagner

North Dakota Pharmaceutical Association: William H. Shelver, Ph.D.

Ohio

Case Western Reserve University, School of Medicine: Kenneth A. Scott, Ph.D.

Medical College of Ohio at Toledo: R. Douglas Wilkerson, Ph.D.

Northeastern Ohio University, College of Medicine: Ralph E. Berggren, M.D.

Ohio Northern University, College of Pharmacy: Joseph Theodore, Ph.D.

Ohio State University, College of Medicine: Robert Guthrie, M.D.

Ohio State University, College of Pharmacy: Michael C. Gerald, Ph.D.

University of Cincinnati, College of Medicine: Leonard T. Sigell, Ph.D.

University of Cincinnati, College of Pharmacy: Henry S.I. Tan, Ph.D.

University of Toledo, College of Pharmacy: Norman F. Billups, Ph.D.

Wright State University, School of Medicine: John O. Lindower, M.D., Ph.D.

Ohio State Medical Association: Janet K. Bixel, M.D.

Ohio State Pharmaceutical Association: J. Richard Wuest, Pharm.D.

Oklahoma

University of Oklahoma College of Medicine: Ronald D. Brown, M.D.

Southwestern Oklahoma State University, School of Pharmacy: W. Steven Pray, Ph.D.

University of Oklahoma, College of Pharmacy: Loyd V. Allen, Jr., Ph.D.

Oklahoma State Medical Association: Clinton Nicholas Corder, M.D., Ph.D.

Oklahoma Pharmaceutical Association: Carl D. Lyons

Oregon

Oregon Health Sciences University, School of Medicine: Hall Downes, M.D., Ph.D.

Oregon State University, College of Pharmacy: Randall L. Vanderveen, Ph.D.

Pennsylvania

Duquesne University, School of Pharmacy: Lawrence H. Block, Ph.D.

Hahnemann University, School of Medicine: Vincent J. Zarro, M.D., Ph.D.

Medical College of Pennsylvania: Athole G. McNeil Jacobi, M.D.

Pennsylvania State University, College of Medicine: John D. Connor, Ph.D.

Philadelphia College of Pharmacy and Science: Alfonso R. Gennaro, Ph.D.

Temple University, School of Medicine: Ronald J. Tallarida, Ph.D.

Temple University, School of Pharmacy: Murray Tuckerman, Ph.D.

University of Pennsylvania, School of Medicine: Marilyn E. Hess, Ph.D.

University of Pittsburgh, School of Pharmacy: Terrence L. Schwinghammer, Pharm.D.

Pennsylvania Medical Society: Benjamin Calesnick, M.D.

Pennsylvania Pharmaceutical Association: Joseph A. Mosso, R.Ph.

Puerto Rico

Universidad Central del Caribe, School of Medicine: Jesús Santos-Martínez, Ph.D.

University of Puerto Rico, College of Pharmacy: Benjamin P. de Gracia, Ph.D.

University of Puerto Rico, School of Medicine: Walmor C. De Mello, M.D., Ph.D.

Rhode Island

Brown University Program in Medicine: Darrell R. Abernethy, M.D., Ph.D.

University of Rhode Island, College of Pharmacy: Thomas E. Needham, Ph.D.

South Carolina

Medical University of South Carolina, College of Medicine: Herman B. Daniell, Ph.D.

Medical University of South Carolina, College of Pharmacy: Paul J. Niebergall, Ph.D.

University of South Carolina, College of Pharmacy: Robert L. Beamer, Ph.D.

South Dakota

South Dakota State University, College of Pharmacy: Gary S. Chappell, Ph.D.

South Dakota State Medical Association: Robert D. Johnson

South Dakota Pharmaceutical Association: James Powers

Tennessee

East Tennessee State University, Quillen College of Medicine: Ernest A. Daigneault, Ph.D.

Meharry Medical College, School of Medicine: Dolores C. Shockley, Ph.D.

University of Tennessee, College of Medicine: Murray Heimberg, M.D., Ph.D.

University of Tennessee, College of Pharmacy: Dick R. Gourley, Pharm.D.

Vanderbilt University, School of Medicine: David H. Robertson, M.D.

Tennessee Pharmacists Association: Roger L. Davis, Pharm.D.

Texas

Texas A&M University, College of Medicine: Marsha A. Raebel, Pharm.D.

Texas Southern University, College of Pharmacy and Health Sciences: Eugene Hickman, Ph.D.

University of Houston, College of Pharmacy: Mustafa Lokhandwala, Ph.D.

University of Texas, Austin, College of Pharmacy: James T. Doluisio, Ph.D.

University of Texas, Medical Branch at Galveston: George T. Bryan, M.D.

University of Texas Medical School, Houston: Jacques E. Chelly, M.D., Ph.D.

University of Texas Medical School, San Antonio: Alexander M.M. Shepherd, M.D., Ph.D.

Texas Medical Association: Robert H. Barr, M.D.

Texas Pharmaceutical Association: Shirley McKee, R.Ph.

Utah

University of Utah, College of Pharmacy: David B. Roll, Ph.D.

Utah Pharmaceutical Association: Robert V. Peterson, Ph.D.

Utah Medical Association: David A. Hilding, M.D.

Vermont

University of Vermont, College of Medicine: John J. McCormack, Ph.D.

Vermont Pharmacists Association: Frederick Dobson

Virginia

Medical College of Hampton Roads: William J. Cooke, Ph.D.

Medical College of Virginia/Virginia Commonwealth University, School of Pharmacy: William H. Barr, Pharm.D., Ph.D.

Medical Society of Virginia: Richard W. Lindsay, M.D.

University of Virginia, School of Medicine: Peyton E. Weary, M.D.

Virginia Pharmaceutical Association: Daniel A. Herbert

Washington

Unversity of Washington, School of Pharmacy: Wendel L. Nelson, Ph.D.

Washington State University, College of Pharmacy: Martin J. Jinks, Pharm.D.

Washington State Pharmacists Association: Danial E. Baker

West Virginia

Marshall University, School of Medicine: John L. Szarek, Ph.D.

West Virginia University, School of Medicine: Douglas D. Glover, M.D.

West Virginia University Medical Center, School of Pharmacy:
Arthur I. Jacknowitz, Pharm.D.

Wisconsin

Medical College of Wisconsin: Garrett J. Gross, Ph.D.

University of Wisconsin, Madison, School of Pharmacy: Chester
A. Bond, Pharm.D.

University of Wisconsin Medical School, Madison: Joseph M.
Benforado, M.D.

State Medical Society of Wisconsin: Thomas L. Adams, CAE

Wisconsin Pharmacists Association: Dennis Dziczkowski, R.Ph.

Wyoming

University of Wyoming, School of Pharmacy: Kenneth F. Nelson, Ph.D.

Wyoming Medical Society: R. W. Johnson, Jr.

Wyoming Pharmaceutical Association: Linda G. Sutherland

Members-at-Large

Norman W. Atwater, Ph.D., Hopewell, NJ

Cheston M. Berlin, Jr., M.D., The Milton S. Hershey Medical
Center

Fred S. Brinkley, Jr., Texas State Board of Pharmacy

Herbert S. Carlin, D.Sc., Califon, NJ

Jordan Cohen, Ph.D., College of Pharmacy, University of
Kentucky

John L. Cova, Ph.D., Health Insurance Association of America

Enrique Fefer, Ph.D., Pan American Health Organization

Leroy Fevang, Canadian Pharmaceutical Association

Klaus G. Florey, Ph.D., Princeton, NJ

Lester Hosto, Ph.D., Arkansas State Board of Pharmacy

Jay S. Keystone, M.D., Toronto General Hospital

Calvin M. Kunin, M.D., Ohio State University

Marvin Lipman, M.D., Scarsdale, NY

Joseph A. Mollica, Ph.D., Montcharin, DE

Stuart L. Nightingale, M.D., Food and Drug Administration

Daniel A. Nona, Ph.D., The American Council on Pharmaceutical Education

Mark Novitch, M.D., Kalamazoo, MI

Charles A. Pergola, SmithKline Beecham Consumer Brands

Donald O. Schiffman, Ph.D., Genealogy Unlimited

Carl E. Trinca, Ph.D., American Association of Colleges of
Pharmacy

INDEX

Brand names appear in italics. Generic or family names appear in standard typeface.

Expertly detailed, pharmaceutical guides
can now be at your fingertips
from U.S. Pharmacopeia

THE USP GUIDE TO MEDICINES
78092-5/$6.99 US/$8.99 Can

- More than 2,000 entries for both prescription
  and non-prescription drugs
- Handsomely detailed color insert

THE USP GUIDE
TO HEART MEDICINES
78094-1/$6.99 US/$8.99 Can

- Side effects and proper dosages for over 400
  brand-name and generic drugs
- Breakdown of heart ailments such as angina,
  high cholesterol and high blood pressure

THE USP GUIDE TO
VITAMINS AND MINERALS
78093-3/$6.99 US/$8.99 Can

- Precautions for children, senior citizens and
  pregnant women
- Latest findings and benefits of dietary supplements